FIFTH EDITION

BROWN'S SKIN
& MINOR SURGERY
A TEXT AND COLOUR ATLAS

EDITED BY JONATHAN BOTTING

AND JULIA SCHOFIELD

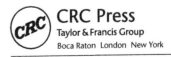

CRC Press
Taylor & Francis Group
Boca Raton London New York

CRC Press is an imprint of the
Taylor & Francis Group, an **informa** business

CRC Press
Taylor & Francis Group
6000 Broken Sound Parkway NW, Suite 300
Boca Raton, FL 33487-2742

First issued in paperback 2020

Version Date: 20140304

ISBN 13 : 978-0-367-57605-9 (pbk)
ISBN 13 : 978-1-4441-3836-8 (hbk)

Library of Congress Cataloging-in-Publication Data

Botting, Jonathan, author.
  Brown's skin and minor surgery : a text and color atlas / Jonathan Botting, Julia K. Schofield, John Brown. -- Fifth edition.
    p. ; cm.
  Skin and minor surgery
  Preceded by Minor surgery / John Stuart Brown. 4th ed. 2000.
  Includes bibliographical references and index.
  ISBN 978-1-4441-3836-8 (hardcover : alk. paper)
  I. Schofield, Julia, 1956- author. II. Brown, John Stuart, author. III. Title. IV. Title: Skin and minor surgery.
  [DNLM: 1. Surgical Procedures, Minor--Atlases. 2. Dermatologic Surgical Procedures--Atlases. WO 517]

RD111
617'.024--dc23

Visit the Taylor & Francis Web site at
http://www.taylorandfrancis.com

and the CRC Press Web site at
http://www.crcpress.com

Contents

VIDEO CLIPS

Video clips are available online to illustrate some of the procedures described in this book. There is a URL in the text wherever a video clip is cited and a panel of QR codes at the end of each chapter for which videos are provided.

To use the QR codes to view the videos you will need a QR code reader for your smartphone/tablet. There are many free QR code readers available, dependent on the device you are using. We have supplied some suggestions below of well-known QR readers, but this is not an exhaustive list and you should only download software compatible with your device and operating system. We do not endorse any of the third-party products listed below and downloading them is at your own risk:

- iPhone/iPad: Qrafter—http://itunes.apple.com/app/qrafter-qr-code-reader-generator/id416098700
- Android: QR Droid—https://market.android.com/details?id=la.droid.qr&hl=en
- Blackberry: QR Scanner Pro—http://appworld.black-berry.com/webstore/content/13962
- Windows/Symbian: UpCode—http://www.upc.fi/en/upcode/download/

Once you have downloaded a QR code reader, simply open the reader app and use it to take a photo of the code. The video will then load on your smartphone/tablet.

If you do not have a smartphone/tablet, you can view the videos online by typing in the URL shown for each video, or following the hyperlink if you are using the ebook edition.

We are interested in your feedback on the QR codes included with this title. If you have any comments on the use of QR codes, please send them to zelah.pengilley@tandf.co.uk.

Foreword

Jonathan Stuart Brown, M.D.

When I wrote the first edition of *Minor Surgery—A Text and Atlas* in 1986, I remember feeling relieved that, as with *Gray's Anatomy*, it would need very little updating, as minor surgical treatments were unlikely to change to any significant degree.

With each subsequent edition, it became obvious that changes were needed; not only had materials and instruments improved, but also many treatments had been modified and improved, and new legislation and advice had been introduced.

Throughout all the editions, the emphasis has been to offer the highest standards of care to the patient; thus, doctors are recommended to seek advice from surgical colleagues, to attend one or more of the many excellent Minor Surgery courses, and only perform those procedures where they feel completely competent and comfortable.

The forewords to the first four editions were all written by consultant surgeons, two of whom were also presidents of the Royal College of Surgeons, and I have been very privileged to be asked to write the foreword to this edition.

When I retired from general medical practice, I felt it was appropriate to ask younger, more up-to-date, and experienced colleagues if they would be willing to update the book. To update one's own book is fairly straightforward, but to update someone else's book is a hugely daunting task, and I am most grateful to Jonathan Botting, Julia K. Schofield, and their small team of experts for the huge amount of hard work they have done on my behalf. I could not have anticipated a better end result and I am truly delighted. To them, I express my everlasting thanks, and I know readers of this edition will find a wealth of information and advice contained within its covers.

Acknowledgements

We gratefully acknowledge and thank those who provided invaluable expertise:

Richard Baxter—General Practitioner, for editorial support.
Andrew Fleming—Consultant, Plastic Surgeon at St. George's Hospital, London, for providing images of Dupuytrens.
Rupert Gabriel—General Practitioner, for electrosurgery advice.
Diane Gilmour—Past President of the Association for Perioperative Practice (AfPP), for her advice on Chapter 3, 'Infection Control'.
Soon Lim—General Practitioner, for editorial support.
David Warwick—Consultant Hand Surgeon at Southampton University Hospitals NHS Trust, for providing information and images for collagenase treatment of Dupuytrens.
Matthew Wordsworth—General Practitioner, for providing carpal tunnel advice.

We are grateful to all who gave permission for the re-use of material; most are credited individually, but we would also like to acknowledge the following:

The video clips are reproduced with kind permission of Limbs and Things.
Much of the text relating to skin lesions and dermatological surgery techniques is reproduced from Schofield J, Kneebone R (2006) *Skin Lesions: A Practical Guide to Diagnosis, Management and Minor Surgery*, 2nd ed., with kind permission of the authors.

Editors

Jonathan Botting, MRCGP,
GP, Barnes, London SW13; GP Trainer; Dermatological Surgeon, Chelsea and Westminster Hospital and Queen Mary's Hospital; Course Organiser for Diploma in Minor Surgery; RCGP Clinical Champion for Minor Surgery 2010–12.

Julia Schofield, FRCP, MRCGP, MBE,
Principal Lecturer, Programme Lead, MSc Dermatology Skills and Treatment, School of Postgraduate Medicine, University of Hertfordshire; Consultant Dermatologist, United Lincolnshire Hospitals NHS Trust.

Contributors

Jonathan Bowling, MBChB, FRCP,
Dermoscopy UK; Consultant Dermatologist and Honorary Senior Clinical Lecturer, Oxford University Hospitals NHS Trust, Oxford, UK.

Simon Eccles, BDS, FRCS, FRCS (Plast),
Consultant Plastics and Craniofacial Surgeon Chelsea and Westminster Hospital, London, UK; President of the Plastic Surgery Section of the Royal Society of Medicine.

Tony Feltbower MB, BChir, LRCP, MRCS, DRCOG, AFOM,
General Practitioner and Vasectomist, Westminster Road Medical Services Ltd., Coventry, UK.

Madeleine Flanagan, RGN,
Principal Lecturer, School of Postgraduate Medicine, University of Hertfordshire, Hertfordshire, UK.

Ian Reilly, FCPodS DMS,
Consultant Podiatric Surgeon, Northamptonshire Healthcare Foundation NHS Trust; Private Practice: BMI and Ramsay Hospital Groups.

Laurel Spooner, MRCP, MRCPG, DRCOG, DCH, ASPC,
Primary Care Surgeon and General Practioner; Immediate Past President of the Association of Surgeons in Primary Care, London, UK.

Tim T. Wang, FRCS,
Imperial College London; Specialist Plastics Registrar, Chelsea and Westminster Hospital, London, UK.

PART 1

Essential background information

Chapter 1

Facilities

INTRODUCTION

This chapter describes the essential facility and resource requirements for performing minor surgery. There are two sections as follows:

- The equipment required to perform minor surgery.
- Staffing needs to support the service.

Facilities should be not only fit for purpose, but also adaptable to meet future demands. Many of the fixtures and fittings will be expensive, and care should be taken when choosing these to ensure that they are fit for the intended purpose. There will be a range of consumable products (such as sutures and sterile gloves) for which it will be possible to evaluate and change suppliers as necessary.

EQUIPMENT REQUIREMENTS

There are core requirements for equipping all minor surgery rooms, and optional facilities dependent upon the level of planned service. It is a mistake to underestimate the facilities, fixtures, and fittings required. Attention to detail as you set up the service will prevent the surgeon from discovering half way through an operation that there is not enough room to move or that a particular instrument, suture, or dressing is missing. This section considers the following equipment needs:

- Room requirements such as size.
- Ancillary equipment, for example electrocautery equipment.
- Surgical instruments, including a review of the advantages and drawbacks of reusable versus disposable equipment.
- Single-use consumables, such as gloves and sutures.
- Drugs, including local anaesthetics.
- Safety equipment.

When considering your facilities and equipment needs, attention to detail in relation to infection control is important. Chapter 3 considers this area specifically, but throughout this chapter there is emphasis on making the minor surgical facility easy to keep clean.

Room requirements

The following important areas will be discussed in relation to the operating room as they are considered essential aspects of the provision of a safe minor surgery service:

- Size.
- Surfaces, floor, walls, and doors.
- Storage.
- Handwashing facilities.
- Operating table/stool.
- Illumination and ventilation.
- Patient preparation area.
- Communication needs.

Readers are directed to their own national guidance and requirements when designing or refurbishing premises to create a minor surgery service. Figure 1.1 shows an illustration of a minor surgery room.

Size

The first requirement of any room used for minor surgery is that sufficient space exists to allow the surgeon *uninterrupted access* around the patient. This is more important than the actual floor size. The recommended size for a consulting room is 13.5–15 m² and that for a treatment/minor surgery room 18–20 m². These are the dimensions recommended for NHS premises in the United Kingdom and built on the following principles, which should be followed when planning a treatment or minor surgery room:

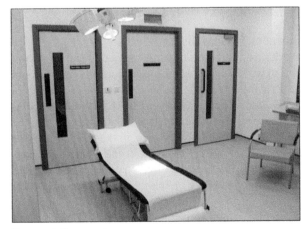

Figure 1.1 Treatment room.

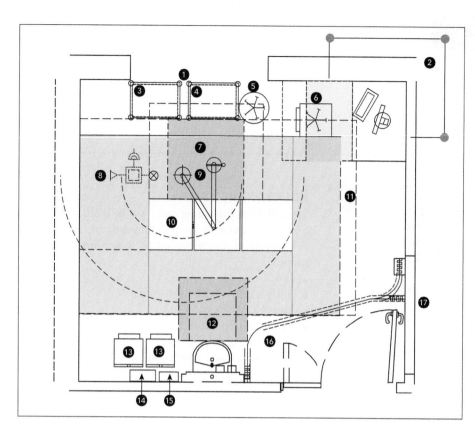

Figure 1.2 Suggested floor plan.
1. Possible window location
2. Engineering services outlet zone
3. Supplies trolley
4. Dressing/instrument trolley
5. Stool
6. Chair
7. Space for changing*
8. Pendant services
9. Ceiling-mounted examination light
10. Couch with paper roll attached
11. Clinical workstation
12. Clinical wash-hand basin
13. Sack holder
14. Glove and apron dispenser
15. Paper towel dispenser
16. Optional privacy curtain
17. Alternative door location

*See DH Health Building Note 00–02 for details

- The average operating couch plinth measures 1.85 × 0.63 m. Around it there needs to be a minimum space for the surgeon to move, say 0.8 m. This means an operating space of 3.45 × 2.23 m.
- Worktops with storage underneath or room to work will average 0.6 m deep on one side of the room, while on the other side of the room there will be washing facilities and waste bins, again 0.6 m deep.
- The operating couch, storage, and washing requirements therefore require an area of about 4 m × 3 m, i.e. 12 m² alone.
- Allowing space for a desk and chairs (for record-keeping, taking consent, etc.) and a patient changing area will increase the floor area by 3–6 m².
- This produces a room size requirement minimum of 15–18 m².

A suggested floor plan is shown in Figure 1.2.

Surfaces, floor, walls, and doors

Work surfaces should be easily cleaned, impervious, and able to withstand chemical disinfectants. All edges should be sealed (Figure 1.3). The floor should be of a seamless, wipe-clean variety, and never carpet. It should be non-slip and sealed around all edges (Figure 1.4). Ideally, the surface coating should continue up the wall surfaces for about 10 cm to allow cleaning of the whole floor area. Walls should be free of unnecessary clutter and in good order. A good supply of splash-proof electrical sockets a reasonable height from the floor should be used. The access door should incorporate some form of lock to stop unauthorised access when necessary.

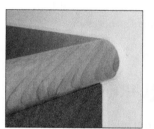

Figure 1.3 Sealed worktops.

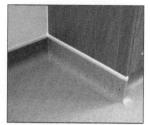

Figure 1.4 Sealed floor finish.

Storage space

Open shelving should be avoided, and contents should be stored in cupboards. Cupboards should be numbered with an easily accessible index of their contents, or the contents should be clearly labelled on the cupboard doors. Cupboards containing chemicals or drugs should be lockable.

Trolley

The equipment to be used for each procedure will be taken from the storage cupboards and needs to be readily available to the surgeon. The best way of achieving this is on a small stainless steel operating trolley on wheels, with two shelves (Figure 1.5). Being stainless steel, it will be easy to clean between cases. Having it on wheels means that the surgeon can place it exactly where it is needed. The lower shelf enables dressings, etc., to be available to the surgeon.

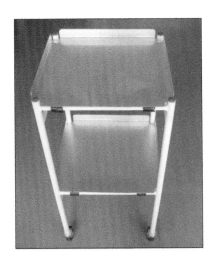

Figure 1.5 Two-layer stainless steel trolley.

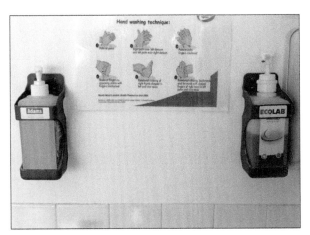

Figure 1.7 Wall-mounted dispensers.

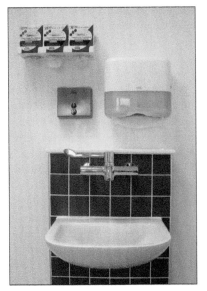

Figure 1.6 Wash basin.

Operating table/stool

The traditional hospital operating table is a very bulky and expensive piece of equipment, and is not required for the majority of minor surgical procedures. The key principles to consider when choosing an operating couch are as follows. It should be:

- Comfortable, accessible, and large enough to meet the patient's needs.
- Height-adjustable to meet the surgeon's needs.
- Possible to lower the head end, in order to manage a vasovagal episode.

A very acceptable alternative is the height-adjustable physiotherapy couch (or plinth) in three sections (allowing either end to be raised or lowered; Figure 1.8). Unlike a traditional operating table, these couches drop low to facilitate access by the elderly or infirm. Being wider than an operating table, they allow patients to feel more secure (and in addition the patient is unlikely to need extra support if the arm is to be operated on). The relative lack of bulk under the 'table' also allows the surgeon to operate sitting with room for their legs. Finally, a 'breathing hole' in the head section allows the patient to lie prone comfortably.

Handwashing facilities

- A designated handwashing basin with mixer, elbow/wrist-operated or automatic proximity-sensing taps, and no plug in the basin is essential (Figure 1.6). Current UK infection control dictates the use of free-standing sinks (not set in a work surface).
- There should be a wall-mounted dispenser containing disposable paper hand towels, and a liquid soap dispenser (Figure 1.7). If nailbrushes are used, they should be single use and disposable (they are not, however, considered necessary; see Chapter 3).
- Standard containers containing surgical scrub solutions for routine washing and hand-scrubbing before each operation should be affixed to a wall-mounted dispenser, mounted above the sink. The two most commonly used agents are Hibiscrub® (chlorhexidine gluconate 4% in detergent base) and Betadine® surgical scrub (povidone–iodine 7.5% in a detergent base).

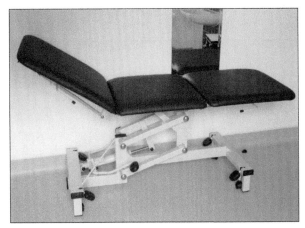

Figure 1.8 Physiotherapy couch with manual hydraulics.

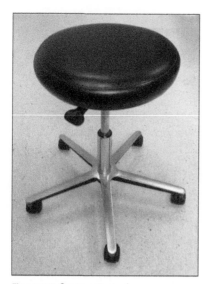

Figure 1.9 Surgeon's stool.

The couch should have an impervious washable surface and be protected with disposable paper towels that are changed between patients. A pillow with waterproof cover under a disposable pillow slip should also be used to aid patient comfort.

The table or plinth must be fitted with lockable wheels because it will occasionally need to be moved if, for example, a wheelchair-bound patient is going to undergo a simple procedure while remaining in their wheelchair. Electrically operated height-adjustable plinths with a foot control are available, but these are much more expensive and have few advantages over a manually operated couch. The surgeon can adjust the latter using his or her feet.

Although many surgeons are used to standing while operating, most minor surgery can be performed seated. The surgeon should have a comfortable stool that is on wheels and can be adjusted for height (Figure 1.9).

Remember though that the operating couch you purchase should be suitable for the procedures you plan to undertake; for example, for advanced procedures such as carpal tunnel surgery, an operating table with arm rests will be best.

Illumination and ventilation
Windows
Natural daylight will make the room more pleasant and inviting but risks loss of privacy. For this reason, windows need screening. Curtains and blinds are not suitable in an operating room due to dust collection (the only exception to this being where blinds may be 'sandwiched' between layers of double glazing). The most suitable screening is opaque glass or coatings. Very effective opaque sheeting can be retrospectively fitted to existing clear glass. This remains easy to clean, provides complete privacy, and also diffuses bright sunlight to avoid glare.

Lighting
The lighting should provide good background illumination and also focused, cool operating lighting. Good surgery warrants good lighting. Small mobile units are considered unacceptable. A dedicated minor surgery light should be capable of providing illumination of up to 50,000 lux at 0.5 m. In addition, the light source needs to be sufficiently large to avoid shadowing and suitably powerful to allow it to be focused from a distance.

For all these reasons, a ceiling-mounted, fully adjustable, dedicated operating light should be considered essential. The light should be fitted with a removable sterilisable handle, and this handle should in turn be fitted with sterile disposable covers. This then allows surgeons to adjust the light exactly as they want it. It is possible to purchase lighting heads with up to six separate light sources, but these can be imposing and bulky. A really good single, double, or triple light source is sufficient (Figure 1.10). Ensure that a spare bulb is kept in stock.

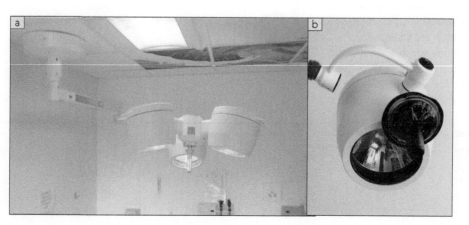

Figure 1.10 (a) Three-head operating light. (b) Single-head operating light with sterile, disposable handle cover.

Ventilation

Minor surgical rooms should have a method of air extraction to the outside using an extractor fan, not by opening windows or doors. Temperature control is important for both patient and staff comfort. Thermostatically controlled heating for winter and air-conditioning (Figure 1.11) in summer are ideal. The air change requirements for a hospital operating room are extremely demanding and not relevant to most minor surgery facilities; again, the specification will be dictated by the level of surgery undertaken.

Patient preparation area

Due consideration needs to be given to where patients are able to prepare for their surgery. It is embarrassing to force patients to undress without privacy, although this is sometimes unavoidable within the theatre. A separate changing area with easily removed (for cleaning or replacement) curtains is ideal. Blankets have become less used due to the theoretical risk of cross-infection, so consideration needs to be given to the use of disposable sterile drapes or simple gowns for patient cover. It is essential that patients are spared embarrassment, but it is equally important that an adequate operating area is prepared. This should be explained to patients at an early stage to allow them to voice any concerns.

Communication

All minor surgery rooms should have a method for summoning assistance, both for routine help and for emergencies. For the former, a telephone and/or intercom system should be used; for the latter, a simple to use, easy to see emergency call system should be fitted and tested regularly.

Making the room work for you and the patient

The room should be ergonomically designed to ensure smooth straightforward movement from the preparation area to the operating area. For example, the surgeon needs to be able to move from washing to drying the hands, thence to application of sterile gloves, and from there to the patient. The assistant needs to be able to have space for anaesthetic preparation, equipment storage, easy access to all disposables, and room for specimens and pathology requests. In addition, there needs to be room for completing notes, etc. Ideally, the roles of the surgeon and the assistant start at opposite ends of the room, akin to production lines meeting in the centre. In this way, the surgeon and assistant are less likely to cross paths.

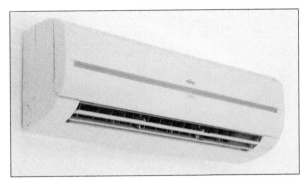

Figure 1.11 Air-conditioning unit.

Ancillary equipment

This section considers other equipment that may be needed to provide a minor surgery service. Measures for ensuring haemostasis are very important and are considered first. Not everyone will want to offer a cryotherapy service, but for those that do, a section on this is included.

Electrocautery

In this technique, a red-hot platinum wire is used to coagulate small blood vessels or to cut through tissue. It differs from diathermy in that it works solely by heat. The use of electrocautery is discussed in Chapter 18. Its main uses are:

- To remove or treat lesions, for example skin tags and spider naevi.
- To control bleeding, especially after curettage or shave excision.
- To destroy residual tissue, for example following curettage of basal cell carcinomas.

Electrocautery machines consist of an electrical source and a range of platinum wire tips.

Electrocautery machines

Standard mains machines consist of a transformer, with a dial to control the current and therefore the temperature, together with a hand-held attachment into which the cautery tip is fitted (Figure 1.12). The advantage of this type of machine is that it allows precise control of the temperature of the tip, but it is rather cumbersome to use.

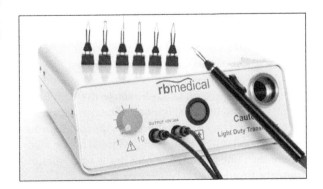

Figure 1.12 Mains cautery machine. (Image copyright RB Medical, reproduced with kind permission.)

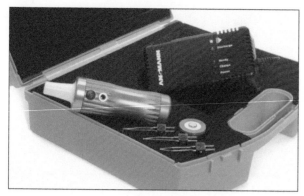

Figure 1.13 Battery-operated cautery device. (Image copyright RB Medical, reproduced with kind permission.)

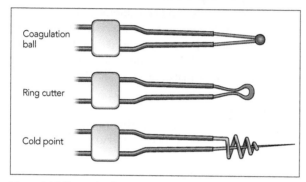

Figure 1.14 Example of cautery tips.

An alternative is a rechargeable machine that is not attached to the mains during use (Figure 1.13). This has the advantage of being portable and more convenient. However, it is not possible to control the temperature since the current is either on or off. Nevertheless, with experience, the temperature of the wire can be varied by altering the time from heating to application. It is important to make sure that the batteries are adequately charged before each session. Disposable machines are expensive but may be convenient for occasional use.

A variety of burner heads should be stocked (Figure 1.14):

- *Flat blade*: For general cautery (e.g., large areas) and cutting; this coagulates and cuts at the same time
- *Simple loop*: As above but for light cutting.
- *Ball-end*: Preferred by some for general cautery; these stop bleeding without cutting through the tissues.
- *Cold tip*: A fine central point with a heating wire around it; this can be used to cauterise single vessels (e.g., a spider naevus).

The burner tips need either to be single use or robust enough to withstand sterilisation. The tips are platinum coated, and excessive heat destroys the coating. You will need a good supply of tips as they should not be used on more than one patient. The heat in the wire will not sterilise the tip adequately between patients.

Diathermy

Diathermy is another technique used to damage tissue in a controlled way. It depends on electricity rather than just heat to produce its effects. Diathermy machines produce a low current at a high voltage and a very high frequency. The standard hospital operating theatre diathermy is *bipolar*. This means that it has two electrodes: a large one in the form of a pad, usually attached to the patient's thigh, and a smaller one used by the surgeon to cut or coagulate the tissue.

Much more suited to minor surgery is the *unipolar* diathermy, capable of cauterising anything from single blood vessels to large wound areas (Figure 1.15a). Unipolar diathermy only uses one electrode. The most widely used machine is the Birtcher hyfrecator®. It may be used in three ways:

- To *coagulate* tissue in a similar way to electrocautery.
- To *fulgurate* tissue using the stream of sparks produced when it is held just above the lesion.
- To *desiccate* tissue by causing drying in a small area around the point of the hyfrecator needle.

The hyfrecator is increasingly used in minor surgery. The cable to the handle needs to be treated with care as it is easily damaged. The diathermy tips are available as sharp (for single vessels) and blunt (for general cauterising) (Figure 1.15b). The tips, which are single use, are available individually sterilised or boxed. The instrument handle should be protected by single-use sterile sheaths (Figure 1.15c).

Figure 1.15
(a) Unipolar diathermy (hyfrecator). (b) Single use diathermy tips (dark grey—blunt, light grey—sharp tipped). (c) Sterile diathermy handle sheaths.

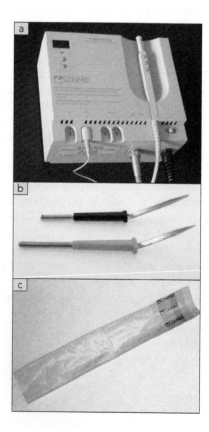

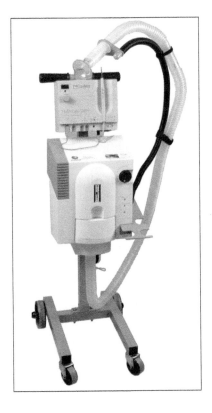

Figure 1.16 Mobile smoke extractor mounted below diathermy unit. (© Schuco International [London] Ltd. Used with permission.)

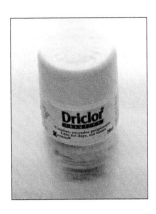

Figure 1.17 Driclor.®

Figure 1.18 Esmarch® bandages/tourniquets. (Image copyright VBM Medizintechnik GmbH, reproduced with kind permission.)

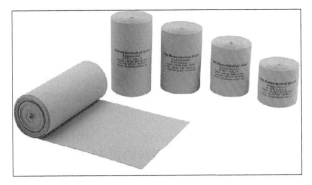

More powerful diathermy units tend to be used in operating theatres rather than minor surgery treatment rooms. Surgeons may feel uncomfortable without full bipolar diathermy. These units require the use of sterilisable bipolar forceps and/or patient electrodes. More details can be found in Chapter 26.

Microwave/radiowave cutting units are becoming more widely available, but they demand specialist training and maintenance.

Smoke removal

Electrosurgery causes burning, which in turn produces smoke. Smoke particles can in theory contain prions and degradation products, so smoke extraction/recovery units are therefore becoming standard equipment in theatres (Figure 1.16). Although not essential in minor operation theatres, their use should be encouraged, especially if regular electrosurgery is to be performed (see Chapter 26).

Other haemostatic agents and other equipment
Chemical cautery

- Driclor® is one brand of aluminium chloride hexahydrate in a 'roll-on ball' antiperspirant container (Figure 1.17). It is an excellent haemostatic agent for use after facial curetting and shave excisions to achieve control of bleeding.
- Silver nitrate sticks are useful for haemostasis, particularly when applied to adventitious tissue developing from a wound, but they should not be applied to facial wounds as there is the theoretical risk of silver tattooing of the skin.

Tourniquet

Where a bloodless operating field is required, such as for ingrowing toenails, excision of ganglia, removal of foreign bodies, or exploration, a tourniquet may be required. For fingers and toes, this need only be a length of rubber tubing, a rubber strip, a wide rubber band, or even a surgical rubber glove with the tip cut off and rolled down the digit. If available, purpose-made rubber Esmarch® bandages (available in a variety of widths) should be used to exsanguinate the area and as a tourniquet (Figure 1.18).

Cryotherapy

Liquid nitrogen boils at −196°C. In order to store this liquid, specialised insulated containers must be used. These are designed to withstand the extreme temperatures and allow controlled venting of nitrogen gas and ease of transfer of the contents. Large volumes can be stored in Dewar flasks; the larger the flask size, the longer the potential storage time.

Liquid nitrogen is poured from the Dewar storage flask into hand-operated equipment as required. Safety is paramount during transfer of liquid nitrogen so storage should be in a well-ventilated area, and the operator should wear eye protection along with insulated gloves to transfer the liquid nitrogen into the hand-operated unit. The hand-operated unit can be either a small insulated flask with a hand-operated trigger or even a simple insulated polystyrene cup. With the latter, liquid nitrogen is applied using a cotton bud. See Chapter 19 for more details on cryotherapy.

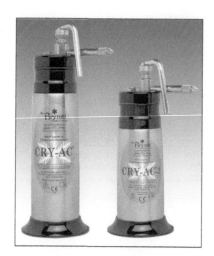

Figure 1.19 Liquid nitrogen cryo-therapy gun, the Cry-Ac™Tracker™ Cam. (Brymill Cryogenic Systems, www.brymill.com. Used with permission.)

Cryo-guns rely upon the pressure produced by the evaporating liquid to propel a fine jet controlled by an adjustable trigger (Figure 1.19). A full hand-operated cryo-gun will remain usable for up to 1 day.

Surgical instruments (reusable or disposable)

Every doctor has a favourite selection of instruments, and what suits one surgeon does not always suit another. One practitioner may prefer small, fine-toothed delicate instruments, whereas another is happier with large, robust instruments.

More stringent requirements for sterilisation have led to a more widespread use of single-use, disposable instruments. These instruments can be of excellent quality, but the need for affordability tends to limit their precision and surgical 'feel'. There are pros and cons to using these instruments (Table 1.1). In addition, there are environmental concerns with single-use instruments being made of metal alloys that are destroyed by incineration and therefore have no recyclable potential. Against this, manufacturers of single-use devices argue that the energy

Table 1.1 Pros and cons of disposable and reusable instruments

For disposable:	For reusable:
• Sterility guaranteed	• High quality
• Scissors always sharp	• Easy to use
• Everything included*	• Finer instruments
• Convenient	• User-defined choice
Against disposable:	**Against reusable:**
• Variable quality	• Blunt/wear with use
• Difficulty in handling fine sutures	• Need for and costs of sterilisation
• Instrument choice not user defined	• Expensive to replace
• Cost and environmental issues	• Swabs and drape supplies needed

Surgical packs are available with all instruments, swabs, drapes, and containers.

costs of resterilising instruments cause more environmental damage.

From a purely practical point of view, high-quality reusable instruments in excellent working order will always outperform single-use equivalents. This is particularly relevant when handling very fine sutures, when using very fine skin forceps, and when requiring very fine tissue scissors.

Whatever the instruments used, it is now essential within the United Kingdom to be able to track and trace those instruments for every patient. All packs should have unique pack codes, and these should be recorded within the lifelong patient notes.

Basic surgical sets

The range of instruments to choose from can seem baffling, and many disposable instrument sets are pre-selected. However, some general principles for instrument choice will be outlined below. The equipment required will depend on the type of surgery being performed, but the minimum surgical instruments required when cutting through skin and suturing should include the following:

- Suture/needle holder.
- Skin forceps, toothed and non-toothed.
- Artery forceps.
- Scissors, fine and suture.
- Skin hook.

Optional equipment will include small retractors and items such as towel clips.

Information about how to hold and use the surgical instruments described below can be found mostly in Chapter 17.

Suture/needle holders

A fine, well-made needle/suture holder can make suturing a pleasure; conversely, a badly made or heavy-duty pair can turn the simplest of procedures into a battle. Suture/needle holders have short powerful jaws, and ideally the surface of each jaw will have criss-cross lines cut into it (Figure 1.20). These jaws can grasp a needle firmly without it slipping round. However, if you use the instrument to pick tissue up, the jaws will crush it and cause damage.

Important points to consider when choosing a suture holder include the following:
- *Length*: If less than about 5 inches (13 cm), they will be difficult to hold in a palm grip. If longer than about 7 inches (18 cm), they will be too unwieldy.
- *Profile*: If they are flat, they will sit well in the palm. If contoured (Kilner), they will be suitable only for finger operation (see below).
- *Latching*: An easily engaged and disengaged ratchet will greatly facilitate suturing. Some suture holders (Gillies) are combined with suture scissors, but these are non-latching and less easily used by most surgeons.

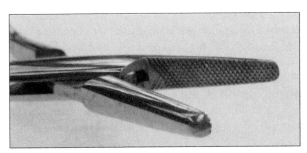

Figure 1.20 Kilner suture/needle holder jaws in detail.

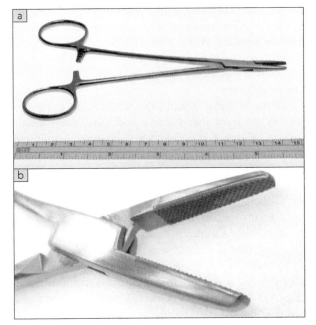

Figure 1.21 (a) Crile–Wood suture holder. (b) Close-up of the tungsten carbide jaws.

Crile–Wood suture holder

As previously described, this style of suture holder is ideally suited to skin surgery, in particular fine sutures. If chosen with a length of 15–18 cm, it can be used both with a traditional and with a palm grip. The precision ratchet allows palm opening and closing of the holder. As it has fine jaws, the instrument manages small needles well.

Kilner suture holder

This is found in many basic sets and is common in disposable packs. With offset handles, these are designed to be held in the traditional 'surgeon's grip', the offset being designed to allow the jaws of the instrument to be in close proximity to the skin while allowing room for the surgeon's hand (Figure 1.22). This suture holder traditionally had a single, large ratchet and was too large to be used with a palm grip. The 12.5 cm Kilner with multiple ratchets and improved jaws that is now widely available in disposable packs has overcome this problem. Avoid the 13.3 cm single-ratchet Kilner as this will not allow an easy palm grip, and the jaws are often coarse and will flatten small curved needles.

Gillies suture holder

The Gillies suture holder incorporates a scissor section as well as a needle grip (Figure 1.23). This allows the surgeon to use just one instrument to both hold and then cut the suture. However, there is no ratchet, and the scissors are not suited for buried knots.

- *Jaws*: The best (most expensive) suture holders will have very fine jaws, and these will be lined on the 'biting' surface with tungsten carbide. This extremely hard but fragile material can be very accurately milled to ensure an excellent needle grip as well as a gentle suture material grip, thereby giving excellent control with less chance of breaking the suture material (which is especially important when using finer sutures). Although disposable tungsten carbide suture holders are available, their cost is usually prohibitive, so single-use disposable suture holders are unlikely to feature the use of this material.

A 15–18 cm Crile–Wood suture holder (Figure 1.21a) with tungsten carbide jaws (Figure 1.21b) is recommended as it is one of the easiest to use needle holders. The length allows the instrument to be held in the palm of the hand, like a screwdriver.

More detail about selected suture/needle holders is included below for completeness.

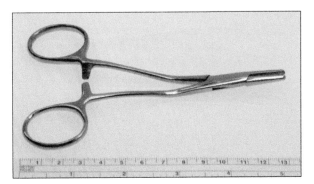

Figure 1.22 Kilner suture holder.

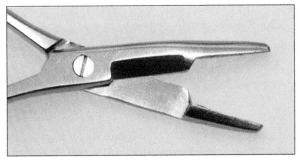

Figure 1.23 Gillies suture holder and scissors.

Skin forceps

Forceps provide a number of functions for the skin surgeon:

- Stabilising skin for cutting and suturing.
- Lifting skin specimens to aid removal.
- Handling needles to avoid 'sharps' injuries.

The more delicate the construction of the forceps, the more precisely they can be handled and the less likely they are to damage delicate structures; however, they will also be more prone to damage by injudicious use. It is important to have both toothed and non-toothed forceps and to understand the different uses of each (Figure 1.24).

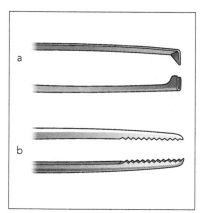

Figure 1.24 The difference between (a) toothed and (b) non-toothed forceps.

Toothed forceps

Toothed forceps are traditionally used for handling skin, which means that the forceps should have very fine teeth to avoid unnecessarily puncturing and damaging the skin. These forceps are particularly helpful when holding wound edges. It is therefore advisable to have fine, light-weight forceps with small teeth that will not damage the skin edges.

Non-toothed forceps

Non-toothed forceps grip a suture needle better than all but the finest-toothed forceps and are very useful for holding needles and sutures. Non-toothed forceps can be used for handling skin but have the potential to do more damage than toothed forceps if the jaws keep slipping off.

Choice of forceps

Of all the available designs, the Adson 12.5 cm forceps remain the most user-friendly and suitable for minor surgery (Figure 1.25). They are lightweight yet blessed with an operating shape that allows easy manipulation. They are neither too long nor too stiff to use. With fine, or micro, teeth, these are very delicate on skin, but are easily damaged by poor handling. They are delicate instruments specifically designed to hold tissue and not crush it. They should be used to hold, stabilise, or lift tissue but should never be used to twist or rotate tissues.

McIndoe or Gillies forceps tend to be too long for skin use, 'turnover end' forceps are too stiff and crude (Figure 1.26), whereas iris forceps tend to be too small and delicate.

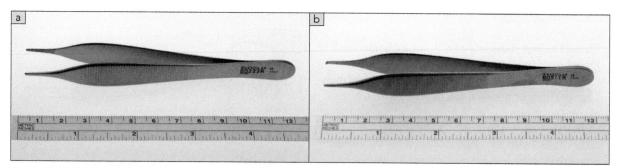

Figure 1.25 (a) Non-toothed and (b) toothed Adson forceps.

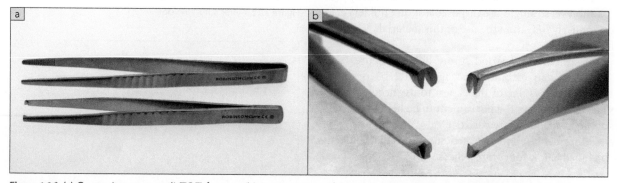

Figure 1.26 (a) Coarse 'turnover end' (TOE) forceps. (b) A comparison of the teeth of the turnover-end forceps (larger) and the Adson forceps (finer).

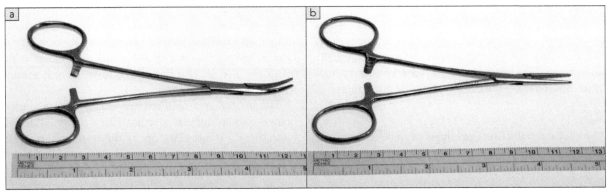

Figure 1.27 (a) Curved and (b) straight artery forceps.

Artery forceps

These forceps can meet a variety of uses in minor surgery. They come in straight and curved profile, both being useful, but for most minor skin procedures the curved shape is most versatile (Figure 1.27). Originally designed to clamp bleeding vessels, these instruments can be used for this function as long as care is taken to avoid crushing the skin edges. They can also be used for blunt dissection, for holding suture ends, and to aid placing scalpel blades on reusable scalpel handles and removing them afterwards. In some cases, artery forceps can be used to hold tissue being removed or resected (as long as the area of clamping is not of histological importance as it will be crushed). The most useful are the small (12.5 cm) curved or flat Halstead mosquito forceps.

Scissors

Scissors are required in minor surgery to:

- Cut tissues.
- Bluntly dissect tissues.
- Separate tissue planes.
- Cut sutures and wound dressing materials.
- Cut nails during podiatric surgery.

Scissors should be used for particular functions and should only be used for their intended actions. Their design, calibre, and profile are determined by the different functional requirements. In particular, much lighter and more precise scissors should be used for cutting tissues. Fine operating scissors should never be blunted by being used to cut dressings. Suitable examples are as follows.

Cutting tissue

For fine cutting of skin and other tissue, a pair of small, sharp-tipped iris scissors is ideal (Figure 1.28). These scissors are invaluable when cutting very delicate tissues and can be used very carefully to initiate blunt dissection.

Blunt dissection

For gently parting tissue layers while avoiding puncturing areas of the tissue, small curved, blunt-tipped strabismus scissors are ideal (Figure 1.29). These curved blunt scissors are useful not only for blunt dissection, but also for separating tissues around cystic lesions (such as epidermoid cysts) as their blunt tips avoid penetration of the cysts. They are available in a wide range of sizes, but the 11 cm length is ideally suited to minor surgery.

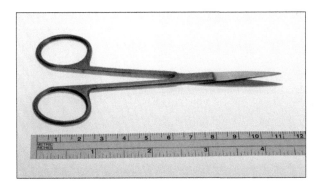

Figure 1.28 Straight iris scissors.

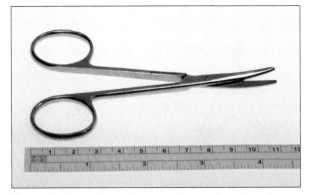

Figure 1.29 Curved blunt-tipped strabismus dissecting scissors.

Sutures and dressings

For more generalised and heavy-duty use, larger, general purpose scissors are appropriate. Suture scissors (Figure 1.30) and general purpose scissors are usually interchangeable, although suture scissors should have blunt tips to reduce the chance of 'needle-stick' injury.

Nails

More substantial scissors or clippers will be required for cutting nails (Figure 1.31). Heavy-gauge, sharp-tipped scissors may be needed for podiatric surgery for cutting nails.

Skin hook

The Gillies or McIndoe skin hook is a useful addition to the minor surgery pack, as it can be very useful in lifting a specimen as it is dissected free, and can enable wound edges to be raised to facilitate undermining and dissection (Figure 1.32a). The instrument allows tissues to be handled delicately. However, the hook needs to have a fine, sharp tip, which means there is a risk of penetrating injuries and very sharp 'needle-stick' injuries; therefore, the skin hook should be handled with caution. It is a relatively expensive item to include within a disposable instrument set, particularly as it is not always needed. Within a reusable set, two skin hooks are a useful inclusion (Figure 1.32b). There is also the possibility of making a fine DIY skin hook as described below.

DIY skin hook

There are several sets of published details for fashioning simple, disposable skin hooks from a variety of needles. One technique uses a disposable diabetic syringe with integrated needle. This fine-tipped instrument is ideally suited to facial skin surgery.

The instruments required are simple—a fine suture holder and a diabetic needle with syringe attached (100 U, i.e., 1 ml). The tip of the needle is grasped towards the end of the needle holder. The needle holder is then smoothly turned through 180° while holding the needle firmly. By grasping the tip of the needle with the fine suture holders, the needle can be bent back 180° into a J-like shape (Figure 1.33).

The skin hook thus produced is ideally suited to hooking through delicate facial tissue. The syringe makes a suitable handle, and as the syringe and needle form a single unit, there is no chance of the needle separating from the syringe handle. In addition, the delicate structure of the needle ensures that if excess tension is applied, the metal will tend to straighten out, releasing the specimen before damage occurs. If this does happen, it is advisable to use a new needle and syringe unit to avoid the possibility of metal fatigue and breakage of the needle tip.

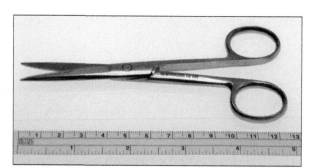

Figure 1.30 Suture scissors.

Figure 1.31 Nail clippers.

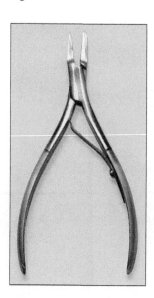

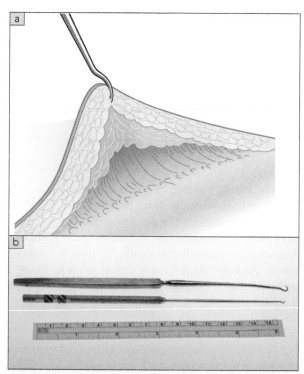

Figure 1.32 (a) Skin hook in skin. (b) Suitable skin hooks.

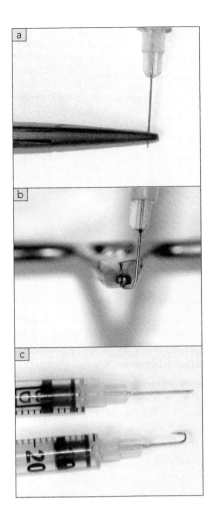

Figure 1.33 How to make a DIY skin hook.

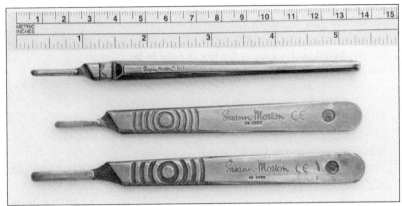

Figure 1.34 Scalpel blade handles. Top: rounded size 3 Beaver handle; middle: size 3 Bard–Parker handle (for blades Nos. 15 and 11); bottom: size 4 Bard–Parker handle (for blades Nos. 20 and 22).

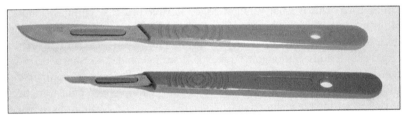

Figure 1.35 Disposable scalpels with integral blade. Top: No. 22; bottom: No. 15.

The advantages of this technique are that it utilises a fine needle firmly attached to a 'handle' (the syringe body). In addition, it can utilise the same needle with syringe unit that has been used to inject anaesthetic around the lesion (as long as it has not been contaminated by handling).

Scalpel

A scalpel is a cutting instrument comprising a blade and a handle. There are a range of different-sized blades with different uses.

Scalpels can be either metal handled with disposable blades or plastic-handled disposable instruments. Using the former requires attachment and detachment of the blade without injury (see Chapter 17 for information about how to apply a scalpel blade safely).

Reusable metal handles and blades

There are two commonly used handles with different profiles. The most common is the traditional size 3 Bard–Parker profile, but some surgeons prefer the less common rounded Beaver handle (Figure 1.34).

One of the advantages of using metal handles is that the surgeon can choose a handle to suit his or her individual needs. The single-use blade will be made of carbon steel and very sharp.

Disposable scalpels

These have a plastic handle and there is less flexibility of choice around the size and shape of the handle and blade. The stainless steel blade is often not as sharp as the disposable blades used with the reusable handle. Disposable (plastic-handled) scalpels (Figure 1.35) have the advantage that there is no blade handling when attaching the blade to and detaching it from the handle. Against this is the matter of cost: single-use scalpels cost more than single blades.

Blade shapes and sizes

When choosing blades (Figure 1.36), the following principles apply:

- The small, curved profile of the No. 15 blade makes it ideal for nearly all skin surgery.
- The sharp-pointed No. 11 blade makes it less stable for skin surgery and more suited to incisional procedures, or for scoring hard structures such as nails.
- Large, curved blades such as the No. 21 tend to be used to shave off skin lesions.

> **DON'T FORGET ▶▶**
> The No. 21 blade requires a different, larger blade handle from the No. 15 and No. 11 blades. The blades and handles are *not* interchangeable.

Other blades

If lesions are to be regularly removed by shave excision, purpose-made blades (e.g., DermaBlade®; Figure 1.37) can be used. This is a flat, straight-edged flexible blade. Mounted in a flexible plastic frame, it is held between thumb and finger and used to very gently 'shave' off raised skin lesions. Although a large No. 21 scalpel blade can do this, the DermaBlade® is more easily controlled and is extremely sharp. Further details of the technique of shave excision are included in Chapter 19.

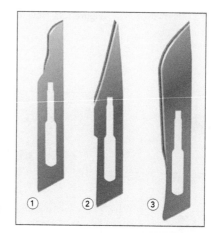

Figure 1.36
Commonly used scalpel blades.
1. No. 15 blade
2. No. 11 blade
3. No. 21 blade

Other useful instruments

Curette

Curettage is a useful surgical procedure when used appropriately (see Chapter 19 for more information about the indications and technique). The curette is generally easy to choose. If instruments are being sterilised, the surgeon has the choice between reusable Volkmann curettes (Figure 1.38) and the more frequently used circular disposable curettes (Figure 1.39), usually of 4 or 7 mm diameter. Although Volkmann curettes can be resharpened, their disadvantage is their relative bluntness compared with the scalpel-sharp single-use instruments. Care needs to be taken when using the disposable items as they will cut skin as easily as a scalpel.

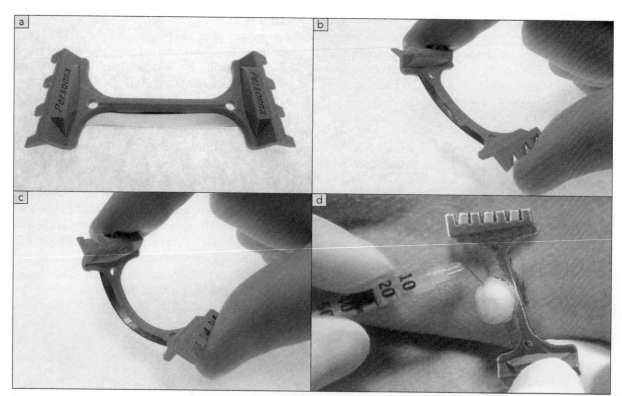

Figure 1.37 DermaBlade®.

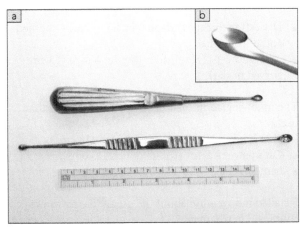

Figure 1.38 (a) Volkmann reusable curettes; (b) detail of blade.

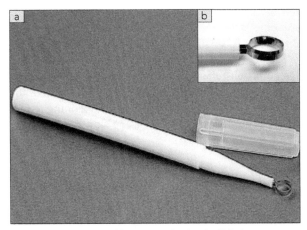

Figure 1.39 (a) Disposable curette; (b) detail of blade.

Biopsy punch

These are single-use, disposable instruments used for taking small specimens for histological analysis using a circular cutting action. The circular diameter of the available punch biopsy varies from 2 to 8 mm in diameter (Figure 1.40a,b). Histopathologists may have difficulty interpreting very small specimens of 3 mm diameter or less, so the smaller sized punch biopsies are not recommended.

The construction may include a small plunger to push out the punched core of skin (which is particularly useful for the smallest diameter punches), and some are designed to allow visualisation of the target as the punch is applied to the skin (VisiPunch™; Figure 1.40c). A punch biopsy of 5 mm diameter or more can sometimes be used to excise small lesions, but orientation of the specimen may not be possible.

The circular punches cut through the skin by the use of a rotating movement. Elliptical biopsy punches are available, which require a rocking action to cut the skin, but these are not recommended. The circular punch is much easier to use and will produce an elliptical scar if the skin is stretched prior to and during cutting. Larger circular punch biopsies with a diameter of 6 mm or more will tend to produce dog-ear wound defects when closed. A supply of 4, 5, and 6 mm punches is recommended.

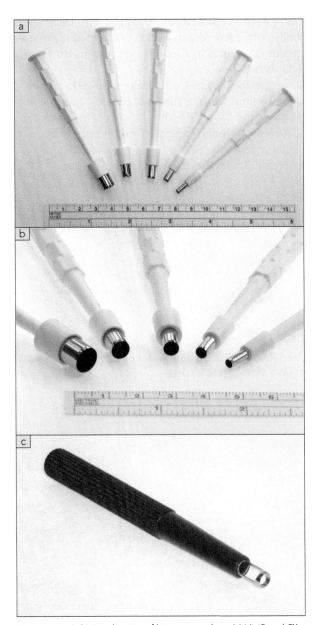

Figure 1.40 (a,b) A selection of biopsy punches. (c) VisiPunch™.

Retractor

At some stage, the practitioner may need some small retractors. A small, double-ended cat's paw retractor is useful (Figure 1.41). A range of others are available, including self-retaining instruments such as the Kocher's thyroid retractor, West Weitlaner 5.5 inch (14 cm), or the baby Kilner/Dickson Wright spring self-retaining retractor. Alternatively, an assistant using skin hooks will be required.

Dissector

Completing the list of small general instruments is the McDonald double-ended 7.5 inch (19 cm) dissector (Figure 1.42), which is extremely versatile and useful for many minor procedures.

Typical surgical set

Below is a list of recommended instruments. Each type is available in many versions, and in practice the differences do not matter much. A basic set of instruments (Figure 1.43) is as follows:

- Scalpel handle size 3 with disposable No. 15 blades.
- Strabismus scissors (curved) 4.5 inch (11.5 cm)—for dissecting.
- Dressing scissors (straight) 5 inch (13 cm)—for cutting sutures.
- Needle holder (Crile–Wood 5.5 inch (14 cm).

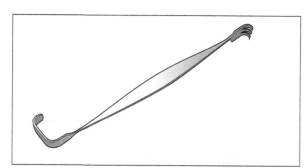

Figure 1.41 Cat's paw retractor.

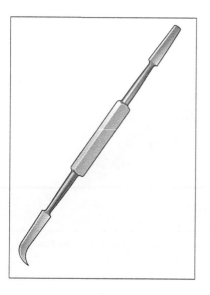

Figure 1.42
Dissector.

- Dissecting forceps (Adson 5 inch (13 cm)—toothed and non-toothed).
- Artery forceps (Halstead mosquito 5 inch (13 cm)—curved or flat).

The following additional instruments are also extremely useful:
- Skin hook (McIndoe single 7.5 inch [18 cm]).
- Cat's paw retractor (Kilner 6 inch [15 cm]).
- Large flat blades for shave excision.

Detailed information about the use of the instruments is contained in Chapter 17.

Single-use consumables/disposable items

There are a range of single-use consumable items that are essential for a skin surgery service, and it is important to have stocks of a range of these necessary items, which include the following:
- Sterile and non-sterile gloves and other items of body protection.
- Gauze/dressing packs.
- Skin preparation solutions.
- Surgical drapes.
- Skin marker pens.
- Needles and syringes.
- Sutures.
- Dressings.

Although some single-use minor operating sets will include some disposable consumables, such as gauze swabs, the supplies will vary depending on the pack.

Gloves

Most minor surgery involves the most superficial layers of the skin. For any skin surgery penetrating the dermis, sterile gloves (Figure 1.44) should be used as the risk of infecting the surgical wound is similar to the risk of an open wound being dressed. For the latter, gloves are worn as much for the protection of staff as to avoid introducing infection. The same can be said of the majority of skin surgery. For many superficial procedures, disposable single-use gloves are sufficient.

Type I latex allergy, causing urticaria in its mildest form and angioedema and anaphylaxis at its most severe, can pose problems for the surgeon, staff, and patients. Most people with latex sensitivity will be aware of their problem, and enquiring about latex sensitivity is an important part of the preoperative assessment. The prevalence of latex sensitivity has increased so it is better to err on the side of caution and ensure that vinyl or latex-free gloves are always available. As a general rule, powder-free gloves should be used. More information can be found about latex sensitivity in Chapter 4.

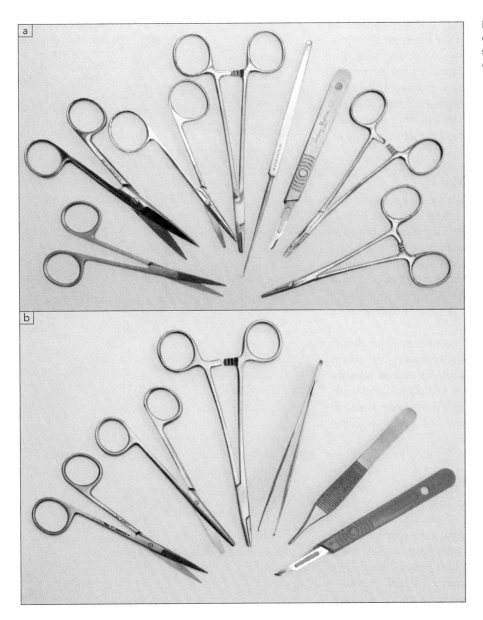

Figure 1.43 (a) Suggested essential surgical instrument set (reusable). (b) Disposable operating pack.

Glove size

All staff in an operating room should know their hand size. Sizes range from extra small (size 5.5) to extra large (size 9), the standard UK and US sizes based on hand circumference:

- Measure with a tape measure around the knuckles on your hand.
- Measure your dominant hand. Your size = the circumference in inches.

For non-sterile gloves, the sizes tend to be small, medium, and large:

- Small equates to sizes 6–7.
- Medium equates to sizes 7–8.
- Large equates to sizes 8–9.

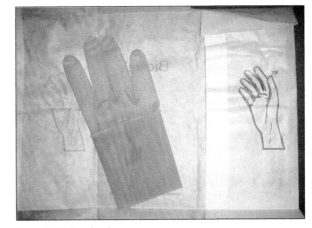

Figure 1.44 Sterile gloves.

A large glove may be easier to put on but runs the risk of poor instrument control and the finger ends projecting loosely and getting in the way of safe operating. Too tight a glove restricts blood circulation to the fingers and movement. All staff should have received instruction on applying gloves in a sterile manner. If their skills are rusty, it would be advisable to seek guidance from a surgical colleague or from the numerous video examples on Web sites such as YouTube.

Gowns, eye protection, masks

There is usually no need to wear a gown or mask; there is little evidence that these affect infection rates. A disposable plastic apron, however, provides useful protection; make sure to change the apron after each patient. Face masks are not usually required in minor surgical procedures—they provide little advantage to either patient or surgeon. To avoid droplet infection, keeping your mouth shut by not talking is much more effective than wearing a mask!

The use of eye protection is recommended for all surgical procedures. It is essential when operating on patients known to have blood-borne infections such as hepatitis and HIV, and in situations where a spurting blood vessel is likely to be encountered. Simple clear glasses or safety goggles provide such protection, are readily available, and are relatively inexpensive.

Surgical drapes

Surgical drapes allow a sterile field upon which to operate. Whereas hospital operating theatres use large secured drapes arranged over the patient, much minor surgical work uses small sterile paper towels. These can be difficult to secure, are rarely waterproof, and are often prepared by tearing a 'hole' for the operating field. They are far from ideal. If smaller drapes are used in minor surgery (Figure 1.45), they should be fenestrated with a small operating area surrounded by adhesive, allowing the drape to be accurately placed and securely fixed to the skin. In many locations, drapes are not feasible and care should be taken to avoid contaminating instruments and sterile gloves during surgery.

Skin preparation

Elaborate skin preparation for simple skin surgery procedures is probably unnecessary. However, it is well recognised that the skin is colonised by various types of bacteria. Up to 50% of these are *Staphylococcus aureus*, and studies have shown that, during open abdominal surgery, wound contamination almost always originates from skin pathogens. In addition, studies have also shown that the use of a preoperative wash containing chlorhexidine decreases the bacterial count on the skin by 80–90%, resulting in a decrease in perioperative wound contamination.

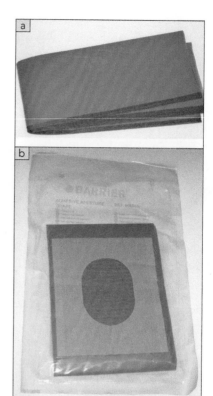

Figure 1.45
(a) Disposable surgical drape.
(b) Disposable fenestrated drape.

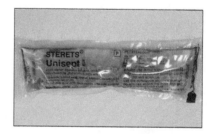

Figure 1.46 Sachet of chlorhexidine.

Skin preparation fluids can be purchased either as single-use sachets or multi-use bottles. Avoiding the use of concentrates that need diluting reduces the potential for error. Iodine-containing preparations are also best avoided as some patients are sensitive to iodine and the solution tends to discolour the skin, making skin markings difficult to see.

Chlorhexidine gluconate solution 0.05–4% is the most universal skin preparation product and is widely available, depending upon manufacturer, as a clear, blue, or pink solution (Figure 1.46). However, reports of chlorhexidine sensitivity are becoming more frequent.

GOLDEN RULE ✳

Because of the potential risk of igniting the skin, flammable skin cleansers should be avoided.

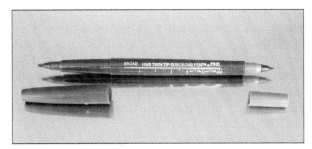

Figure 1.47 Skin marker pen.

Skin markers

A good, fine skin marker is essential and can be either sterile or non-sterile (Figure 1.47). It should be specifically designed for surgical wound marking. The traditional ink is Bonney's blue, which does not stain the skin or have any systemic effect. The most versatile marker pens will have two tips—a very fine tip and a slightly broader one. The marker pen should include a measure, either on the body of the pen or as a separate paper disposable measure. This will enable the surgeon to accurately measure the appropriate surgical margin.

Needles and syringes

Local anaesthesia will be required for all but the most minor of procedures. This can be administered by a syringe attached to a separate needle, by a combined needle and syringe (such as a 1 ml diabetic needle and syringe), or via a dental syringe and needle (Figure 1.48). Table 1.2 summarises the advantages and disadvantages of these. The majority of skin anaesthesia can be achieved with small volumes of anaesthetic. Where larger volumes of anaesthetic are required (e.g., for ring blocks

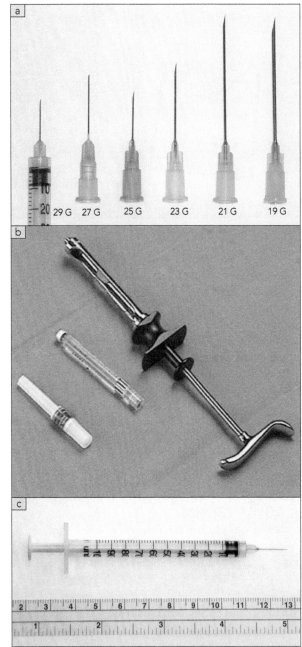

Figure 1.48 (a) Suggested needles: 29 G (0.33 mm) diabetic needle, ideal for intradermal anaesthesia; 27 G (0.4 mm) needle, ideal for digital ring blocks; 25 G (0.5 mm) alternative for intradermal use; 23 G (0.6 mm) needle, ideal for sub-dermal anaesthesia; 21 G (0.8 mm) needle for drawing up solutions; 19 G (1.1 mm) for aspiration (b) Dental syringe and cartridge. (c) Diabetic needle and syringe (29 G).

Table 1.2 **Pros and cons of needle and syringe combinations**			
	Separate needle and syringe	Diabetic needle with attached syringe	Dental needle and syringe
Advantages	• Large volumes are possible • Variable needle lengths • 'Drawing back' before injecting is possible	• Very fine needles • Small volumes, easily injected • No chance of leakage or detachment • No need to 'draw back'	• Sealed dental cartridges aid sterility • No drawing up • Long, fine needles
Disadvantages	• Large volumes and risk of toxicity • Leakage/detachment • Larger bore needles	• Fixed needle length • Limited volume	• Fixed ratio of anaesthetic (more adrenaline [epinephrine]) • Cannot draw back • Cost of dental syringe

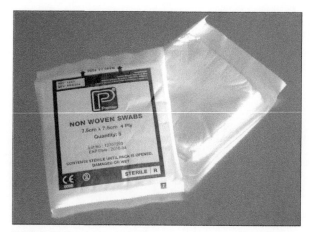

Figure 1.49 Sterile gauze swabs.

and other nerve blocks), a variety of syringe sizes should be stocked along with suitable needles. Wherever possible, fine-bore needles should be used (27 G needles are readily available)

Gauze/dressing packs

Gauze should be available in sterile packs (Figure 1.49) and also in larger multi-use 100-pad packs, the most useful size being 10 × 10 cm. A standard dressing pack with gauze, sterile drape, and gallipot is useful and should be part of the stock held. Some surgeons will use a dressing pack for simple procedures such as curettage and cautery.

> **GOLDEN RULE** ✳
> Additional gauze is essential. Be prepared for excessive bleeding even if it never happens.

Sutures (and other skin closures)

A large number of different sutures are available so it is important to get to know a small selection. The ideal suture is totally inert, provides ease of use, and does not require removal. No such suture exists, but many materials come close to some of those characteristics. One of the greatest suture developments of the twentieth century was the attached needle. Prior to this, needles required threading.

In choosing a suture, the following factors need to be considered: type of material (braided or monofilament, biological or synthetic), absorbability, diameter of material, size and shape of needle, and cutting profile. These factors are considered below.

Type of material

Historically, sutures made from biological tissues, such as silk and catgut, were widely used. Biological sutures are now rarely used, having been superseded by those made from synthetic materials. These newer synthetic sutures may consist of a single strand (monofilament; e.g., Prolene™) or of many fine strands braided together (multifilament; e.g., Vicryl™).

Braided multifilament sutures

The most common braided biological multifilament suture is silk, and the most common synthetic multifilament suture is Vicryl™ (polyglactin 910). There is really only one advantage to a braided suture such as silk—it is easier to knot. A braided material acts more like string in a surgeon's hands. One or two throws produces an initial knot that will hold and not slip. Another throw in the opposite direction creates a secure knot. In addition, braided material may exhibit greater tensile strength than an equivalent monofilament suture.

However, braided sutures display some significant disadvantages. Braided material provides a surface that can be colonised, thereby providing a method for bacteria to travel down the length of the suture. The surface of the material tends to induce a more active tissue response, with the potential for greater scarring. For this reason, non-absorbable braided skin sutures should be avoided; silk skin sutures have no place in skin surgery. Multifilament braided absorbable sutures such as polyglactin (Vicryl™) and polyglycolic acid (Dexon™) may still have a place in skin surgery, where their strength and knot characteristics can facilitate closing large wounds, but although tissue reactions are unlikely, deep sterile stitch abscesses can occur due to a foreign body reaction.

There is also sometimes a place for the use of rapidly absorbed braided multifilament sutures (e.g., Vicryl Rapide™) in certain locations. Here, because the knot bulk is outside the skin, stitch abscesses tend not to be a problem. They may be used where suture removal may be troublesome or embarrassing, or where the individual may be traumatised by removal (e.g., children).

Monofilament sutures

These sutures consist of a single strand of smooth, nylon-like material. This glides smoothly through the tissue, is inert, and excites virtually no tissue reaction. These sutures are excellent for most uses, including subcuticular closures. Their disadvantage is that they are more difficult to tie. Because they are less pliable than silk, they tend to come undone. However, it is worth learning to use them as they produce excellent results. An example is Prolene™.

Absorbable versus non-absorbable sutures

Absorbable sutures are used for suturing deeper layers or for tying blood vessels. Catgut is no longer available and should not be used. Polyglactin (Vicryl™) and polyglycolic acid (Dexon™) are multifilament absorbable sutures. They are reabsorbed within about 4–6 weeks and usually produce little in the way of tissue reaction. In minor skin surgery, they can also be used for subcuticular stitches, where they have the advantage that they do not need to be removed.

When using non-absorbable interrupted skin sutures, many clinicians like to insert absorbable sutures in the deeper tissues to reduce the tension in the surface sutures. It is argued that the superficial skin sutures can then be more confidently removed because the immediate subcutaneous tissue will be held together by the deeper sutures. Most surgeons believe that this gives a better cosmetic result and that the wound is less likely to open, particularly in areas of tension such as the back. Absorbable sutures can be used if a deep suture is required for haemostasis.

There are several important points to be remembered when selecting absorbable or non-absorbable sutures:

- In general, interrupted skin sutures need to be non-absorbable because of the time taken for absorbable sutures actually to be absorbed (4–6 weeks). The longer the material penetrates the skin, the greater the likelihood of scarring.
- Where sutures are to be buried under the skin, they need to be absorbable (the only exception being some subcuticular sutures designed to be withdrawn). The most important characteristics for buried sutures are their rate of absorption and their rate of loss of tensile strength. In some areas (face and mucous membranes), the suture material needs to be absorbed rapidly. In other areas, especially over the back, the greatest requirement is for sustained tensile strength to avoid wound stretching, so here a very slowly absorbed suture is preferable.

> ### GOLDEN RULES ✳
> - Deep buried sutures = absorbable sutures.
> - Skin sutures = non-absorbable. There are exceptions, such as some areas of genital skin where suture removal may be embarrassing and possibly the scalp where the sutures may be difficult to find.

Table 1.3 Commonly used suture gauges					
Standard gauge	6-0	5-0	4-0	3-0	2-0
Metric gauge (mm)	0.7	1.0	1.5	2.0	3.0

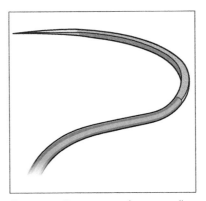

Figure 1.50 Suture swaged onto needle.

Diameter of material/suture size

There are two systems for describing the thickness of a suture: metric and traditional.

Metric

The number of the suture is equivalent to its diameter in tenths of a millimetre. A No. 2 suture, for example, is 0.2 mm in diameter.

Traditional

Although less rational than the metric system, the traditional system is still widely used. Suture thickness is expressed by an appropriate number of zeroes, for example 3-0, 4-0, 5-0, and so forth. The greater the number of zeroes, the finer the gauge of the suture. For the procedures described in this book, 3-0 is the thickest and 6-0 the finest suture that you will need (Table 1.3).

Size and shape of needle

The suture is swaged directly into a channel or hole in the butt end of the needle (Figure 1.50).

Most needles used for skin surgery are curved, although the size of the needle and its degree of curvature can vary. In almost all situations, a needle of three-eighths of a circle will be suited to skin surgery (Figure 1.51). The size of the needle is recorded in millimetres, this measurement referring to the diameter of

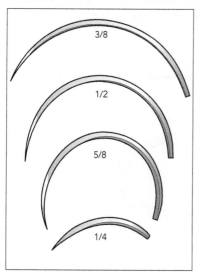

Figure 1.51 Degree of curvature of common suture needles.

the needle if it were a complete circle (Figure 1.51). As the size increases, so the calibre of the needle shaft tends to increase.

In minor surgery, two main sizes of needle are used:
- 16 mm needles are used for small incisions, particularly for the smaller 5-0 and 6-0 suture material. It is also a useful size for placing deep sutures in small wounds.
- 19 mm needles are used for almost all other skin suturing.

There are very rare occasions when a larger (25 mm needle) might be useful to close a large haemorrhaging scalp wound. Conversely, very fine and small 13 mm needles can be useful for facial surgery.

Cutting profile of needle

The final aspect of needle design is the profile (cross-section) of the needle tip. Needles originally had a simple tapering point. The disadvantage of this type of needle in skin, however, is that there is no cutting action, so the needle has to be forced through the skin. For this reason, skin surgery tends to use cutting or reverse-cutting needles, where the cross-sectional shape of the needle is triangular rather than round.

The most conventional of these needles has a cutting edge that runs along the inside, concave surface (see red triangle in Figure 1.52 [1]). By reversing this profile and using the outer, convex surface to cut (as in Figure 1.52 [2]), a reverse cutting needle is stronger and more resistant to bending. In areas where the insertion of the needle is difficult, a reverse cutting needle may avoid the needle and suture pulling or tearing through the skin to the wound edge. In practice, either sort of cutting needle may be used. There is no need for round needles in skin surgery.

Manufacturers produce variations on the triangular cross-section to improve their passage through the skin (e.g., Ethilon 'Prime' needles).

Information on the suture pack

The following information will be listed on the suture pack (Figure 1.53):
- Type of material.
- Diameter of material.
- Size and shape of the needle.
- Cutting profile of the needle.
- Total length of the suture material—on average 45 cm for skin sutures.
- Expiry date.

Other skin closures

It is worth considering keeping supplies of the following to be used instead of or alongside conventional sutures:
- *Surgical adhesives* (such as cyanoacrylate). To simplify skin closure.
- *Fibrin-based tissue adhesives*. These are useful for haemostasis and can seal tissues. Although without the tensile strength needed to close the skin, fibrin tissue adhesives can be useful when fixing skin grafts.
- *Stainless steel staples*. Staples are more expensive than traditional sutures and also require great care in placement, especially in ensuring the eversion of wound edges, so are unlikely to be needed.
- *Porous paper tapes*. For example, Steri-Strips™ are useful to ensure proper wound apposition and to provide additional reinforcement to sutures. Skin adhesives (e.g., OpSite™ spray or tincture of benzoin) aid tape adherence.

Further information about additional skin closures is included in Chapters 17 and 21.

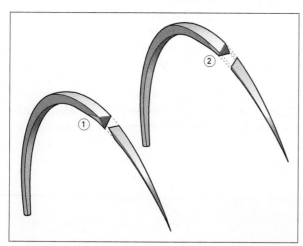

Figure 1.52 Needle profiles: (1) Conventional cutting needle. (2) Reverse cutting needle.

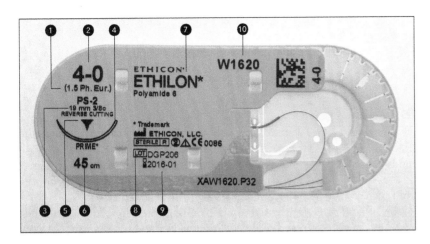

Figure 1.53 Information on suture pack:
1. Size (metric)
2. Size (traditional)
3. Needle length
4. Needle shape
5. Point shape
6. Suture length
7. Suture material
8. Lot number
9. Expiry date
10. Reference number for ordering

Dressings

The functions of a wound dressing are usually to keep the wound clean, to absorb any exudate or blood, and possibly to keep the wound dry and under pressure. The most convenient dressings to stock incorporate a pad with surrounding adhesive (Figure 1.54). Where dressings are to be used, they should be of adequate size and function. A range of sizes should be stocked:

- Total size 5 cm × 7 cm, pad size 2.5 cm × 4 cm.
- Total size 9 cm × 10 cm, pad size 4.5 cm × 6 cm.
- Total size 9 cm × 15 cm, pad size 4.5 cm × 10 cm.

It is also important to stock a range of adhesive tapes such as Elastoplast® and Micropore™. These are used to apply extra pressure to wounds likely to bleed. In addition, crêpe bandages should be stocked along with a small range of 'spot' plasters for very small wounds (such as small punch biopsies).

More information about wound care is included in Chapter 8.

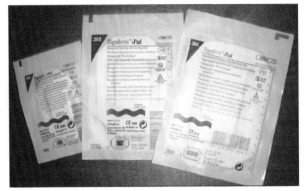

Figure 1.54 Suitable dressings.

Drugs

Local anaesthetic agents

Anaesthetics used in minor surgery will tend to be either injected (intradermally or subdermally) or applied topically. More detail about local anaesthetic agents is included in Chapter 7.

Injectables

The ideal injected local anaesthetic will be rapid in onset of action and rapidly cleared (lidocaine) or of a more sustained action (bupivacaine). Lidocaine is available in concentrations of 1% or 2%. Lidocaine is most commonly used combined with adrenaline (epinephrine). It is important that lidocaine preparations with and without adrenaline are both stocked and clearly marked to ensure that adrenaline is never inadvertently injected into end-organs (see Chapter 7).

Other injectable agents include:
- *Buffering solutions.* Sodium bicarbonate 8.4% in ampoules allows the acidic anaesthetic to be prepared as a pH-neutral injection.
- *Normal saline.* This should be stocked in sterile ampoules to enable lidocaine to be diluted down to 0.5% strength, which creates a near isotonic solution.

Topical anaesthetics

Emla® cream, containing 25 mg lidocaine and 25 mg prilocaine per gram, and Ametop™ (4% amethocaine gel), are effective for anaesthesia of the skin prior to needle puncture, for superficial cautery, or for split-skin grafting.

Emergency drugs

The following should be available to manage emergencies.

Anaphylaxis treatment

In case of allergic responses to the anaesthetic agents or to other chemicals:

- Intramuscular adrenaline (autoinjectors are convenient but expensive). Remember that adrenaline has a short shelf-life.
- Intramuscular/intravenous antihistamine such as chlorpheniramine.
- Intramuscular/intravenous corticosteroid such as hydrocortisone.

Cardiac drugs

- Intravenous atropine (in case of bradycardia).
- Intramuscular/intravenous diamorphine/morphine in case of acute myocardial infarction (plus an antiemetic).
- Aspirin (soluble) and nitrolingual spray for acute myocardial ischaemia/angina.

Central nervous system drugs

- Diazepam (Diazemuls®) for intravenous or rectal administration or buccal midazolam.

Respiratory drugs

- Inhaled/nebulised beta-2 agonist (in case of bronchospasm).

Safety equipment

The surgeon should be in a position to assess a patient in an emergency and provide immediate support for life-threatening situations. The drugs and equipment required will reflect the emergencies the surgeon might face and the local facilities. Some clinical facilities, for example, are within a few minutes' reach of a fully equipped ambulance staffed by highly trained paramedics. Others may be much more remote. Possible emergencies include:

- Vasovagal attack.
- Convulsion (from a vasovagal attack, the anaesthetic, or epilepsy).
- Acute anxiety, hyperventilation, or psychotic episode.
- Myocardial infarction/cardiac arrest.
- Anaphylaxis or allergic reaction to the drugs or chemicals used.
- Haemorrhage.

Assessing a patient appropriately requires the following equipment:

- Sphygmomanometer.
- Stethoscope.
- ECG monitor.
- Pulse oximeter.

The minimum equipment necessary to provide immediate emergency support is:

- Intravenous cannulae, a giving set, and intravenous fluids (both colloid and crystalloid), including adhesive skin tape.
- Essential drugs including adrenaline, hydrocortisone, and chlorpheniramine (see above).
- Plastic airways.
- An oxygen cylinder with a giving set (2–4 l per minute).
- A bag and face masks.
- Suction (either mains or mechanically operated).

Other equipment that is desirable but not essential is:

- A defibrillator.
- A laryngoscope and endotracheal tubes.

Further detail on resuscitation is included in Chapter 16.

Miscellaneous
'Sharps' containers

Needles, broken glass ampoules, and other 'sharps' need to be disposed of safely. They should be placed in a plastic receptacle such as a 'burn-bin', which is subsequently incinerated (Figure 1.55). These should be sealed and placed in a lockable clinical waste container when no more than three-quarters full. The sharps bin should be either wall-mounted or placed on the work surface so that it is not accessible to children. The location should be chosen close to where the surgical trolley is cleaned to avoid carrying sharps around the room.

Clinical waste disposal

Bloodstained and contaminated dressings and paper drapes should be collected in plastic bin liners (usually yellow or more recently orange) within a foot-pedal-operated bin (Figure 1.56a) separate from non-clinical soiled waste. For non-soiled waste (hand towels, etc.), ordinary black bin liners, again in a pedal-operated bin, should be provided close to the basin (Figure 1.56b).

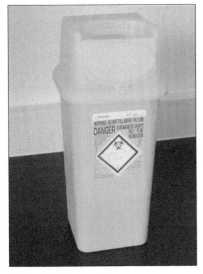

Figure 1.55 Sharps bin.

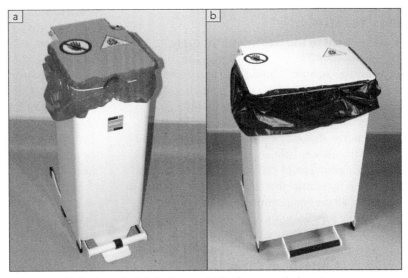

Figure 1.56 (a) Bin for soiled clinical waste. (b) Bin for non-soiled waste.

First aid box

In the United Kingdom, under the Health and Safety (First Aid) Regulations 1981, even doctors' surgeries need to have first aid provisions. There should be a named first aider to take charge of any accident, ensure that it is reported and recorded, and make sure a simple first aid box is always within the building. It is not a good idea to rely on treatment room first aid supplies.

The first aid box should contain:

- A guidance card on resuscitation.
- Individually wrapped sterile adhesive dressings.
- Triangular bandages.
- Medium-sized sterile wound dressings.
- Large sterile wound dressing.
- Safety pins.
- Sterile eye pads and bandages.

First aid boxes should not contain medications of any kind.

Music system

For many patients, there is no such thing as a minor operation—it is a major event and can create considerable anxiety. Playing relaxing music quietly in the background can be of immense benefit for both patient and staff. Within the United Kingdom, a licence from the Performing Rights Society will be required to do this. Some doctors provide a personal stereo and ask patients to bring along their favourite music. Decide in advance whether someone else's music will be a help or a hindrance to the surgeon!

STAFF REQUIREMENTS

Competent, suitably trained support staff are essential for the smooth running of the operating room, and for the safety and comfort of the patient. Their role is vital and is becoming increasingly skilled. Often with a nursing background, health-care professionals taking on this role possess additional skills in minor surgery and the care of instruments. They may be a practice nurse, an operating theatre assistant, or a health-care assistant, but appropriate training is the key feature. For the purpose of this section, the role will be referred to as the theatre assistant(s). Important details of the skills required for a theatre assistant are discussed at the end of the section.

It is preferable to have the same team of surgeon and assistant working regularly together so that the surgeon's individual preferences and surgical techniques are known in advance. The best assistants work with the surgeon as a team, each being able to predict what the other will do or need. This leads to safe, efficient surgery. Enthusiastic amateurs should be limited to observation only. Any surgeon who has performed minor operations without the help of a competent assistant will realise what an essential role the trained theatre assistant plays in the smooth and safe running of the procedure and care of the patient.

Roles and responsibilities of the theatre assistant(s)

Management of the treatment room/ operating theatre

The theatre assistant should be responsible for the smooth running of the operating area. This will include the following key operational responsibilities:

- Supervising and ensuring that there is adequate cleaning of all floors, walls, working surfaces, and operating theatre lights.
- Checking equipment and reporting any defects or faults. It is essential that the assistant knows how to operate all the equipment.
- Checking supplies of sutures, dressings, drugs, dressing packs, and instrument packs, and reordering supplies when stocks are low. There should be a supplies checklist to ensure that the theatre does not run out of supplies, and a system to ensure this continues during times of leave.
- Ensuring that all policies are up to date and implemented effectively.

Some 'protected time' is essential for checking, cleaning, and restocking the treatment room. It also allows for unexpected emergencies and encourages safe practice.

Time management and booking arrangements

Planned operating sessions are preferable to random ad hoc sessions. A planned session also enables the theatre assistant to prepare the room in advance for each procedure and to check essential equipment. In addition, it reduces the risk of possible cross-infection if the operating room is being used as a multi-treatment room. A good assistant will also be able to liaise with booking and administrative staff to predict how long individual procedures are likely to take and organise operating lists accordingly.

Communicating with the patient and surgeon

The theatre assistant will be involved in the four phases of the communication process:

- Introduction.
- Consent.
- Operation.
- Postoperative instructions.

Supporting the communication needs of the patient and surgeon through each of these stages instils confidence and reassures the patient. Further information about the importance of communication skills is included in Chapter 14, as this is considered to be an important essential generic skill.

Positioning the patient correctly

Both the patient and the surgeon must be comfortable during any operation, and the assistant can help with positioning the patient correctly. For the majority of surgical procedures, it is better to have the patient lying down rather than sitting upright in order to reduce the possibility of fainting. Lesions on the face, the front of the body, and the limbs can be treated with the patient lying comfortably on their back, with the head supported by a pillow. However, if the lesion is on the back of the head, back, buttocks, thighs, or back of the lower limbs, the patient may have to lie face down. In this situation, it is worth spending time making sure the patient is comfortable and able to keep still, as well as ensuring good exposure of the lesion to be treated, without causing undue tension on the skin in any direction. Additional pillows or supports are helpful when it is necessary to have patients in a semi-prone position or on their side.

Preparing the local anaesthetic

Almost all minor operations will be performed using local anaesthetic, and each surgeon will have preferred anaesthetic agents and means of administration.

The assistant should be aware of preferences and be able to prepare any ampoules, syringes, and needles. For simple infiltration anaesthesia to the skin, some surgeons may be happy for a suitably trained and licensed assistant to perform this while they are handwashing, thereby saving time. Both the surgeon and the assistant should check that the correct drug is being administered, and that the maximum dose for that particular anaesthetic agent is not exceeded.

Preparing instruments and instrument packs

One of the essential roles of any assistant is preparing all necessary instruments and instrument packs that are likely to be used for the operation. The choice of sutures may be discussed in advance, or at least the likely sutures can already be prepared for use by the assistant, together with surgical drapes and any postoperative dressings and bandages. The assistant will also be responsible for setting up any monitoring equipment such as a pulse oximeter, blood pressure monitor, or electrocardiograph that might be required, and for explaining the reasons for this to the patient.

The role of the assistant during an operation

As well as reassuring the patient at all times, the assistant will be required to assist at some operations. This may involve holding simple skin retractors, applying pressure to bleeding vessels, cutting sutures, inserting sutures if appropriate, cleaning the skin at the end of the operation, or applying skin-closure strips, aerosol skin cover, and/or dressings and bandages.

Scrubbed or unscrubbed?

For most minor operations, it is not necessary for the assistant to be scrubbed and wearing sterile gloves, but for procedures where an additional pair of hands is necessary, the assistant should wash their hands and don sterile gloves exactly as the surgeon would do. In this situation, it can be helpful to have a third 'unscrubbed' person on hand in case an additional instrument, suture, or anaesthetic is needed.

Postoperative information leaflets, recovery, and aftercare

The following are important responsibilities once the procedure has been completed:

- Ensuring a good supply of readily available, up-to-date patient information leaflets to give to each patient at the end of the procedure.
- Providing the patient with postoperative care instructions and offering to answer any questions.
- Organising any follow-up appointments for suture removal or dressings.
- Providing patients with contact details for if they have any concerns, in particular including advice on how to seek help out of hours.

Role of the assistant at the completion of an operation

Following any surgical procedure, the assistant should clear away any instruments and dressings and then escort the patient from the operating couch to an adjacent recovery area. With regard to the disposal of sharps, many surgeons prefer to dispose of the sharps themselves to avoid risking a needle-stick injury to the assistant. However, other surgeons argue that this is something that the assistant is capable of doing safely as he or she will have a clear record of the sharps provided. Whatever the preferred choice, it is essential that the surgeon and the assistant are clear between them who is responsible for this very important task.

Documentation and record keeping

The assistant is responsible for ensuring the following:

- Keeping a log of the procedure, either computerised and/or as a hard copy.
- Making sure that all samples are sent for histopathological examination.
- Documenting the samples sent to the histopathology laboratory and checking that the details on the histopathology request form match those on the specimen pot and in the log.

- Implementing a fail-safe system with the surgeon to ensure that all reports are received back in a timely fashion and are acted upon appropriately.
- Checking that all the required documentation has been completed by the surgeon.

More detail on documentation can be found in Chapter 2.

At the end of the 'list'

At the end of the operating list, the assistant should be responsible for sorting the instruments, cleaning them if appropriate, packing them ready to send for sterilisation, completing all paperwork, cleaning and sterilising any surfaces which may have been contaminated, and leaving any specific advice or requests for the cleaners.

Staff training and continuing professional development

All surgeons have their own idiosyncrasies; good assistants know these and work with them. Surgeons, on the other hand, need to recognise that they are but one part of a successful team. There is no place for a prima donna within a surgical theatre. Look no further than the example of a Formula 1 motor-racing team undertaking a pit stop to realise the importance of teamwork. It is no accident that some enlightened surgical units have looked to racing teams to understand teamwork. Each person knows their own role, but they also know each other's and can in this way predict errors before they occur.

Within minor surgery, it is essential that the assistant is kept fully involved within the surgical process, and it is also essential that their time during an operating list is protected. Safe surgery ensures that the assistant does not have to leave to answer the phone, provide a result, or carry out some other non-theatre task. Regular training in basic resuscitation skills, including cardiopulmonary resuscitation, is essential. In addition, within the theatre, the assistant should know the location of all the emergency drugs, dressings, and other equipment and know how to use them. Assistants should be trained to identify common surgical complications such as haemorrhage or vasovagal attacks and predict what will be required. Both surgeon and assistant should ensure that continuing educational needs are met.

Recommended competency framework

The following describes a recommended competency framework for a surgical assistant.

Knowledge

- The purpose of minor surgery.
- Types of minor surgery.
- Types and uses of different local anaesthetics.
- The explanation to give to the patient about to undergo minor surgery.
- How to care for a patient about to undergo minor surgery.
- Information to give to patients on how to care for their wound.
- Methods of storage and dispatch of specimens following minor surgery.
- The records kept of minor surgery having taken place.
- How to obtain the necessary equipment.
- How to obtain/complete the necessary forms to accompany the specimens.
- How to dispose of the equipment used.
- How to dispose of faulty equipment.
- Where the emergency drugs are stored.

Skills

- Demonstrate laying up a trolley for minor surgery.
- Demonstrate the care of a patient undergoing minor surgery.
- Demonstrate assisting the doctor carrying out minor surgery.
- Demonstrate knowledge of the correct specimen pots to place different specimens in and their disposal.
- Demonstrate how to give patients advice on how to care for their wound.
- Demonstrate how to dispose of the dirty equipment safely.

Chapter 2

Informed consent, record keeping, documentation, and audit

INTRODUCTION

The first section of this chapter discusses obtaining informed consent, which is an essential part of the interaction between clinician and patient before a procedure is performed. The second section describes the need to keep good records of any procedure, to ensure optimal patient care, and to enable clinical practice to be audited and constantly reviewed against national and local guidance. The final sections consider policies that need implementation if surgery is to be offered in an environment that is safe for staff and patients (e.g., infection control) and emphasise the importance of audit to measure performance and support the provision of safe, high-quality care.

INFORMED CONSENT

Principles
The principles underlying consent are laid out below.

What is meant by consent?
The principle of consent is that individuals must give their permission before they undergo an investigation or receive any type of medical treatment. Consent is required however large or small the procedure, investigation, or treatment involved. This principle of consent is clearly laid down in international human rights law, so although reference is made in this section to UK law on this subject, the principles represent good clinical practice. However, the law and codes of practice will vary between one country and the next—you need to be up to date and compliant with the ones where you work.

There is international variation in legal meaning between the terms *informed consent* and *valid consent*, and in some texts *valid consent* is also referred to as *real consent*. Informed consent places an emphasis on the communication of all possible risks to the patient, whereas valid consent focuses on the patient's comprehension of an adequate and appropriate level of information. In the United Kingdom, the emphasis is on informed consent.

When is consent valid?
If consent is to be valid, it must meet the following criteria:
- *Voluntary:* In other words, the decision must be made by the patient alone and not in response to undue pressure from health-care professionals, friends, or family.
- *Informed:* The individual must have received sufficient information to fully understand the implications of the investigation or treatment, in particular its benefits and risks. Equally, information about the consequences of not having the investigation or procedure performed should have been provided and alternative options discussed.
- *Capacity:* The person should have the mental capacity to understand the full range of information provided and to be able to make an informed decision based on that information.

Who can consent?
An appropriately informed person who has the required mental capacity is able to consent. This person can be the patient or someone authorised by law to make this decision on behalf of the patient. There are specific issues relating to children and young adults, which will be discussed below.

Are there ever any situations when treatment can go ahead without consent?

Only in exceptional circumstances can treatment go ahead without consent. These are as follows:

- In an emergency where life-saving treatment is required and where it is not possible for consent to be obtained, for example if the patient is unconscious.
- If the person lacks the mental capacity to understand and use the information provided to make a decision, then the health-care professionals can give the treatment provided that it is believed that this is in the best interests of the patient.

What is meant by having the mental capacity to consent?

Capacity is simply the ability of an individual to use and understand information sufficiently to make a decision about their medical treatment, at the time that it needs to be made. Capacity is absent when this ability is lost, either permanently or transiently, through an impairment of function of the brain or mind. This dysfunction may impair one or more of the following: comprehension, retention, reasoning, and communication (in any form), and capacity will then be lost. There are a range of situations where this may occur, for example:

- Mental health conditions such as schizophrenia or bipolar disorder.
- Dementia.
- Conditions causing confusion, drowsiness, or loss of consciousness.
- Intoxication caused by drugs or alcohol.

The key questions to consider when deciding whether someone has the capacity to consent to a treatment or procedure are:

- Does the person understand the information that is being discussed relating to the decision?
- Can the person remember the information that is being discussed?
- Is the individual able to use the information to inform the decision-making process?
- Can any decision be effectively communicated?

It is also important to remember that people's capacity may change over time. In addition, it is important to recognise that some people may have the capacity to make simple straightforward decisions but struggle with more complicated problems.

What comprises adequate information?

The patient should be given adequate information, in a form that can be readily understood, with the aim of empowering the patient to make a decision on whether or not to proceed with an action. Individual patients will indicate their preference for different levels of information or involvement in decision-making. Health-care professionals should not prejudge or assume the patient's want or need for information, in particular in relation to pre-existing knowledge and comprehension.

With regard to the types of procedure considered in this book, this is the type of information you should discuss:

- The diagnosis of the condition being treated and its prognosis.
- The options for the treatment of the condition, including the option to not treat.
- What is involved in any procedure proposed.
- The benefits, risks, and likelihood of success for the range of treatments/procedures discussed.

For any surgical procedure, the specific issues that will need to be covered are:

- The use of a local anaesthetic.
- The possibility of bleeding and wound infection.
- The wound produced and the time scale for healing.
- A discussion of the likely scar.
- Potential complications likely at specific sites, for example the risk of hypertrophic scar formation on the chest.
- The possibility of additional procedures becoming necessary (for example, you indicate that you will perform a curettage and cautery of a skin lesion but, as a result of excessive bleeding, suturing is required).

Declining information

Some patients express their preference to receive no information at all. The reason behind this choice should be explored and discussed, and wherever possible a basic set of essential information should be provided. If even this minimal information is declined, the possible consequences, including the invalidity of the consent, should be discussed with the patient. A procedure cannot be undertaken if the patient has not given informed consent, and the patient needs to know this and be clear about the consequences of not having the procedure performed. Accurate documentation of this type of discussion and outcome is essential.

Withholding information

Information should only be withheld if the clinician believes that giving it will cause the patient serious harm. It is not unknown for a relative, partner, friend, or carer to request that information is withheld from the patient in the event that the patient becomes upset by the information or decides to refuse treatment on learning the risks. This is considered to be an inadequate cause for withholding information from the patient.

Facilitating comprehension

Information, no matter how comprehensive and accurate, is useless if the patient cannot understand, retain, use, or weigh up the information needed to make the decision of whether to agree to or refuse an examination, investigation, or treatment.

In the United Kingdom, national guidance recognises the legal presumption of capacity to make decisions and warns of the following:

- Assumptions that a patient lacks capacity must not be made on the basis of age, disability, appearance, behaviour, medical condition (including mental illness), personal beliefs, an apparent inability to communicate, or the fact that the patient makes a decision that you disagree with.
- An irrational decision may be the result of either a different value system or a warped perception of reality. Capacity is preserved in the former but not the latter.
- Capacity can fluctuate, so time and support may be needed to maximise the patient's ability to make decisions for him- or herself.

It is very easy for time pressures to compromise the quality of consent. The manner and circumstances in which information is presented affect the chance of this information being understood and retained by the patient. Some patients want another person, such as a relative, partner, friend, carer, or advocate, to be involved in discussions or to help them make decisions. Supportive material in the form of written or audiovisual aids can be very helpful, but it is easy to forget to check that they are up to date and accurate. The importance of time for reflection is also increasingly being recognised, especially when the risks are significant and the information is complex.

Additional procedures

When performing the types of surgery described in this text, it is unlikely that additional procedures will become necessary, so this is much less of an issue than for larger surgical procedures. It may, however, occasionally be relevant. For example, you may decide to curette and cauterise a lesion, such as a pyogenic granuloma. If during the procedure it might become clear that you are going to need to use sutures to control haemostasis, you should have discussed this with the patient beforehand as a potential additional procedure.

Who can obtain consent?

The person obtaining consent for a treatment or procedure should usually be the health-care professional directly responsible for the treatment or procedure, or a member of the team who has received appropriate training in obtaining consent. In order to be able to do this, the health-care professional must:

- Have the ability to recognise whether the patient has the mental capacity to make the decision about the treatment or procedure.
- Be able to provide the patient with enough information to provide informed consent, particularly in relation to the risks and benefits of the treatment/ procedure.
- Recognise the importance of the voluntary nature of consent.
- Know about the particular issues relating to obtaining consent from children and young adults and the issue of parental responsibility where appropriate.
- Be familiar with any required documentation relating to the obtaining of informed consent.

How can consent be given?

Consent can be given verbally, non-verbally, or in writing. In much day-to-day clinical practice, consent is implied, for example when we measure a patient's blood pressure. Written consent is good clinical practice for any surgical procedure and is therefore recommended for the procedures described in this text.

DON'T FORGET ▶▶

Written consent is of no value whatsoever in the following circumstances:

- Where the consent was not given voluntarily.
- Where the patient was not fully informed about the procedure and its risks and benefits.

[NHS organisation name] consent form 3

Patient identifier/label

Patient/parental agreement to investigation or treatment

(procedures where consciousness not impaired)

Name of procedure (include brief explanation if medical term not clear)

....

Statement of health professional (to be filled in by health professional with appropriate knowledge of proposed procedure, as specified in consent policy)

I have explained the procedure to the patient/parent. In particular, I have explained:

The intended benefits ....

....

Serious or frequently occurring risks ....

....

I have also discussed what the procedure is likely to involve, the benefits and risks of any available alternative treatments (including no treatment) and any particular concerns of those involved.

The following leaflet/tape has been provided ....

Signed .... Date..

Name (PRINT).. Job title...

Statement of interpreter (where appropriate)

I have interpreted the information above to the patient/parent to the best of my ability and in a way in which I believe s/he/they can understand.

Signed .... Date .... Name (PRINT)...............................

Statement of patient/person with parental responsibility for patient

I agree to the procedure described above.

I understand that you cannot give me a guarantee that a particular person will perform the procedure. The person will, however, have appropriate experience.

I understand that the procedure will / will not involve local anaesthesia.

Signed .... Date..

Name (PRINT) .... Relationship to patient ....

Confirmation of consent (to be completed by a health professional when the patient is admitted for the procedure, if the patient/parent has signed the form in advance)

I have confirmed that the patient/parent has no further questions and wishes the procedure to go ahead.

Signed .... Date ....

Name (PRINT) .... Job title ....

Top copy accepted by patient: yes / no (please ring)

Figure 2.1 UK Department of Health sample consent form.

Other advantages of obtaining written consent for the patient and practitioner are as follows:

- The documentation can be used as a checklist to ensure that all the relevant information has been provided.
- A copy confirming the areas discussed can be offered to the patient.
- The signed document can be stored in the lifelong patient record.

Examples of consent forms are available for download from the Department of Health Web site (Department of Health, 2009a [archived site]). The downloaded rich text format (.rtf) version allows modification (Figure 2.1). You may prefer to develop your own consent documentation (see the Appendix at the end of this chapter for an example).

Respecting the patient's decision
Refusing treatment
Provided you are sure that the patient has the capacity to make a decision and that you have provided them with accurate, unbiased information, the patient has the right to refuse treatment, no matter how wrong or irrational the decision seems. The patient's decision must be respected, but you must be sure to express your concern about the decision and discuss the possible consequences of the refusal of treatment. You should also document such discussions and the outcome in detail.

Requesting a different treatment
If the patient requests a different treatment that is felt to be of greater risk than benefit compared with the suggested treatment, the health-care professional does not have to provide the treatment. In these circumstances, it is helpful for the clinician to explain the reasons for his or her decision, as well as the risks and benefits of the alternatives, and suggest that the patient seek a second opinion.

Absence of coercion
Coercion can take a range of forms. Patients are sometimes coaxed, cajoled, and even bullied into seeking a medical opinion and/or surgical procedure by friends or families. Similarly, undue external pressure may be put on patients to accept or refuse a particular investigation or treatment. It is important to be aware of this and to be able to advise patients of their need to come to their own decision and of their legal right to refuse treatment should they so wish. Coercion invalidates consent.

Specific issues in children and young people
Principles
- Unnecessary surgical procedures leading to permanent scarring should be avoided in children and young adults. The clinician should ask the question 'Is this procedure medically indicated?' Children and young adults should be involved in decisions about their treatment and should not be coerced into having unnecessary surgery. Cosmetic excisions are to be avoided wherever possible in children and young adults.
- The health-care professional should, as with adults, determine whether the child or young adult has the 'capacity' to give consent to the procedure or treatment.
- People over the age of 16 years may be competent to consent to treatment and procedures, and the law in the United Kingdom recognises this competence.
- If a child or young adult is not competent to consent to treatment, consent must, except in an emergency, be obtained from someone with parental responsibility.
- Once a child reaches the age of 18, no one can consent on their behalf.

Children aged 16 and 17
The clinician should explain the proposed procedure and the risks and benefits and make a judgement about whether the young adult is competent to give consent by assessing the following:
- Has the patient understood the consequences of the procedure, particularly in relation to potential lifelong scarring?
- Is he or she able to use this information sensibly and thoughtfully to come to a decision?
- Is the patient able to communicate his/her wishes?

There will be one of two outcomes:
- In some situations, the clinician will determine that the young adult meets the criteria of having the capacity to give informed consent.
- For others, this will not be the case, and someone with parental responsibility will need to provide consent to treatment.

Where there is any uncertainty about how to proceed and there is no medical need to perform the relevant surgical procedure urgently, a period of reflection is recommended, and any decision should be deferred.

Children under the age of 16
Children under the age of 16 can be deemed legally competent to consent to treatment, without the need for parental permission or knowledge, provided that they have 'sufficient understanding and maturity to enable them to understand fully what is proposed'. In England and Wales, this is called Gillick competency.

Gillick competency
Gillick competency relates to a decision taken in the House of Lords in 1985. Victoria Gillick challenged a circular from the Department of Health in England which suggested that parental consent was not required to prescribe contraception for under-16s (*Gillick* v. *West Norfolk and Wisbech Area Health Authority*, 1986). Mrs Gillick argued that prescribing contraception to this age group was illegal because consent lay with the parent, so the issue before the House of Lords was whether the minor involved could give consent.

The House of Lords judgment made clear that parental rights exist only to safeguard the best interests of the minor, and that in certain circumstances (where the minor has 'sufficient understanding and maturity to enable them to understand fully what is proposed') the minor can consent to treatment, and the parent cannot veto this consent.

Gillick competency is binding in England and Wales, and has been approved in Australia, Canada, and New Zealand. In Scotland, the same provision is incorporated in *The Age of Legal Capacity (Scotland) Act 1991*. There is separate legislation in Northern Ireland, but it is presumed that the same decision would be followed by the courts there.

Gillick versus Fraser competency

There is widespread confusion regarding the term 'Gillick competency', which many refer to as 'Fraser competency'. Lord Fraser was involved in the Gillick judgment but was responsible for publishing guidelines relating specifically to contraception and the importance of involving parents in decisions about contraception in minors. There were rumours that Victoria Gillick resented having her name associated with the ruling relating to the assessment of children's mental capacity and consent to treatment. There is no evidence to support this (Wheeler, 2006).

Parental responsibility

Parental responsibility provides parents with the right to consent to treatment when the child (under the age of 18) is deemed, after consideration of the issues above, not able to consent him- or herself (General Medical Council, 2007). In the United Kingdom, The Children Act 1989 outlines who has parental responsibility for a child. If a clinician is in any doubt about whether the adult attending with the child has appropriate parental responsibility in a specific case, advice should be sought.

Consent in the United Kingdom

In the United Kingdom, there is very specific national guidance in two important documents:

- *General Medical Council guidance.* The GMC document *Consent: Patients and Doctors Making Decisions Together* (General Medical Council, 2008), which is directed at medical practitioners, makes very specific recommendations on the information a medical practitioner should provide as part of the consent process. It advises that the risks discussed should include the common, less serious complications and the rare serious ones. However, it makes clear the importance of tailoring the information provided to the needs of individual patients.
- *Department of Health guidance.* The Department of Health document *Reference Guide to Examination or Treatment* (Department of Health, 2009b) places an emphasis on reference to UK case law, and health-care professionals are advised that information about all significant possible adverse outcomes is given, and that a record of the information given is made.

Summary

Consent is a process that should reflect the legal requirements of seeking permission, thereby avoiding the healthcare professional being accused of assault or battery. It should also be viewed as reflecting an optimal patient–doctor relationship cemented by trust and mutual respect.

The two 'rules of 3' that inform valid consent are:

- The *key elements* of consent: capacity, appropriate information, and voluntariness.
- The *process* of consent: disclosure of information to the patient, receiving of information from the patient, and documentation.

RECORD KEEPING

It is essential to make written records of every minor procedure carried out. The system used, be it hard copy or electronic, does not matter as long as it is effective and fail-safe. At its simplest, this can be a combination of clinical notes and a minor procedure book. Increasingly, however, software systems exist to collect information electronically, and this has the advantage that a template can be used to collect the necessary important information.

Logically, any such system should be linked to the whole patient record. Stand-alone systems to collect information about patients should be developed with consideration of patient confidentiality and data protection. A compromise is to develop a specially designed form for collecting relevant information. The information from such forms can then easily be processed, and if appropriate entered onto a computer system for analysis.

The clinical records of procedures are extremely important for medicolegal reasons. If a problem arises years after the actual procedure was carried out, it may be impossible to defend a claim in the absence of accurate written records. In some circumstances, accurate record keeping is a condition of service, and records may be required when making claims for payment.

The patient
Information required

The following information should be collected and documented clearly:

- The patient's details: name, address, date of birth, contact telephone numbers, and e-mail address if appropriate.
- The date of the initial consultation and the date of the procedure (recording whether there were any delays, and if so, why).
- The clinical diagnosis and indications for the procedure.
- The relevant current or past medical history.
- Regular medications and any allergies.
- Whether the patient has given signed informed consent. Any specific issues discussed, such as infection, bleeding, and scarring, should be documented.

The procedure

Two separate areas of documentation are relevant to the procedure. The first is the patient's medical record and the second is the procedure log, which records the procedures performed on a particular day by a particular surgeon and theatre assistant. Completing the clinical notes is usually the responsibility of the surgeon, and the assistant will usually complete the procedure log.

The World Health Organization checklist

The World Health Organization (WHO) has been active in a number of initiatives to improve the safety of surgical procedures, most recently through the Second Global Patient Safety Challenge: Safe Surgery Saves Lives. The World Alliance for Patient Safety started work on this in January 2007, and a key output of this project is the WHO Safe Surgery Checklist, which is now being implemented worldwide.

The checklist identifies three phases of a surgical procedure: prior to anaesthesia (sign in), before the incision of the skin (time out), and before the patient leaves the operating room (sign out). A list of tasks is identified for each of the three stages, and a checklist coordinator must confirm that the tasks have been completed at each stage of the operation. A manual is available which provides suggestions for implementing the checklist. It is anticipated that use of the checklist will standardise care and minimise common and avoidable risks that occur during surgical procedures.

Although the recommended checklist (Figure 2.2) is not entirely suited to the minor surgical procedures carried out under local anaesthetic that are described in this text, the principles of the documentation are useful and can be readily modified. Figure 2.3 shows an example of the WHO checklist that has been modified for use as a minor surgery record for documentation in the patient's notes. Appendix 2 shows a practical checklist designed and used by the author.

Figure 2.2 World Health Organization generic checklist.

Documenting details of the procedure

Whatever type of documentation is used, the following information should be clearly documented in the patient's records:

- The date of the procedure and the name of the surgeon.
- The local anaesthesia used (strength, type—with or without adrenaline [epinephrine]) and its quantity.
- The suture materials used and the number of sutures.
- Whether haemostasis has been achieved.
- Where any perioperative problems occurred.
- The type and number of specimens sent for histology.
- Details of the postoperative care and arrangements for suture removal; whether information leaflets have been provided.
- Arrangements for communicating any results to the patient.

Procedure log

The procedure log may be hard copy or electronic and completed by either the surgeon or the theatre assistant. It should record the following:

- Brief description of the procedure.
- The local anaesthetic used, including batch numbers and expiry dates.
- The sutures used.
- The number of specimens sent for histopathological examination.
- It is also useful to have a column to complete when the histopathology report is returned: gaps in this column highlight missing reports.

World Health Organization

SURGICAL SAFETY CHECKLIST (FIRST EDITION)

Before induction of anaesthesia ▶▶▶▶▶▶▶▶▶ Before skin incision ▶▶▶▶▶▶▶▶▶▶▶▶▶▶▶▶ Before patient leaves operating room

SIGN IN

- [ ] PATIENT HAS CONFIRMED
  - IDENTITY
  - SITE
  - PROCEDURE
  - CONSENT

- [ ] SITE MARKED/NOT APPLICABLE

- [ ] ANAESTHESIA SAFETY CHECK COMPLETED

- [ ] PULSE OXIMETER ON PATIENT AND FUNCTIONING

DOES PATIENT HAVE A

KNOWN ALLERGY?
- [ ] NO
- [ ] YES

DIFFICULT AIRWAY/ASPIRATION RISK?
- [ ] NO
- [ ] YES, AND EQUIPMENT/ASSISTANCE AVAILABLE

RISK OF >500ML BLOOD LOSS (7ML/KG IN CHILDREN)?
- [ ] NO
- [ ] YES, AND ADEQUATE INTRAVENOUS ACCESS AND FLUIDS PLANNED

TIME OUT

- [ ] CONFIRM ALL TEAM MEMBERS HAVE INTRODUCED THEMSELVES BY NAME AND ROLE

- [ ] SURGEON, ANAESTHESIA PROFESSIONAL AND NURSE VERBALLY CONFIRM
  - PATIENT
  - SITE
  - PROCEDURE

ANTICIPATED CRITICAL EVENTS

- [ ] SURGEON REVIEWS: WHAT ARE THE CRITICAL OR UNEXPECTED STEPS, OPERATIVE DURATION, ANTICIPATED BLOOD LOSS?

- [ ] ANAESTHESIA TEAM REVIEWS: ARE THERE ANY PATIENT-SPECIFIC CONCERNS?

- [ ] NURSING TEAM REVIEWS: HAS STERILITY (INCLUDING INDICATOR RESULTS) BEEN CONFIRMED? ARE THERE EQUIPMENT ISSUES OR ANY CONCERNS?

HAS ANTIBIOTIC PROPHYLAXIS BEEN GIVEN WITHIN THE LAST 60 MINUTES?
- [ ] YES
- [ ] NOT APPLICABLE

IS ESSENTIAL IMAGING DISPLAYED?
- [ ] YES
- [ ] NOT APPLICABLE

SIGN OUT

NURSE VERBALLY CONFIRMS WITH THE TEAM:

- [ ] THE NAME OF THE PROCEDURE RECORDED

- [ ] THAT INSTRUMENT, SPONGE AND NEEDLE COUNTS ARE CORRECT (OR NOT APPLICABLE)

- [ ] HOW THE SPECIMEN IS LABELLED (INCLUDING PATIENT NAME)

- [ ] WHETHER THERE ARE ANY EQUIPMENT PROBLEMS TO BE ADDRESSED

SURGEON, ANAESTHESIA PROFESSIONAL AND NURSE REVIEW THE KEY CONCERNS FOR RECOVERY AND MANAGEMENT OF THIS PATIENT

THIS CHECKLIST IS NOT INTENDED TO BE COMPREHENSIVE. ADDITIONS AND MODIFICATIONS TO FIT LOCAL PRACTICE ARE ENCOURAGED.

WHO Surgical Safety Checklist:
For Dermatology Interventions ONLY
(adapted from the WHO Surgical Safety Checklist)

National Patient Safety Agency

National Reporting and Learning Service

NHS

PATIENT DETAILS

*If the NHS Number is not immediately available, a temporary number should be used until it is

NURSE/DOCTOR SIGN IN
Before injection of LA

☐ Have all team members introduced themselves by name and role? **Yes**

☐ Has the patient confirmed his/her identity, site, procedure and consent? **Yes**

☐ Is the surgical site marked? **Yes/not applicable**

Is the patient on an anticoagulant?
☐ **Yes**...
☐ **No**
If yes, what is INR? ....

☐ Is the patient on dipyridamole/aspirin? **Yes/No**

☐ Allergies:..
....

☐ Does the patient have a pacemaker fitted? **Yes/No**

☐ Has the sterility of the instrumentation been confirmed (including indicator results)? **Yes**

☐ Are there any patient-specific concerns?
....
....
....

☐ Are there equipment issues or concerns?
....
....
....

Name:	
Signature of Registered Practitioner:	

NURSE SIGN OUT
After the procedure
Before any member of the team leaves the operating room

☐ Has haemostasis been achieved? **Yes/No**

☐ Dressing:...
....

Registered Practitioner verbally confirms with the team:
☐ Have instruments been checked and signed the ASDU return sheet? **Yes/No**

☐ Have sharps been disposed of as per Trust Policy? **Yes/No**

☐ Have details of the procedure been recorded in the operations record book? **Yes/No**

☐ Have any equipment problems been identified that need to be addressed **Yes/No**

Histology:
☐ How many specimens?...................................

☐ Have they been labeled and do the specimen labels match the patient details? **Yes/No**

Surgeon and Registered Practitioner—Aftercare
☐ Has wound management been discussed with the patient ....**Yes/No**

☐ Has the patient been given information on the procedure.....................................**Yes/No**

☐ Has the patient been given the practice nurse letter ....**Yes/No**

☐ Date of suture removal.......................

☐ Does the patient require a follow-up appointment ....**Yes/No**

☐ If **yes** has the appointment been arranged ....**Yes/No**

Name:	
Signature of Registered Practitioner:	

Label from CSSD pack:

Date:

This checklist is for Dermatology Interventions ONLY

This modified checklist must not be used for other surgical procedures

Figure 2.3 Modified World Health Organization checklist for dermatology surgery.

WHO Surgical Safety Checklist:
For Dermatology Interventions ONLY
(adapted from the WHO Surgical Safety Checklist)

National Patient Safety Agency
National Reporting and Learning Service

NHS

DOCTOR TO COMPLETE

LOCAL ANAESTHETIC
☐   Type used...
☐   Quantity ....

Operation notes:

Date of operation:	

Name:	
Signature of Surgeon:	

This checklist is for Dermatology Interventions ONLY
This modified checklist must not be used for other surgical procedures

Figure 2.3 (Continued) Modified World Health Organization checklist for dermatology surgery, reverse side.

Histopathology requests and reports

It is good practice to send every specimen for routine histological examination. There must be a fail-safe system to ensure that all the specimens are sent, successfully received in the laboratory, and reported upon, and that the results are received back. The system should ensure that histology reports are seen by the doctor who carried out the procedure and who is responsible for any necessary further action.

Completing the request form

The histopathology request form should be labelled and completed before any surgery is started, making sure to include the following:

- The patient's identity (name, number) and date of birth.
- The date of surgery.
- The type of procedure, for example excision or incision biopsy, curettage, punch, or shave excision.
- The clinical details, the location, and the suspected clinical diagnosis or differential diagnosis. The more clinical information provided, the better; for example, you may wish to include skin type, which can be helpful for small punch biopsy samples.
- If more than one specimen is sent from the patient, the site of each lesion should be made clear and each lesion numbered, matching the number to each specimen pot using a diagram if necessary (remember that pathologists tend to use A, B, C, rather than 1, 2, 3) (Figure 2.4).
- Do not use abbreviations for locations. State Left or Right, not L or R; likewise, use Upper or Lower, not U or L, and so on. Remember that it's the patient's left or right and not yours!
- Give clear information about from where and whom the sample has been sent.
- Indicate clearly to where and whom the report should be sent. Provide your contact address, phone number, and even e-mail address.

The specimen pot

- Indicate the patient's name and date of birth and site of the lesion on the pot; check this against the patient and the request form.
- Wherever possible, use patient labels, and always write with permanent ink or ballpoint pen, avoiding marker pens that may smudge.
- For multiple specimens, indicate the site on the pot and alphabetically number the pot to match the request form.
- Each specimen should have its own individual pot; there is absolutely no place for putting multiple specimens in one pot.
- Screw the top on tightly to prevent leakage.
- Ensure that there is sufficient volume of preservative to cover the specimen completely.

Keeping a record of specimens sent

- The name, address, and date of birth of every patient, together with the nature of the specimen, should be entered into a register, procedure book, or computerised log.
- Ideally, this should be done at the time of the operation, or immediately afterwards.
- To ensure that no sample is lost in transit, consider sending a printed histology log to the pathology department with the specimens.
- This log should state the patient's details and what samples (and numbers of samples) have been sent. This can be checked by the receiving pathology staff, signed, and returned promptly (by fax or e-mail) to the sender so that any discrepancies are reported immediately.
- In this way, there will be no doubt that the specimens have reached the pathology department; it is too late to find a specimen has 'gone missing' weeks after the surgery.

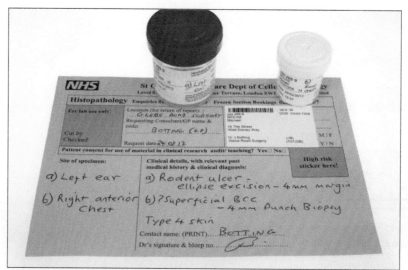

Figure 2.4 Histopathology request form and specimen pot.

When the report is received

When the histology results return, this must be entered in the log, and any omissions noted and acted upon promptly. The system must identify when results have not been received within a specified time so that the report can be chased up. Only by doing this will you be able to ensure the timely management of any unexpected clinical problems (such as a malignancy).

It is essential that the logged result is acted upon. This should be actioned by the surgeon or in their absence a suitably trained deputy.

Postoperative information

The final stages of documentation in the patient record will be completed once any histopathology report has been received and/or the patient has returned for post-operative review. The following should be documented at this stage:

- The outcome of the procedure.
- Any postoperative complications.
- The date any histopathology report was received, and any consequent action taken.
- The final diagnosis.
- If the patient is referred on, whether this was urgent or routine, the date of referral, and who they were referred to.

GOLDEN RULE ✳

The patient-care episode and record can only be considered to be completed once the histology result has been received, documented, and acted upon.

DOCUMENTATION POLICIES AND PROTOCOLS

The role of policies and protocols is that they define good practice based on clinical evidence and national guidance, and set standards for particular areas of care. A good policy will also include a list of key standards against which to audit, thereby ensuring their effective implementation. There are a range of policies that require development and implementation for any organisation offering minor surgery. Some examples are as follows:

- Infection control.
- Needle-stick injuries.
- Decontamination.
- Consent.

More details of these can be found in the relevant chapters, and sample policies are available from professional organisations.

AUDIT

Clinical audit is the process by which health-care professionals regularly and systematically review their own practice against best practice and, where necessary, change it. Its purpose is to help practitioners, both personally and within the teams in which they work, to achieve the best possible quality of care for patients. The philosophy underlying clinical audit is one of self-assessment and peer review. The simple collection of data is often called audit. True audit should be based on sound principles. *Audit is not research*: research determines *what* constitutes good care, whereas audit determines *how* well that good care is practised.

What are the benefits of audit?

A well-planned audit will bring some or all of the following benefits:

- Improvement in outcomes and quality of care for patients.
- Team building.
- Education.
- Efficiency in the use of resources.
- The involvement of patients in the work of the practice.
- Building on links with other providers of care.

Who should be involved?

- Anyone who is involved in the delivery of health-care services: for example, doctors, nurses, administrative and managerial staff.
- Audits may cross the interface between primary and secondary care (generalists and specialists), particularly as part of a multidisciplinary team.
- Users—the views and experiences of the patients are important in informing the provision of services.

General principles

Audit should:

- Improve outcomes and quality of care for patients.
- Be simple.
- Be based on a set of standards.
- Involve and have the commitment of all relevant members of the team, and be owned by them.
- Involve self-assessment.
- Form part of routine everyday practice, whether clinical or organisational.
- Be seen as an educational process.
- Never be threatening.
- Be completely confidential at the level of the individual patient, practitioner, or practice.
- Be informed by the views of patients (where appropriate).

- Be discussed promptly after the data have been analysed.
- Lead to implementation of change if appropriate.
- Be positive.

Audit *should not*:
- Judge individuals.
- Just be a data collection exercise.
- Gather dust.
- Be an academic exercise.
- Be tedious.

The audit cycle

Audit compares local practice with identified goals or best practice. Where local practice does not meet the standard agreed, the team can identify reasons for this and implement changes accordingly. Completing a successful audit involves the use of the audit cycle, whose stages are shown in Figure 2.5. Each stage is covered in more detail below. It is essential at the outset to agree a suitable topic and the standards toward which you are aiming, and to make sure that the objectives of the audit are clear. Audits are most likely to fail if the objectives of the study are not clear at the outset. All too often, interesting but irrelevant (to the audit subject) items become included, measured, or observed. The next section gives advice about how to choose a suitable topic and understand the process of audit.

Selecting a suitable topic
Some guiding principles are:
- Keep it simple.
- Is a problem suspected?
- Is it relevant to your practice?
- Is it common/important?
- Can you measure it?
- Are standards definable?
- Is it amenable to change?
- If you or other members of the practice are new to audit, is it interesting?

If you have started out with a broad topic, you will need to focus on a particular aspect of the topic for the audit. This can be helped by a brain-storming session and then applying the following very simple checks (which is best done as a group to avoid personal bias):
- *First check*: Is there a suspected problem, and is it amenable to change? If the answer is 'yes', continue to the second check; if it is 'no', choose another topic.
- *Second check*: Complete the table in Figure 2.6 to score your proposed audit project. Then, using the scores, you can decide whether the project is suitable.

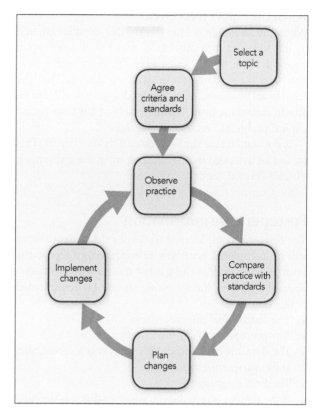

Figure 2.5 Audit cycle.

	No ——→ Yes		
	0	1	2
Common?			
Problem definable and measurable?			
Standard definable?			
Outcome likely to be important?			
Total score			

Significance of score:
7–8 Very suitable
5–6 Suitable
3–4 Questionable
<3 Unsuitable

Figure 2.6 Establishing the suitability of an audit project.

Some important definitions: standard, criterion, target
One of the classic audit errors is to fail to understand the definitions of the words used.

The word 'standard' can be used either to define a measure of good quality care, the degree to which the quality should be met and the exceptions, or more narrowly to mean the level that a criterion of care should reach. For this reason, it is more consistent to think in terms of a *criterion*-based audit.

Specifying a criterion

Each criterion consists of a component and a yardstick (Table 2.1):

- Component = measurable aspect of care.
- Yardstick = desired time frame/quality level.

For example, take the following statement: '*All melanoma patients should have a mole check annually*'. The component in this statement is '*All melanoma patients should have a mole check*'. The yardstick is '*annually*'. (So, all melanoma patients is not the component and should have a mole check annually is not the yardstick!)

Once the criterion or criteria have been agreed, it is necessary to agree a level of quality to aim at for each criterion. This might, for example, be 100% of specimens to be sent for histology. Whatever the level we expect to reach for our audit, this then becomes the target.

The audit standard or target

This is the level to which we expect our population to reach the criterion. It is clearly important to set the standard (target) before observing practice. There can be a number of justifiable standards:

- *The gold standard*: This will often be 100%, i.e., all should meet the yardstick.
- Alternatively, we can look at the *best practice* available. For example, research might show that the best that any unit achieves for taking a swab of potentially infected wounds is 95%.
- We might agree locally what our target should be through debate—a *locally agreed* standard or target.

Standards (or targets) can have a time frame. For example, we might expect 98% of patients to have the result of their histopathology report actioned within 1 week—this is a sensible time frame for most histology results. As explained earlier, the word 'standard' is in many instances used to wrap up not only the criterion and target, but also the exceptions (Table 2.2).

Table 2.1 Examples of components and yardsticks in audit criteria

Component	Yardstick
All excised specimens are sent	Histological analysis
All histology requests	State site of lesion
Any postoperative wound infection	Has a swab been sent for culture and sensitivity?
All histology results are actioned	Within 7 days

Observe practice

The audit may observe practice retrospectively or prospectively. If you choose to look at practice retrospectively, try to make the sample period recent as practitioners and practice may well have changed in the intervening time.

Identifying the population

In an ideal audit, the whole of the relevant population will be audited, for example all melanoma patients. However, where populations are large, it may be necessary to sample unless the search can be undertaken electronically. This is again where many audits can fail as sampling parts of a large population can be complex if one is to avoid bias. Better therefore to choose an easily identifiable, representative population, for example:

- '*On all histology request forms* (the component) *record the suspected clinical diagnosis* (the yardstick)'.
- As the number of samples sent may be high and the recording of the advice may not be suitably coded, it is likely that every request form sent will need to be manually inspected.
- By specifying the component '*On all histology requests sent in January*', the numbers become manageable.

Table 2.2 Some examples of audit standards

Criterion		Target (standard)	Exception
Component	Yardstick		
All melanomas excised	Referred for discussion by a multidisciplinary team	100% of patients	Patient refusal
Postoperative wound	Infection	0%	Incised abscesses
Junk mail received by GPs	Should not exceed 1 ton per year	95%	GPs in training may receive up to 2.5 tons
No patient will be kept waiting for their appointment more than:	10 minutes	80%	Those who arrive after their appointment time

Collect information

Decide which items of information are needed to inform your objectives and determine the best means of obtaining this information. Try not to collect additional information that does not relate to your objectives, however tempting this may seem, as it will only add to the work and cloud the issues. Remember the *KISS principle*—keep it simple, stupid! You should ideally test your method with a small pilot study. And remember to *ensure complete confidentiality for* **all patients (always)** *and practitioners (if appropriate)*.

Some methods of data collection

- *Data collection forms* are useful for audits of structure and process, or for the measurement of a clear-cut outcome.
- *Structured questionnaires* may be used to gain insight into patients' views and experiences. They may be for self-completion or for face-to-face or telephone interview. Questions may be open-ended or may use pre-coded prompt lists or rating scales.
- *Computer searches* may be helpful (where available), for example to identify all patients in the practice with skin cancer who are not receiving appropriate review.

Compare practice with standards

There should be careful planning of how to analyse the information collected in order to inform the objective of the study. Analysis can be carried out by hand or by computer, and the findings should be presented clearly and simply. Ensure that all relevant information is included, with graphical presentations, and that all findings are anonymous to ensure complete confidentiality for patients (and practitioners if necessary). The findings should be made available to all who took part in the audit, with an opportunity to discuss the implications.

Plan and implement change if needed

There are several levels of change that can be implemented. These changes may be one-off or sustained.

- *Unsustained change*: All patients with skin cancer are to have an annual skin review. The change might be to send a letter and appointment to all skin cancer patients who have not been reviewed. This is a one-off, unsustained change.
- *Sustained change*: If, however, a template is developed and all patients coded with skin cancer will automatically have a computer template reminding clinicians that a skin check is due, this will be a sustained change.

If changes are needed, they should be:

- Discussed with all concerned.
- Acknowledged by everyone as being necessary.
- Owned by everyone.
- Open to modification.
- Able to fit with the current situation.
- Satisfying.
- Measurable.

Re-audit

Returning to the start of the audit cycle adds some more questions:

- Have the changes been implemented?
- Have any problems been identified that have hindered the process of change?
- Is the criterion still up to date?
- Should the target (standard) be changed?
- Could the audit method be improved upon?
- Have new topics for audit emerged during the course of this project?

When re-auditing, remember to *audit the whole population*: do not limit your re-audit to just those identified first time round. Doing this ignores any new individuals who may have entered the target population. Try to keep at least some aspects of the re-audit in common with the first audit to allow a comparison.

Suggested topics for audit in minor surgery

Some levels of detail may already be required as part of a doctor's contractual obligations. Data collected at the time of attendance and suitably computer coded will be much easier to analyse than retrospectively obtained data. Table 2.3 shows some suggested audit topics.

Table 2.3 Suggested minor surgery audit topics

Component	Yardstick
All specimens	Signed; recorded in notes
All specimens sent	Results received; results actioned; patient informed
All team members introduce themselves	By name; wear name badges
All excised lesions	Excised completely
All wounds	Remain infection-free
All request forms	State presumptive diagnosis, name of surgeon, site of excision, skin type
Presumptive diagnosis and actual diagnosis	Should be the same

```
┌─────────────────────────────────────────┐
│         AUDIT: KEY MESSAGES              │
│                                          │
│              SUBJECT                     │
│  Is there a problem?  Is it common?  Is  │
│         it measurable?                   │
│         Can it be changed?               │
│                                          │
│              CRITERION                   │
│    Each has a Component and a Yardstick  │
│                                          │
│              STANDARD                    │
│       The target for each criterion      │
│                                          │
│             POPULATION                   │
│       Avoid samples if possible          │
│                                          │
│              CHANGES                      │
│  Sustainable. All involved need to have  │
│         ownership                         │
│                                          │
│              RE-AUDIT                     │
│       Audit the whole popluation         │
│                                          │
└─────────────────────────────────────────┘
```

Figure 2.7 Audit: Key messages.

Figure 2.7 reflects the key important messages that are relevant to audit.

REFERENCES

Department of Health (2009a) Consent forms. Available from: http://webarchive.nationalarchives.gov.uk/+/www.dh.gov.uk/en/Publichealth/Scientificdevelopmentgeneticsandbioethics/Consent/ConsentGeneralInformation/DH_4015950 (accessed April 2012).

Department of Health (2009b) Reference guide to examination or treatment (2nd edn). Available from: www.dh.gov.uk/prod_consum_dh/groups/dh_digitalassets/documents/digitalasset/dh_103653.pdf (accessed July 2012).

General Medical Council (2007) 0 to 18 years: Guidance for all doctors. Available from: www.gmc-uk.org/static/documents/content/0-18_0510.pdf asp (accessed July 2012).

General Medical Council (2008) Consent: Patients and doctors making decisions together. Available from: www.gmc-uk.org/guidance/ethical_guidance/consent_guidance_index.asp (accessed July 2012).

Gillick v. *West Norfolk and Wisbech Area Health Authority and Another* (1986) [1986] 1 AC 112, [1985] 3 All ER 402, [1985] 3 WLR 830, [1986] 1 FLR 224, [1986] Crim LR 113, 2 BMLR 11.

Wheeler R (2006) Gillick or Fraser? A plea for consistency over competence in children. *British Medical Journal* 332: 807.

APPENDIX 1: EXAMPLE MINOR SURGERY CONSENT FORM

This part to be completed by the patient/parent/guardian, nurse or doctor

Patient's surname: ....

Other names: ....

Date of birth:.. Sex (please tick) ☐ Male ☐ Female

This part to be completed by the doctor or nurse

Type of operation/procedure:...

I confirm that I have explained the operation and such appropriate options as are available and the type of anaesthetic proposed, to the patient in terms which in my judgement are suited to the understanding of the patient and/or to one of the parents or guardians of the patient.

Signature: .... Date: ....

Name of doctor/nurse:..

This part to be completed by the patient, parent or guardian

I am the patient/parent/guardian (delete as necessary).

I agree to what is proposed and has been explained to me by the doctor/nurse and to the use of the type of anaesthetic that has been discussed.

I understand that any procedure in addition to the investigation or treatment described on this form will only be carried out if it is necessary and in my best interests and can be justified on medical grounds.

I have told the doctor about any additional procedures I would not wish to be carried out straight-away without my having the opportunity to consider them first.

Signature: .... Name: ....

Address (if not the patient): ....

....

Example minor surgery consent form *reverse*

When you attend for your appointment the doctor will examine you and discuss with you the treatment that is recommended for you. The doctor will then:

- Explain what the recommended surgical procedure is (its nature and aftercare).
- Explain how a local anaesthetic is given.
- Mention any possible complications.
- Discuss any possible mark or scar that may remain after the surgery.
- Discuss alternative treatments.

It is important that you understand everything that is explained to you. Therefore:

- Don't be afraid to ask!
- If it would help bring a friend or relation with you.
- Bring or ask for a translator/interpreter if you need one.
- Ask for more detail if there is anything you don't understand.

Once you and the doctor are both happy, the doctor will complete this consent form and ask for your signature. Please take this opportunity to read the consent form and to think of any questions you may wish to ask the doctor at the time.

PLEASE REMEMBER TO BRING THE FORM WITH YOU TO THE APPOINTMENT

Make notes below of any questions you may have:

....

....

....

....

....

....

....

....

....

....

APPENDIX 2: EXAMPLE PREOPERATIVE CHECKLIST

NHS/patient number:	Surgery date:
Date of birth:	Surgeon:
Surname:	
Forenames:	
Address:	
Next-of-kin:	
Tel. No.:	

Assistance

Speech/language problem?	☐	Visual loss?	☐
Translator required?	☐	Wheelchair bound?	☐
Hearing impediment?	☐	Unable to lie flat?	☐

MINOR OPS. ASSESSMENT CHECKLIST *Tick as appropriate*	Yes	No	N/A	Comments
Doctor and nurse introduced to patient by name?				
Identity of patient checked (name + DOB + address)?				
Antithrobotic medications Warfarin ☐ Aspirin ☐ Clopidogrel/dysopyramide ☐	Date of last INR test .... Date last taken... Date last taken...			
Site confirmed with patient?				
Patient/representative signed consent?				
Does the patient have a pacemaker?				
Does the patient have a history of fainting?				
Name of the procedure recorded?				
Specimen pot and form: name, DOB, location, date, requesting doctor?				
Operation log completed?				
Post-op advice sheet given?				
Follow-up arrangements confirmed with patient?				

Name of nurse:	Name of doctor:
Signature:	Signature:

Chapter 3

Infection control

INTRODUCTION

This chapter discusses the key issues that are relevant to infection control, beginning with reference to useful guidance documents pertinent to the development and implementation of an infection control policy. There then follow a description of some important definitions and a discussion of a range of practical aspects as they relate to the provision of minor surgery in the context of the equipment used and the safety of staff and patients.

KEY PRINCIPLES

In developed countries, infections linked to patients' health care (health-care-associated infections [HCAIs]) affect 5–15% of hospitalised patients. Approximately 5 million HCAIs are estimated to occur in acute care hospitals in Europe annually, representing around 25 million extra days of hospital stay. Although figures for HCAI in community, non-hospital, settings will be much lower, the need for meticulous care remains paramount. To maintain high standards, all those offering minor surgery services should have robust systems in place for infection control that reflect available evidence and national guidance and be clearly stated in an infection control policy. The aims of infection control in minor surgery are as follows:

- To reduce the likelihood of introducing infection to the patient from the surgeon, assistant, or any equipment in the surgery room, such as surgical instruments, during the procedure.
- To reduce the transmission of infection from the patient to the health-care professionals involved in performing procedures on the patient, such as blood-borne infections.

Guidance documents

Although there may be specific requirements for different countries, there are some useful UK documents that set good evidence-based standards that will be relevant in other countries, as they reflect good clinical practice. For example, guidance published in the United Kingdom by the National Institute for Health and Clinical Excellence (NICE) entitled *Infection Control, Prevention of Healthcare-Associated Infections in Primary and Community Care* (NICE, 2003) is a helpful reference document reviewing the evidence for, and making recommendations on, the following:

- Hand hygiene.
- The use of personal protective equipment.
- The safe use and disposal of 'sharps'.

Additionally in the United Kingdom, the Department of Health has published a code of practice on the prevention and control of infections relevant to health-care professionals providing minor surgery entitled *Code of Practice on the Prevention and Control of Infections and Related Guidance* (Department of Health, 2008). The principles contained within these two documents are applicable to the problem of infection control worldwide.

The infection control policy

Anyone providing minor surgery should have a properly implemented infection control policy. It is recommended that there is a designated person responsible for managing and monitoring the control of infection and that there is a clear policy that states:

- What infection prevention and control measures are needed.
- What policies, procedures, and guidance are needed and how they will be kept up to date and monitored for compliance.
- What initial and ongoing training staff will receive.
- A list of contacts who can be approached for advice.

The policy should require the preparation of an annual statement that will be available to anyone who asks to see it. This should detail:

- Infection rates in specific areas (e.g., skin surgery wound infection rates) compared with national and/or local figures.
- Known infection transmission events and actions arising from this (e.g., related to hepatitis B or C, and HIV).
- Audits undertaken and subsequent actions.
- Risk assessments undertaken for the prevention and control of infection.
- Training received by staff.
- Review and update of policies, procedures, and guidance.

Decontamination policy

Decontamination is defined as the use of a combination of the processes of cleaning, disinfection, and sterilisation to make a reusable item safe for further use on service users and for handling by staff (Department of Health, 2008). In addition to an infection control policy, it is recommended that there is a decontamination lead (who can be the same person as the infection control lead) with responsibility to devise a decontamination policy and monitor all aspects of the decontamination cycle. In the United Kingdom, this is a recommendation of the Department of Health code of practice, which states the following:

- The decontamination policy should be consistent with national guidelines and legislation.
- Premises should be cleaned and managed to facilitate infection control. (The UK National Patient Safety Agency [NPSA] has published detailed guidance for maintaining cleanliness in primary care facilities.)
- Records of decontamination should be kept (NPSA, 2010).
- Decontamination of reusable medical devices should follow national policy where available. Single-use medical devices should not be reused. Equipment used for decontamination should be routinely inspected, maintained, and validated.

THE MINOR SURGERY ROOM AND SURGICAL EQUIPMENT

Definitions

Within a minor surgery room, some items will need to be cleaned, some disinfected, and some, particularly instruments, sterilised. It is essential that those who use and maintain the minor surgery room understand the important distinctions between cleaning, disinfecting, and sterilising. Absolute sterility cannot be guaranteed even in the cleanest of operating environments; what should be guaranteed, however, is the sterility of instruments that come into direct contact with patients and staff.

Cleaning

Cleaning is the process that removes contaminants including dust, body tissues, large numbers of microorganisms, and body fluids (e.g., blood or vomit). It is an essential prerequisite to disinfection and sterilisation. It also removes the organic matter that would provide a substrate for microorganisms. Premises should be cleaned and managed to facilitate infection control. (The UK National Patient Safety Agency [NPSA] has published detailed guidance for maintaining cleanliness in primary care facilities.)

Disinfection

Disinfection is a process used to reduce the number of microorganisms, including inactivating viruses, fungi, and vegetative bacteria. Bacterial spores may, however, survive. The process does not therefore kill or remove all microorganisms, but reduces their number to a level that, in normal circumstances, should not be harmful to health.

Sterilisation

Sterilisation is the complete destruction or removal of microorganisms and their spores. Contrary to popular belief, an item may only be sterile or non-sterile—it cannot be nearly sterile. The skin is the main defence against infection. Any organism, even if it is normally of low pathogenicity, can cause infection if it breaches this barrier.

> **GOLDEN RULE** *
> When carrying out procedures that breach the patient's skin, you must use sterile instruments.

Decontamination and levels of risk

The need for cleaning, disinfection, and/or sterilisation is determined by the likely risk to the patient of contracting an infection from contact with a medical instrument and from the procedure being performed on the patient. There are three levels of risk, and minor surgery rooms will tend to have a mix of low- and high-risk items.

Low risk

Low-risk items only come into contact with normal intact skin—for example, stethoscopes and examination couches. *Cleaning and drying* is usually adequate for this group.

Intermediate risk

Intermediate-risk items are those which come into close contact with mucous membranes or will be contaminated with particularly virulent or readily transmissible organisms. This includes items of respiratory equipment including laryngoscope blades and laryngeal mirrors. *Disinfection* is required for this group.

High risk

High-risk items come into close contact with a break in the skin or mucous membranes or are introduced into a normally sterile body area, for example surgical instruments, needles, sutures, and urinary and other catheters. *Sterilisation* is required for this group.

Cleaning, disinfection, and sterilisation in the minor surgery room

Cleaning

The treatment room should be cleaned before and after each operating session. This will include mopping the floor and cleaning the work surfaces and wash basins. It goes without saying that all clinical and non-clinical waste should be cleared from the room at the end of the operating session.

Before each patient enters the minor surgery room, the treatment couch and instrument trolley should be wiped down with a simple surface cleaner (usually containing a surfactant and mild antiseptic). There are single-use antiseptic wipes readily available for this purpose. Even though the couch and trolley will be covered by disposable paper for each patient, this extra cleaning of surfaces helps to avoid any possible patient-to-patient contamination.

Disinfection

Disinfection is suitable for equipment of intermediate risk and, as such, is of little relevance to most minor surgery units. It is most simply achieved by moist heat such as boiling in water (100°C for 10 minutes at sea level), which will kill all organisms except for a few bacterial spores, but remember that boiling items of equipment in water will *not* achieve sterilisation. Disinfection can also be achieved by using a range of chemicals, some

of which are quite toxic. In practice, the choice of disinfectant is usually directed by local infection control policies. The chemicals available are a compromise between human toxicity and microbial toxicity. In order to reduce microbial resistance, it is sensible to rotate the choice of disinfectants. Further information about a range of chemical disinfectants is included at Appendix 1 at the end of the chapter.

Sterilisation

Sterilisation, the complete destruction of microorganisms and their spores, can be achieved by steam (autoclave), steam plus formaldehyde, hot air, ethylene oxide, or irradiation. A brief description of each of these techniques follows.

Autoclaving

This uses steam under pressure and is the most reliable way to sterilise instruments. A temperature of 134°C for 3 minutes or 121°C for 15 minutes is recommended. When the heated steam cycle is complete, vacuum autoclaves dry the instruments under a partial vacuum. This enables hollow-bore instruments to be dried and also allows the items to be sterilised within sealed packs, so that the instruments remain sterile until needed (Figure 3.1).

Hot air sterilisation

This process takes a long time, and items must be able to withstand temperatures of at least 160°C for periods of 2 hours or more.

Ethylene oxide

This is a colourless gas that is toxic on inhalation. It is effective against all organisms and does not damage equipment. The operating cycle ranges from 2–24 hours so the turnaround time is prolonged and it is a relatively expensive process.

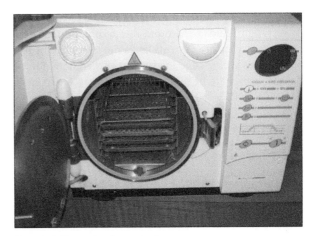

Figure 3.1 Example of an autoclave.

Irradiation

This is an industrial process particularly suited to the sterilisation of large batches of products. Irradiation can cause serious deterioration of materials and is therefore not a suitable method for the resterilisation of equipment. Gamma irradiation is normally used. The particle accelerator used to generate the gamma rays is lethal to life and requires the construction of high-density irradiation chambers.

Formaldehyde

Formaldehyde is irritant to the eyes, respiratory tract, and skin. It can also be absorbed by some materials and subsequently slowly released, with potentially hazardous results. As a result, this technique of sterilisation is now rarely used.

Variant Creutzfeld–Jakob disease and minor surgery

Variant Creutzfeld–Jakob disease (vCJD) is a transmissible spongiform encephalopathy first described in 1996. The condition causes degeneration of the nervous system and is invariably fatal. It is thought to be due to accumulation of an abnormal 'prion' protein in the brain. A clear link has been established between vCJD and certain medical treatments including contaminated pituitary hormone, corneal transplants, and brain surgery involving contaminated instruments.

Prion proteins are very resistant to both chemical and physical decontamination methods, and abnormal prion protein may not be fully inactivated by normal sterilisation procedures. Evidence suggests that effective cleaning of instruments prior to sterilisation is very important to reduce the risk of transmission of vCJD by surgical procedures (NICE, 2008a). Infectivity is highest in relation to any procedure related to the brain or related tissues, whereas the risk of transmission of infection from minor surgical and podiatry instruments is thought to be very low provided optimal standards of infection control and decontamination are maintained (Health Protection Agency North West, 2011).

The issue of vCJD and the potential transmission of prion proteins has been responsible for the introduction of very tight guidance around the decontamination of reusable surgical instruments and a move toward the use of single-use disposable instruments, where any potential risk is likely to be removed completely (Department of Health, 2003).

Sterile instruments

Obtaining a ready supply of sterile instruments is essential when providing a minor surgery service, and information about the types of instrument required is included in Chapter 1. There are three possibilities:
- Single-use disposable instruments (Figure 3.2).
- Purchase of sterile packs from a central sterilisation service department (CSSD) (Figure 3.3).
- In-house sterilisation.

This section discusses each of these options and includes a comparison of the advantages and drawbacks of in-house sterilisation and CSSD supplies of sterile packs (Table 3.1).

Single-use disposable instruments

With the concerns about blood-borne infections and the potential for transmission of prion proteins, there has been a move towards the use of single-use disposable instruments. The instruments can be packaged individually or within operating packs that may include rigid instrument containers, swabs, surgical drapes, and even scalpels and gloves.

The advantages and disadvantages of single-use disposable instruments are discussed in Chapter 1.

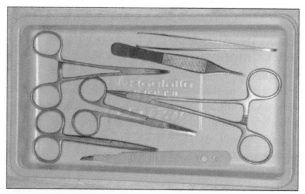

Figure 3.2 Example of single-use operating pack.

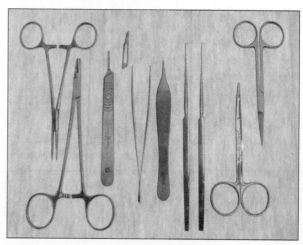

Figure 3.3 Reusable instrument set.

Table 3.1 Comparison of the benefits and disadvantages of central sterilisation service department (CSSD) versus in-house sterilisation

	Benefits	Disadvantages
CSSD	• No expensive equipment to maintain • Always prepared to current standards • Packing can include all necessary extras (gauze swabs, gallipot, etc.) • Packaging confirms sterility	• Equipment may be lost or substituted with inferior instruments • Double the number of sets of instruments are required • May experience delivery problems • Unable to sterilise equipment urgently or as required • May be expensive in the long run
In-house sterilisation	• Equipment always remains on site • Rarely used instruments can be sterilised as required • Always able to adapt to demand	• Need to maintain equipment • May need to change equipment if standards change • Limited pack contents are possible (pouches, not complete operating trays) • Needs staff to operate • Needs space

Transmission of infection is considered unlikely to occur if single-use instruments are used. If single-use instruments are used alongside reusable instruments, it is essential that instrument labelling ensures segregation after use so that no single-use instrument is inadvertently reused.

Central sterilisation service department

CSSDs are usually attached to large local hospitals, but sterilisation services may also be provided by private companies not attached to hospitals. Purchasing a sterilisation service from a local provider confers the advantage that there is no need to keep and maintain the expensive equipment required for in-house sterilisation. It is sometimes possible to arrange sterilisation of your own equipment, and it should be possible to agree a specification for the instrument packs that includes swabs and drapes (Figure 3.4).

Before entering into an arrangement for sterilisation services, it is important to clarify the following:

- Can the service ensure an appropriate turnaround time for sterilisation and return of the instruments?
- What arrangements will be made for collection and delivery?
- How many sets of instruments will be required in total, so that routine lists are included, and delays, losses, or urgent procedures are allowed for?
- What labelling arrangements are in place to be sure that the instruments (if they are your own) are not lost?
- Who is responsible for lost instruments?
- What is the overall charge for the specified contract?

An essential requirement will be that sufficient instrument packs are available. This means either building in a buffer (around a whole week's worth of spare instruments) or having an emergency supply of disposable instruments. Both options involve expense and storage requirements.

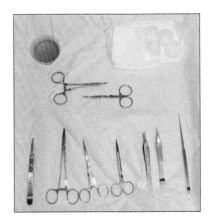

Figure 3.4 Reusable pack with swabs, drape, and galley pot.

In-house sterilisation

If in-house sterilisation is to be undertaken, there will need to be investment in equipment, space, training, maintenance, and supplies. Meeting the standards of sterilisation provided by a CSSD requires the following:

- Dirty and clean instrument rooms.
- Mechanical instrument washer.
- Ultrasonic cleaner.
- Vacuum autoclave.

It is essential that instruments are adequately cleaned before sterilisation as gross debris (such as blood and scraps of tissue) remaining on an instrument during the sterilisation process will act as a barrier to the steam and can thus prevent sterilisation. Proteins, including prions, are not susceptible to steam sterilisation but are removed by proper washing and disinfection procedures. Dirty instruments should be cleaned in a dirty instrument area, which will usually be a dirty sluice fitted with a sink, a dedicated instrument washer, and an ultrasonic bath.

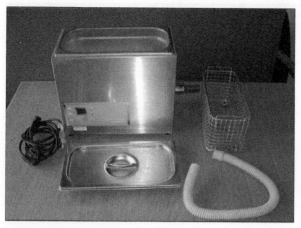

Figure 3.5 Ultrasonic cleaner.

Ultrasonic cleaning

Ultrasonic cleaners require water, a cleaning detergent, and often either a chemical enzyme solution or a disinfectant. Instruments need to be submerged in this solution. The unit then provides a combination of heat and ultrasonic vibration to dislodge any remaining particles. The ultrasonic cleaner uses high-frequency radiowaves (Figure 3.5) to generate air bubbles in the detergent that 'implode' when the pressure changes from positive to negative. This process, known as acoustic cavitation, releases the debris from the surface of the instruments. Ultrasonic cleaner function can be confirmed and logged by the use of test materials in the bath, and the fluid needs to be regularly replaced.

Cleaned instruments then need to be passed through a hatch to the clean instrument sluice, complete with clean sink, work surface for pack preparation, and autoclave for sterilisation.

Drying

Drops of water from a presterilisation washing process remaining on an instrument or within the packaging will act as a barrier to the steam and can thus prevent sterilisation. The cleaned instruments must therefore be dried after cleaning and before being placed in the autoclave for sterilisation.

Autoclave

A vacuum autoclave is recommended that allows instruments to be sterilised in sealed pouches. This is also required for sterilising hollow instruments (such as implant trocars). The autoclave will need to be serviced with a maintenance contract, and also be fitted with a data recorder producing a record of the sterilisation cycle. The instruments should be kept within identifiable packs, and a record made of which pack was used for which patient.

Specific issues in the United Kingdom

Very specific requirements have to be met in the United Kingdom in relation to the decontamination of surgical instruments for community settings, including GP surgeries. The Medicines & Healthcare products Regulatory Agency produces relevant Medical Devices Directives (previously Health Technical Directives) that lay down stringent standards for the medical devices used for sterilisation and instrument cleaning. The changes in NHS sterilisation standards in the United Kingdom have meant that the majority of GP practices have ceased their own autoclaving and instead use local hospital CSSD services or disposable instruments.

PATIENTS AND STAFF

The earlier section concentrated on aspects related to reducing the transmission of infection by effective decontamination of premises and equipment. The first part of this section describes ways to reduce transmission of infection between staff and patients, for example by following good hand hygiene. The second part discusses the risks of blood-borne infections and how to prevent their transmission.

Hand hygiene: 'Your 5 moments for hand hygiene'

It is thought that many HCAIs are preventable through good hand hygiene (NICE, 2003). As part of its global campaign to reduce HCAIs, the World Health Organization (WHO) has developed and publicised a programme to improve hand hygiene among health-care workers entitled 'SAVE LIVES: Clean Your Hands'. The aim of the programme is to improve the hand hygiene practices of health-care workers at the right times and in the right way in order to help reduce the spread of potentially life-threatening infections in health-care facilities.

The WHO has produced some good resources to support the programme. The first of these is the principle of 'Your 5 moments for hand hygiene' (WHO, undated), which identifies the key points at which health-care workers should perform hand hygiene (Figure 3.6):

1. Before touching a patient.
2. Before clean/aseptic procedures.
3. After body fluid exposure risk.
4. After touching a patient.
5. After touching the patient's surroundings.

Your 5 moments for
HAND HYGIENE

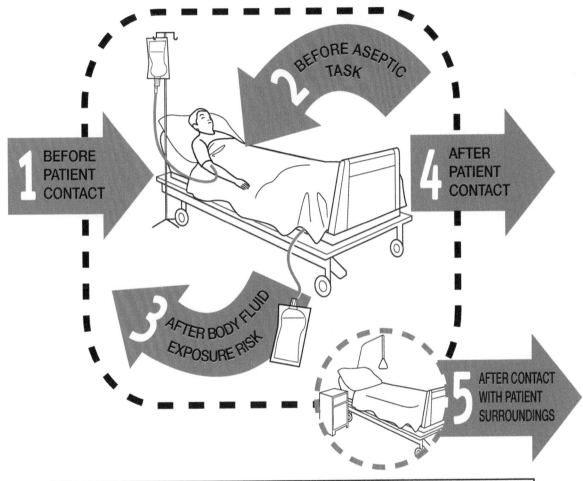

1	BEFORE PATIENT CONTACT	WHEN?	Clean your hands before touching a patient when approaching him or her
		WHY?	To protect the patient against harmful germs carried on your hands
2	BEFORE ASEPTIC TASK	WHEN?	Clean your hands immediately before any aseptic task
		WHY?	To protect the patient against harmful germs, including the patient's own germs, entering his or her body
3	AFTER BODY FLUID EXPOSURE RISK	WHEN?	Clean your hands immediately after an exposure risk to body fluids (and after glove removal)
		WHY?	To protect yourself and the health-care environment from harmful patient germs
4	AFTER PATIENT CONTACT	WHEN?	Clean your hands after touching a patient and his or her immediate surroundings when leaving
		WHY?	To protect yourself and the health-care environment from harmful patient germs
5	AFTER CONTACT WITH PATIENT SURROUNDINGS	WHEN?	Clean your hands after touching any object or furniture in the patient's immediate surroundings, when leaving – even without touching the patient
		WHY?	To protect yourself and the health-care environment from harmful patient germs

Figure 3.6 World Health Organization's 'Your 5 moments for hand hygiene' poster.

Patients and staff

Hand hygiene and minor surgery

Two kinds of bacterial flora affect the skin: *resident* and *transient*. The resident bacteria live deep in the skin and cannot be removed. In general, resident flora are less likely to be associated with infections (but they may cause infections in sterile body cavities, in the eyes, or on non-intact skin). These resident flora protect the skin from colonisation by bacteria with greater infectious potential.

Transient flora that colonise the superficial layers of the skin are picked up very easily but can be removed equally easily by routine hand hygiene including simple washing with liquid soap and water and/or alcohol-based antibacterial handrubbing preparations. Scrubbing the skin in an attempt to get rid of resident flora only makes matters worse by bringing them to the surface.

As a minimum, hands should be cleaned before surgical gloves are put on and after a patient exits the operating room. Evidence has shown that alcohol handrubs are more effective at removing transient flora than handwashing with liquid soap; however, applying surgical gloves after using an alcoholic handrub can be challenging as the gloves tend to stick to the skin.

The WHO has produced useful posters showing how to use alcohol rub and how to handwash (Figures 3.7–3.9). In practice, the choice is usually between an alcohol handrub or washing with an antimicrobial skin cleanser containing chlorhexidine gluconate 4% such as Hibi-scrub® in a minor surgery setting.

Many studies have shown that even when people wash their hands carefully, they often omit some areas, especially the skin creases and the areas between the fingers. Hands should be scrupulously washed using the technique shown in the WHO posters. The hands should at all times stay above the elbows when washing before surgery. When using a handwash, wetting the hands thoroughly before applying the handwash can sometimes reduce the likelihood of the hands getting sore. Hands should be dried carefully with disposable paper towels, which may or may not be sterile, depending on the procedure. Finally, an alcohol-based handrub may be applied and allowed to dry completely, but this is probably not essential.

Chapter 1 provides a list of the requirements for handwashing in the minor surgery area, which include the following:

- Clear access to a clean hand sink with elbow or proximity-sensor mixer taps.
- Paper towels available at all sinks.
- Alcohol handrub and an antibacterial handwash available for use at all sinks.

Further information and more detailed useful recommendations about hand hygiene, reproduced from *Infection Control, Prevention of Healthcare-associated Infections in Primary and Community Care* (NICE, 2003), are included in Appendix 2 at the end of the chapter.

Protective clothing and minor surgery

During most minor surgical procedures, there is no need to wear special theatre clothing; however, a short-sleeved surgical top is a sensible choice. It is not necessary to wear surgical gowns, caps, and shoes, but the following items should be used for all procedures:

- Single-use disposable plastic apron.
- Single-use disposable sterile latex (or latex-free) gloves for surgery.

The following items should be available for use when excessive splashing of body fluids is anticipated:

- Plastic goggles.
- Single-use face masks.

Further information and more detailed useful recommendations about protective clothing, reproduced from *Infection Control, Prevention of Healthcare-Associated Infections in Primary and Community Care* (NICE, 2003), are included in Appendix 3 in the end of the chapter.

Skin preparation and cleansing
Shaving

It is usually unnecessary to shave the patient. If you are operating on a particularly hairy area, for example the scalp, remove the surrounding hair with sharp scissors or a clipper. Shaving large areas is unnecessary: it traumatises the skin, is unsightly, and is uncomfortable for the patient.

It is also now recognised that shaving damages the skin and that the risk of infection increases with the length of time between shaving and surgery (Cruse and Foord, 1980). In one study, shaving more than 2 hours before surgery resulted in a wound infection rate of 2.3%. However, if patients had not been shaved but their body hair had been clipped, the rate was 1.7%, and if they had not been shaved or clipped the rate dropped to 0.9% (Cruse, 1992).

If shaving is essential, it should be performed as close to the time of surgery as possible. Depilatory creams provide an alternative to shaving or clipping. Above all, *never shave the eyebrows*—they may not grow back! For further details, refer to NICE (2008b).

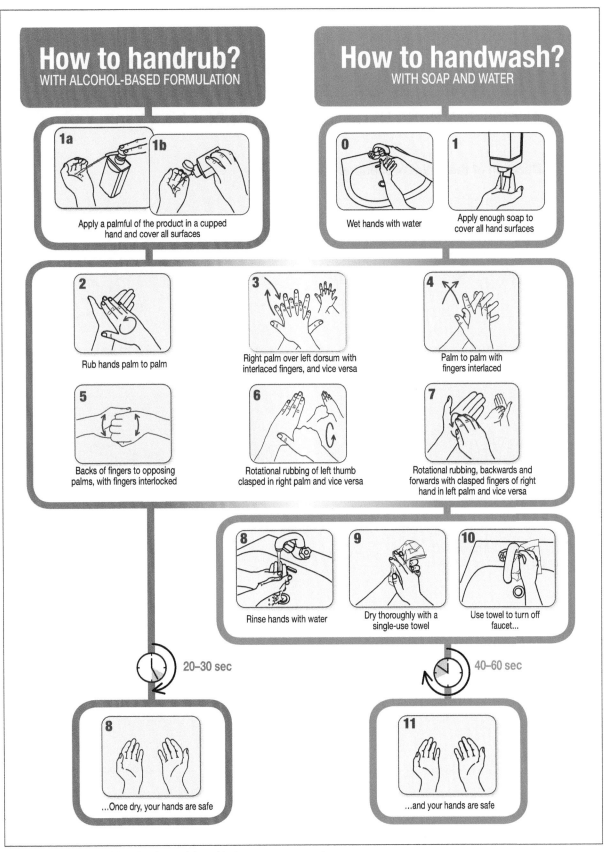

Figure 3.7 Handrub and handwash (World Health Organization poster).

How to handrub?

RUB HANDS FOR HAND HYGIENE! WASH HANDS WHEN VISIBLY SOILED

🕐 **Duration of the entire procedure: 20–30 seconds**

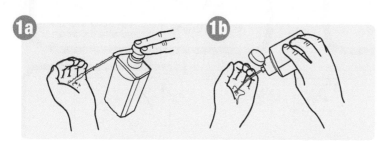

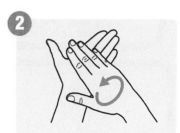

Apply a palmful of the product in a cupped hand and cover all surfaces

Rub hands palm to palm

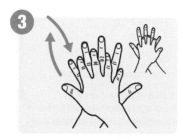

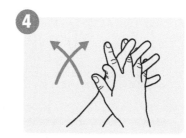

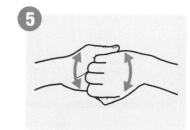

Right palm over left dorsum with interlaced fingers, and vice versa

Palm to palm with fingers interlaced

Backs of fingers to opposing palms with fingers interlocked

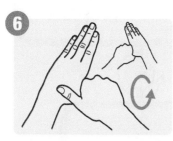

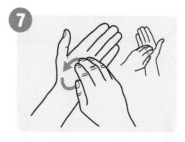

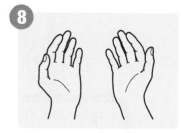

Rotational rubbing of left thumb clasped in right palm and vice versa

Rotational rubbing, backwards and forwards with clasped fingers of right hand in left palm and vice versa

Once dry, your hands are safe

Figure 3.8 How to handrub (World Health Organization poster).

How to handwash?

WASH HANDS WHEN VISIBLY SOILED! OTHERWISE, USE HANDRUB

Duration of the entire procedure: 40–60 seconds

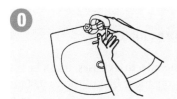

0 Wet hands with water

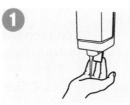

1 Apply enough soap to cover all hand surfaces

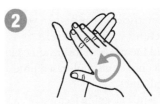

2 Rub hands palm to palm

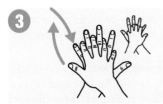

3 Right palm over left dorsum with interlaced fingers and vice versa

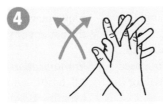

4 Palm to palm with fingers interlaced

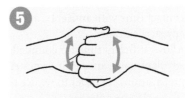

5 Backs of fingers to opposing palms with fingers interlocked

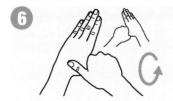

6 Rotational rubbing of left thumb clasped in right palm and vice versa

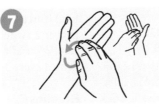

7 Rotational rubbing, backwards and forwards with clasped fingers of right hand in left palm and vice versa

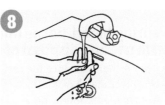

8 Rinse hands with water

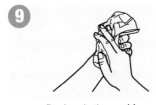

9 Dry hands thoroughly with a single-use towel

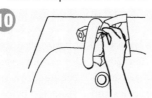

10 Use towel to turn off faucet

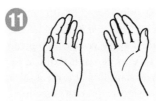

11 Your hands are now safe

Patients and staff

Figure 3.9 How to handwash (World Health Organization poster).

Cleaning the skin

Cleaning the skin prior to operating reduces the bacterial count of transient flora. For most straightforward skin procedures, simple cleaning with a water or alcohol-based antiseptic preparation is adequate. Any of the standard proprietary solutions is satisfactory. These contain antibacterial agents such as chlorhexidine or povidone-iodine. The skin should be cleaned from the operation site outward, and brisk rubbing should be avoided (as it can be painful, is likely to produce an inflamed skin, and releases resident bacteria).

Important points to note are as follows:

- Use normal saline to prepare burned, denuded, or traumatised skin and when working close to sensitive structures such as the eye.
- Avoid the use of chlorhexidine gluconate and/or alcohol or alcohol-based products on mucous membranes.
- Use gentle cleaning techniques when preparing fragile skin, for example in individuals with diabetes or who are elderly or have ulcerated skin.
- To achieve maximum effectiveness, allow sufficient contact time with antiseptic agents before applying any sterile drapes.
- Allow sufficient time for complete evaporation of any flammable antiseptic agent (e.g., alcohol-based preparations) in order to reduce the potential for fire (from electrocautery).
- Consider anaesthetising broken skin prior to cleansing to avoid pain.

Preventing blood-borne infections: the safe use and disposal of sharps

It has been recognised since the early 1990s that health-care workers are at risk of contracting blood-borne infections from patients following a so-called 'needle-stick' injury. These injuries expose workers to blood-borne pathogens such as hepatitis B, hepatitis C, and HIV, which can cause infection in the person injured. The USA has 8 million hospital-based health-care workers and a total of between 600,000 and 800,000 needle-stick or percutaneous injuries every year, which give rise to at least 1000 cases of HIV or hepatitis B or C a year (Bandolier, 2003).

The safe handling and disposal of sharp instruments to protect staff is therefore essential. Sharps injuries and transmission of blood-borne infections are preventable. When discussing the prevention of transmission of blood-borne infections, the emphasis is often on the risk to staff from patients, but it is also important to remember that staff can present a risk to patients. The average risk of transmission of blood-borne pathogens following a single percutaneous exposure from a positive source has been estimated to be (NICE, 2003):

- 33.3% (1 in 3) for hepatitis B virus.
- 3.3% (1 in 30) for hepatitis C virus.
- 0.31% (1 in 319) for HIV.

Definitions

Needle-stick injury

A needle-stick injury is defined as occurring when blood or other potentially infectious material is introduced into the body of a health-care worker (during the performance of his or her clinical duties) by a needle or sharp instrument such as a lancet or scalpel, or by contaminated broken glass.

Sharps

The term 'sharps' is used to describe hollow-bore needles and any other sharp instrument such as other needles, lancets, or scalpels.

Common blood-borne infections

Hepatitis B

This is one of the more infective viruses; it can be transmitted from patient to patient by as little as 0.0001 ml of infected blood. The virus remains active for up to 6 months in dried blood, so instruments that have been poorly cleaned or disinfected may be responsible for infecting other patients. In addition, poor surgical technique may result in the doctor becoming infected from the patient or vice versa.

Immunisation of health-care workers

All health-care workers should be immunised against hepatitis B. After an initial course of three immunisations, the level of immunity should be checked and non-responders (with a titre <100 IU/l) should receive further booster injections. Failure to respond to five injections in total (three in the initial course and two boosters) should trigger a switch to an alternative manufacturer as there can be variations in response. Immunity should be confirmed every 3–5 years.

Hepatitis C

Some patients infected with hepatitis C will experience spontaneous viral clearance, but the virus persists in about 85% of those infected, causing liver fibrosis and cirrhosis. Medical treatment results in viral clearance in about 50% of individuals overall (although the figure may be higher depending on the subtype); this may, however, rise to over 90% with treatment in the acute phase of infection. Many patients worldwide were infected by blood products before routine screening was developed, and infection through needle-stick injuries remains a constant threat.

GOLDEN RULES ❊

- Always check hepatitis B immune response after a course of immunisation.
- Consider a single hepatitis B booster immunisation after 5 years (NHS recommendation).

HIV infection

The acquired immune deficiency syndrome (AIDS) was first described in 1981, and the human immunodeficiency virus (HIV) was first identified in 1983. In 1986, a second strain, HIV-2, was isolated. Like hepatitis B the virus is present in blood and body fluids, but unlike hepatitis B it is relatively easily destroyed outside the body and is not as infectious as the hepatitis B virus. Infection of the surgeon can occur from contamination from infected blood or body fluids, either through an open wound, from aerosol sprays, or from a puncture wound or needle-stick injury.

Following infection, there is an asymptomatic period during which antibody to the virus is not yet present in the blood, and thus HIV tests will be negative. After approximately 6 months, the infected individual may seroconvert, and the HIV antibody may be detected.

Preventing needle-stick injuries

Safe clinical practice assumes that every patient is potentially infectious, so the same standards of care and sterility should be used for all procedures for all patients. In this way, the unsuspected HIV-positive patient will not put the doctor, the staff, or other patients at risk. Most organisations will have a so-called 'sharps policy' that summarises the essential requirements for the safe use and disposal of sharps. The following is recommended (which includes recommendations from NICE, 2003):

- For all patients, the surgeon should wear latex/vinyl gloves and a plastic apron for any procedures in which exposure to blood and/or body fluids is anticipated.
- Sharps should not be passed directly from hand to hand, and handling should be kept to a minimum.
- All sharps must be discarded into a good-quality plastic sharps container (which should never be more than three-quarters full). Needles must never be resheathed, bent, broken, or disassembled before use or disposal.
- Syringes should not be broken but syringe and needle discarded in one piece.
- When a needle or blade needs to be removed, a pair of artery forceps (never a delicate needle holder) should be used. If a blade needs to be mounted onto a handle, it should be attached using forceps and not by hand.
- Used sharps must be discarded into a sharps container (which must not be overfilled) at the point of use by the user, and this must be located close to the clinical procedure.
- Sharps containers in public areas must be located in a safe position and must not be placed on the floor. The containers should be disposed of by the licensed route in accordance with local policy (usually incineration).
- Specimens from patients infected with HIV or hepatitis should be placed in a sealed plastic bag and marked with warning tape.
- Contaminated dressings and waste material should be placed in a yellow plastic bag for incineration.
- Any linen contaminated with blood or body fluids should be handled with gloves and washed in a washing machine at the highest temperature setting.
- A person dealing with any spillage of blood or body fluids should wear an apron and gently pour undiluted Milton solution or similar hypochlorite bleach over the spillage, cover this with paper towels, leave it for 30 minutes, and wipe it up with disposable towels. Alternatively, granular sodium dichloroisocyanurate, for example Presept® granules, may be sprinkled over the spillage and wiped up with paper towels or a disposable cloth.
- Any cuts or abrasions should be covered with a waterproof dressing.

There is often debate about whether the responsibility for the disposal of sharps following a minor surgery procedure lies with the surgeon or the assistant. In *Infection Control, Prevention of Healthcare-Associated Infections in Primary and Community Care* (NICE, 2003), it is made clear that sharps must be discarded at the point of use by the user, and most policies now include this statement. The potential flaw with this policy is that unless surgeons are clearing away all the used instruments and material themselves, it is not they who stand to be injured by a failure to clear all sharps.

Procedures in the event of an injury and accidental contamination

Certain steps that should be taken after a needle-stick injury:

- Suspend the operation briefly.
- Remove the gloves and inspect the wound.
- Encourage the puncture wound to bleed (to expel contaminants introduced by the needle).
- Wash the wound well under cold running water without soap (or alcohol hand cleanser).
- Cover the wound with a dry, clean dressing.
- Conclude the operation wearing fresh surgical gloves.

Any health-care worker experiencing an occupational exposure to blood or body fluids needs to be assessed for the potential risk of infection by a specialist practitioner, such as a physician or occupational health nurse, and offered testing, immunisation, and post-exposure prophylaxis if appropriate.

Patients and staff

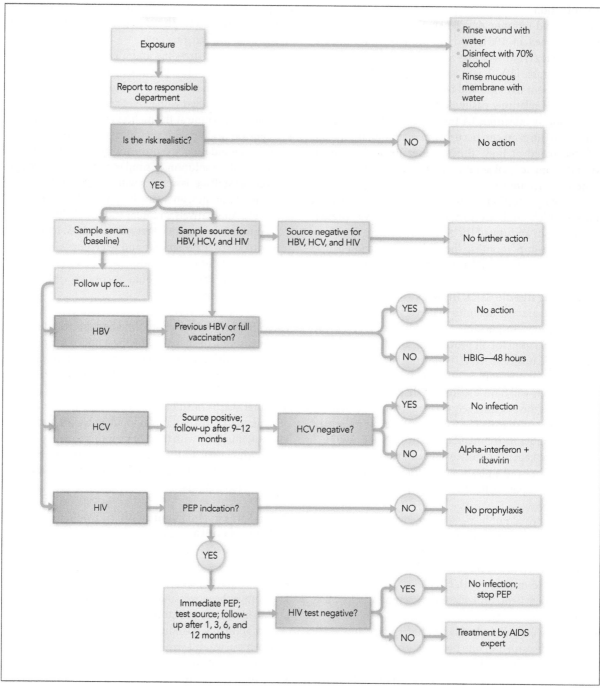

Figure 3.10 Post-exposure assessment and post-exposure prophylaxis, following guidance from the World Gastroenterology Organisation (www.omge.org). HBIG, hepatitis B immunoglobulin; HBV, hepatitis B virus; HCV, hepatitis C virus; HIV, human immunodeficiency virus; PEP, post-exposure prophylaxis.

Post-exposure assessment and post-exposure prophylaxis

Following any exposure, the surgeon needs to make an assessment of the possible risk of transmission of infection, as this will determine the course of action. The flowchart in Figure 3.10 reflects guidance from the World Gastroenterology Organisation (http://www.omge.org/).

Occupational health experts are usually involved in the risk assessment and make any necessary decisions about post-exposure prophylaxis (PEP). It is imperative that any surgeon undertaking minor surgery procedures knows how to access urgent occupational health services, either through the local hospital department or through the nearest accident and emergency department. The surgeon must explain what has happened to the patient—it will nearly always be necessary to take a sample of the patient's blood as their serology may well influence the post-exposure treatment plan.

Health and safety enforcement

Organisations have a responsibility to protect staff and patients against blood-borne infections contracted by needle-stick injuries. In 2010 in the United Kingdom, the Health and Safety Executive used their enforcement powers when they prosecuted an NHS trust after a health-care worker contracted hepatitis C virus after injuring herself on a needle used to take blood from an infected patient. The trust was fined £12,500 plus £9000 costs.

REFERENCES

Bandolier (2003) Needlestick injuries Bandolier Extra. Available from: www.medicine.ox.ac.uk/bandolier/Extraforbando/needle.pdf (accessed July 2012).

Cruse PJE (1992) Classification of operations and audit of infection. In: Taylor EW, editor. *Infection in Surgical Practice*. Oxford: Oxford University Press, pp. 1–7.

Cruse PJ, Foord R (1980) The epidemiology of wound infection. A 10-year prospective study of 62,939 wounds. *Surgical Clinics of North America* 60: 27–40.

Department of Health (2003, updated 2010) Joint ACDP/SEAC Working Group Guidance Transmissible Spongiform Encephalopathy: Safe working and the prevention of infection. Available from www.dh.gov.uk/ab/ACDP/TSEguidance/DH_098253 (accessed July 2012).

Department of Health (2008) Code of practice on the prevention and control of infections and related guidance. London: DH.

Health Protection Agency North West (2011) Transmissible spongiform encephalopathy (TSE/CJD): Guidance for healthcare workers working in primary care & community settings. Health Protection Agency North West.

National Institute for Health and Clinical Evidence (2003) Infection control, prevention of healthcare-associated infection in primary and community care. Available from: www.nice.org.uk/guidance/CG2 (accessed July 2012).

National Institute for Health and Clinical Evidence (2008a) Patient safety and reduction of risk of transmission of Creutzfeldt—Jakob disease (CJD) via interventional procedures. Available from: http://publications.nice.org.uk/patient-safety-and-reduction-of-risk-of-transmission-of-creutzfeldtjakob-disease-cjd-via-ipg196 (accessed July 2012).

National Institute for Health and Clinical Evidence (2008b) Surgical site infection: Prevention and treatment of surgical site infection. Available from: http://publications.nice.org.uk/surgical-site-infection-cg74 (accessed July 2012).

National Patient Safety Agency (2010). The national specifications for cleanliness in the NHS. Available from: www.nrls.npsa.nhs.uk/resources/?EntryId45=59818 (accessed July 2012).

World Health Organization (Undated) Evidence for hand washing. Available from: www.who.int/gpsc/country_work/en/http://www.who.int/gpsc/tools/Five_moments/en/ (accessed July 2012).

FURTHER READING

British Medical Association. Minor surgery—Specification for a direct enhanced service. Available from: www.bma.org.uk/employmentandcontracts/independent_contractors/enhanced_services/DESsurgery.jsp (accessed August 2011).

APPENDIX 1: CHEMICAL DISINFECTANTS

Chemical disinfectants can be toxic if in contact with skin or inhaled. For example, the aldehyde disinfectant Cidex® has been implicated not only in the development of occupational asthma among users, but also in anaphylactic reactions in patients after multiple exposure to equipment cleaned with Cidex® (e.g., cystoscopes). Chemicals can also be corrosive and flammable, so protective clothing (gloves, apron, and a face mask) should be worn. Chemical disinfectants decay and lose their activity over time, and this decay is more rapid at high temperatures and in the presence of impurities. Remember that all disinfectants take time to work.

Clear soluble phenolics (e.g., Stericol® [xylenol] at 1%)

These are good for killing most bacteria, including those causing tuberculosis, but they have limited activity against viruses.

Phenol is the gold standard for disinfectants and was the first to be used in clinical practice when Joseph Lister used it to prevent infection of his surgical wounds. Surgeons first wore rubber gloves not to prevent wound infections in patients but to stop their hands from being burned by the phenol that was sprayed over the wounds during operations. Phenol acts by causing cell disruption and denaturing proteins. It is highly corrosive and toxic to humans.

Because of its undesirable properties, many less toxic derivatives of phenol have been developed. Among the most popular are hexachlorophene and chlorhexidine. Chlorhexidine can be used in an isopropanol solution for skin disinfection, or as an aqueous solution for wound irrigation. It is often used as an antiseptic handwash. When used regularly, it may become mildly irritant and increasing levels of sensitivity are being noted.

Hypochlorites (e.g., Milton or Presept® granules)

These have a wide range of activity against bacteria, fungi, viruses, and bacterial spores, and can be used for decontaminating any area with blood spillage. They are corrosive to metals and must be applied at the correct concentration. In addition, they are inactivated by organic matter and decay on storage.

Alcohols (e.g., methanol, ethanol, isopropanolol)

Alcohols have good activity against bacteria and viruses. They should only be used after all the visible surface dirt has been removed from the area to be disinfected. Alcohols dehydrate cells, disrupt membranes, and cause coagulation of protein. A 70% (v/v) aqueous solution is more effective at killing microorganisms than are absolute alcohols: because the primacidal effect of alcohols is membrane disruption, bacterial endospores and many viruses are unaffected by alcohols.

Aldehydes (e.g., glutaraldehyde and formaldehyde)

These substances are active against bacteria, viruses, and fungi. They have a slow action against tubercle bacilli and are irritant to skin and eyes. Aldehydes react with nucleic acids and proteins, causing them to denature, and this is the mechanism underlying their lethal effects. Both are used in solution but may become inactivated in the presence of organic matter.

Halides (e.g., chlorine and iodine)

Halides are very powerful oxidising agents and are widely used for sterilisation and disinfection. Despite their rapid germicidal action, they may, however, become rapidly inactivated in the presence of organic matter.

Both chlorine and iodine are highly irritant to humans. Chlorine is used in low concentrations to prevent microbial growth in mains water supplies. In higher concentrations, it is used to disinfect swimming pools. The most commonly used chlorine preparation is sodium hypochlorite—household bleach. Tincture of iodine, an old-fashioned antiseptic, is a solution of 2.5% iodine in 90% alcohol. In addition, 2% iodine in isopropanol was also widely used at one time. However, these preparations were very irritant and rapidly inactivated.

It is now usual to use iodophores to ameliorate the irritation that iodine usually causes. Iodophores comprise iodine in an organic polymer. They permit slow release of the iodine, reducing the irritation and prolonging the effective use of the antiseptic. A commonly used iodophore is povidone-iodine.

Quaternary ammonium compounds (e.g., cetrimide and benzalkonium chloride)

These act as cationic detergents. They are widely used as disinfectants for domestic use and in hospitals. In dilute solution, they are also sold to control acne. One appeal of these compounds is their pleasant smell.

However, bacteria of the genus Pseudomonas can metabolise these compounds, using them as a carbon, nitrogen, and energy source. Indeed, cetrimide agar is used as a selective medium for the laboratory isolation of pseudomonads.

APPENDIX 2: FURTHER INFORMATION ON HAND HYGIENE

The following is a list of recommendations reproduced from *Infection Control, Prevention of Healthcare-Associated Infections in Primary and Community Care* (NICE, 2003):

- Hands must be decontaminated immediately before each and every episode of direct patient contact or care and after any activity or contact that could potentially result in hands becoming contaminated.

- Hands that are visibly soiled, or potentially grossly contaminated with dirt or organic material, must be washed with liquid soap and water.

- Hands must be decontaminated, preferably with an alcohol-based handrub unless hands are visibly soiled, between caring for different patients or between different care activities for the same patient.

- Before regular hand decontamination begins, all wrist and ideally hand jewellery should be removed. Cuts and abrasions must be covered with waterproof dressings. Fingernails should be kept short, clean, and free from nail polish.

- An effective handwashing technique involves three stages: preparation, washing and rinsing, and drying. Preparation requires wetting hands under tepid running water *before* applying liquid soap or an antimicrobial preparation. The handwash solution must come into contact with *all* of the surfaces of the hand. The hands must be *rubbed* together vigorously for a minimum of 10–15 seconds, paying particular attention to the tips of the fingers, the thumbs, and the areas between the fingers. Hands should be rinsed thoroughly before drying with good quality paper towels.

- When decontaminating hands using an alcohol handrub, hands should be free from dirt and organic material. The handrub solution must come into contact with all surfaces of the hand. The hands must be *rubbed* together vigorously, paying particular attention to the tips of the fingers, the thumbs, and the areas between the fingers, until the solution has evaporated and the hands are dry.

- An emollient hand cream should be applied regularly to protect skin from the drying effects of regular hand decontamination. If a particular soap, antimicrobial handwash, or alcohol product causes skin irritation, an occupational health team should be consulted.

APPENDIX 3: PERSONAL PROTECTIVE CLOTHING

The following is a list of recommendations reproduced from *Infection Control, Prevention of Healthcare-Associated Infections in Primary and Community Care* (NICE, 2003):

- Selection of protective equipment must be based on an assessment of the risk of transmission of microorganisms to the patient, and the risk of contamination of the health-care practitioners' clothing and skin by patients' blood, body fluids, secretions, or excretions.

- Gloves must be worn for invasive procedures, contact with sterile sites and non-intact skin or mucous membranes, and all activities that have been assessed as carrying a risk of exposure to blood, body fluids, secretions or excretions, or sharp or contaminated instruments.

- Gloves must be worn as single-use items. They must be put on immediately before an episode of patient contact or treatment and removed as soon as the activity is completed. Gloves must be changed between caring for different patients, and between different care or treatment activities for the same patient.

- Gloves must be disposed of as clinical waste and hands decontaminated after the gloves have been removed. Gloves that are acceptable to health-care personnel and that conform to European Community (CE) standards must be available.

- Sensitivity to natural rubber latex in patients, carers, and health-care personnel must be documented, and alternatives to natural rubber latex gloves must be available.

- Neither powdered gloves nor polythene gloves should be used in health-care activities.

- Disposable plastic aprons should be worn when there is a risk that clothing may become exposed to blood, body fluids, secretions, or excretions, with the exception of sweat.

- Full-body fluid-repellent gowns must be worn where there is a risk of extensive splashing of blood, body fluids, secretions, or excretions, with the exception of sweat, onto the skin or clothing of health-care personnel (e.g., when assisting with childbirth).

- Plastic aprons should be worn as single-use items, for one procedure or episode of patient care, and then discarded and disposed of as clinical waste.

- Face masks and eye protection must be worn where there is a risk of blood, body fluids, secretions, or excretions splashing into the face and eyes.

- Respiratory protective equipment, for example a particulate filter mask, must be used when clinically indicated.

Chapter 4

Professional and legal issues, and health and safety at work

INTRODUCTION

The first half of this chapter looks at important issues that are relevant if things go wrong and patients are unhappy with their treatment. The second half describes the important health and safety issues that are appropriate to minor surgery.

COMPLAINTS AND MALPRACTICE

Complaints are an integral part of medical practice. They can arise from clinical, organisational, or patient-generated factors. Complaints usually focus on three areas:

- The alleged failure of performance on the part of the health-care professional.
- An error or omission in the service.
- Any financial loss as a result of the above.

Where a complaint cannot be resolved in a timely fashion or in a manner satisfactory to the complainant, the issue may proceed to a legal claim of malpractice for financial damages. This section explores:

- Managing complaints.
- Malpractice and medicolegal issues.
- The factors that commonly lead to complaints in minor surgery.
- Professional liability insurance.
- Escalation to regulatory bodies.

Complaints

Complaints cause stress and anxiety. All complaints should be acknowledged and answered in a professional manner—they should never be ignored or dismissed. Most can be resolved by sympathetic communication, but some will unfortunately progress to a legal medical malpractice claim.

Patients complain for a variety of reasons, including the following:

- The provision of substandard, improper, or negligent medical or non-medical care by the health-care professional or the organisation to which the worker belongs.
- Non-medical factors including lapses in professionalism or common courtesy on the part of the staff at the practice.

In addition, it is important to recognise that complaints are sometimes due to perceived rather than actual substandard treatment. This can arise either from a failure of communication or from unrelated idiosyncratic problems in the patient's life that lower the threshold for unrealistic expectations or the perception of insult or mistreatment. It is therefore never wise to dismiss any complaint without thought or further investigation.

Complaints may be made directly to the health-care provider or to the administrative body under which the provider operates. Ideally, there should be an existing agreed-to complaints procedure, implemented uniformly across health-care communities, and this will vary from one country to another. The aim of any complaints handling procedure is not to delay or dissuade the complainant with administrative barriers but to achieve:

- Ease of access for patients and complainants.
- A simple straightforward procedure, with common features across the health-care community.
- Separation of complaints from disciplinary procedures.
- An ability to extract lessons on quality from complaints in order to improve services for patients.
- Fairness for staff and complainants alike.
- Rapid, open, and transparent processes.
- An approach that is honest and thorough, with the prime aim of resolving the problems and satisfying the concerns of the complainant.

The emphasis is on resolving complaints as quickly as possible. This is usually achieved through an immediate informal response by an identified front-line member of staff or practitioner, and subsequent investigation and conciliation in an open and non-defensive way. This should reduce the likelihood of a medical malpractice claim.

Important points related to complaints

- Never dismiss or ignore complaints, however trivial or unreasonable they may seem.
- Have a clear process for managing complaints with clear time scales for response.
- Always acknowledge any complaint promptly and politely.
- Make sure there is an identified individual with a lead role for managing complaints.
- Successful complaint resolution at a local level should prevent escalation to a medical malpractice claim.

Medical malpractice claims

Some complaints that are not resolved in a timely fashion or in a manner satisfactory to the complainant will result in a legal claim of malpractice for financial damages. The impact of such legal action can be devastating to the person against whom the claim is made as it challenges their competence and may have a financial impact (legal costs and compensation or damages payments to claimants).

Many countries have regulations in place for medical and nursing practitioners to take out professional liability insurance to meet such financial costs should a claim be successful and/or to gain access to medicolegal expertise to challenge malpractice claims, and if necessary, defend the health-care professional in court. It is essential that health-care professionals performing surgical procedures understand their local requirements for professional liability insurance, also known as malpractice insurance or medicolegal indemnity.

For malpractice claims to be successful, the claimant and the claimant's legal representatives have to demonstrate *all* of the following:

- That there was a '*duty of care*' to the patient. Such a duty of care exists whenever a health-care provider undertakes to care or treat a patient.
- That the '*duty of care was breached*'. In other words, that the quality of medical care has been below that of a reasonable standard. In many countries, this 'reasonable standard' is that recognised as proper by a responsible body of medical opinion, with the proviso that this opinion should be reasonable and responsible, having some basis in logic. If a doctor is found to have provided an adequate standard of care, there has been no medical negligence and no medical malpractice.
- *Causation of damage*. That the breach of 'duty of care' caused injury or damage. Damage can be pecuniary or emotional. There needs be a clear demonstration that the inadequate standard of care has resulted directly in an unsatisfactory result ('damage') for the patient. This is usually determined by the opinion of an expert witness, who, depending on each jurisdiction, may be put forward by the claimant or the defendant, or may act impartially with a duty to the court.

> **DON'T FORGET** ▶▶
> In the absence of any 'damage' as a result of the breach of the duty of care, there is no basis for a claim, irrespective of whether the health-care provider was negligent.

Claims must be initiated before any time limitation period lapses. The starting point for this period varies from one country to another and can be when an incident occurs, when treatment ends, or when the patient discovers the negligence. Similarly, the duration of this period also varies.

Professional liability insurance

In medical practice, there are several variations of professional liability insurance, otherwise known as malpractice indemnity. These differ in actual costs as well as in the detail of the benefits and services offered by the company. They can be divided into the following.

Personal and organisational

Some large health-care organisations put aside a budget for medical indemnity to meet the costs of successful claims of malpractice against their employees and the costs of legal expertise to deal with these complaints. In the United Kingdom, this is called Crown Indemnity. In addition, most health-care professionals, mainly doctors, subscribe to medical defence organisations (MDOs) at their own expense, either exclusively if they are not covered by Crown Indemnity because they are self-employed, or to cover Good Samaritan acts outside their normal employed role. However, MDOs will usually not advise on or provide financial indemnity for complaints arising from care given in one's employed role when Crown Indemnity applies.

'Claims made' or 'incident-based'

Policies with commercial companies are made under a legally binding contract, with a maximum cover and on a 'claims made' basis. The insured doctor is only covered for claims arising from incidents that both occur and are reported while the policy is in force. When this expires, so does the cover, unless a run-off payment is made.

Policies with mutual companies are discretionary on a decision of their boards, with unlimited cover and on an 'occurrence or incident basis'. The doctor is covered for claims arising from incidents that have occurred during the subscription period no matter when they are reported, even if it is many years after that subscription period has ceased and even if the doctor has retired or died. It is particularly important on changing MDOs to confirm in writing whether that new company or organisation takes on previous risk. This is not always the case, and 'run-off' cover may need to be bought from the previous MDO.

Escalation of claims: the independent regulator

Some complaints, that cannot be resolved at a local level, result in the health-care professional being reported to the recognised independent regulator of these professionals. In the United Kingdom, the General Medical Council (GMC), established under the Medical Act of 1858, fulfils this role for doctors; its purpose is to 'protect, promote and maintain the health and safety of the public by ensuring proper standards in the practice of medicine.'

In the United States, state medical boards monitor and licence the competence and professional conduct of physicians and take appropriate action against a physician's license if the complaint is upheld. The structure and authority of medical boards vary from state to state. Other countries will have different structures.

The UK GMC declares that: 'We are not here to protect the medical profession—their interests are protected by others. Our job is to protect patients. Where any doctor fails to meet those standards, we act to protect patients from harm—if necessary, by removing the doctor from the register and removing their right to practise medicine.' Although it does advise that most complaints are more effectively resolved by making them locally to the place where the care had taken place, it does accept direct referrals in cases where there are, among other factors:

- Repeated or serious mistakes in carrying out medical procedures.
- Failure to respond to a patient's medical need.

However, any patient who feels the need to complain will consider a mistake serious and a need unmet.

On receiving the complaint, the GMC will decide whether it is appropriate for it to investigate the case on the basis of a set of criteria for taking action against the doctor, and if so, it will initiate an investigation. This can be an extremely stressful and lengthy process, and every effort should be made to prevent complaints from reaching the stage of being reported to the regulatory body. If such a situation arises, access to experienced medicolegal expertise, usually through an MDO, is invaluable.

Common complaints in minor surgery

Data from the MDOs show that it is unusual for complaints to arise from minor surgery activity. The more invasive procedures give rise to the most complaints; just under half of all successful claims arise from the excision of lesions, with cryotherapy and vasectomy ranked next. The most common reasons for complaint are scarring (including keloid formation), depigmentation (from cryotherapy), and postoperative surgical site infection.

Most of these complaints can probably be avoided by better information being provided for patients. Some patients hold the belief that cutting surgery can be carried out without scarring in the best hands, and that leaving a scar indicates incompetence. It is good clinical practice to draw the size of the lesion on paper and describe the marking procedure and the size of the final scar once the clinical margins and a 3:1 ellipse have been added.

Knowledge of areas with a high risk of a poor cosmetic outcome and skill in techniques for minimising scarring are essential for good patient care and are also satisfying for pride in a job well done. These are described elsewhere in this book, but it must be remembered that sometimes a longer, less noticeable scar is superior to a short, more obvious one that gives rise to functional sequelae. Finally, the least noticeable scar is an absent one from avoiding surgery, and the option to do nothing should always be discussed, particularly when there is no medical need or indication for surgery to be performed.

Guidance and advice on the prevention and treatment of surgical site infections is considered elsewhere in this book. However, patients go home following surgery to environments beyond our control, and infections, although rare, will always be a risk. This should therefore be discussed as part of the consent process.

How to avoid complaints

There is no foolproof way of avoiding complaints from patients. However, the process of obtaining informed consent prior to a minor surgery procedure provides the opportunity to explain and document the procedure's risks and benefits, making clear what has been explained to the patient. You should always offer the patient a copy of the consent form. Demonstration that a patient has provided written consent to a procedure can be a key piece of documentary evidence if there is a complaint following a surgical procedure. Remember, however, that this written consent is only valid where the criteria for patient competence, voluntariness, and provision of adequate information have all been satisfied.

Several factors will help to reduce the number of complaints you receive, and other factors will help to support your defence in the event of a complaint:

- *Good communication skills.* This extends beyond verbal skills, with a good understanding of the patient's language and the ability to pick up non-verbal clues indicating that the patient is anxious or angry. Care should be taken when there are language barriers and when time pressures risk leading you to ignore signs that the patient is not happy with what is going on at the time.
- *Common courtesy and professionalism.* Patients attending for minor surgery are invariably nervous. This can alter their perception of what is being said and done, and lower their pain threshold and tolerance. The balance of relaxed confidence and professionalism is sometimes difficult to achieve, and what is required differs from one patient to another. This comes with experience, but this author finds the motto to 'Do unto others as you would others unto you' usually works.

- The *World Health Organization surgical safety checklist* (see Chapters 2 and 5) is a simple tool for surgical teams to use to improve the safety of their surgical procedures.
- *Meticulous note keeping and documentation.* It is very easy to write too little, but the documentation forms the most important piece of objective evidence if any complaint is investigated, either locally or externally. Minimum standards for documentation are described in Chapter 2.
- *Standardisation of the preoperative information and postoperative instructions* given helps significantly by demonstrating your usual standard of care.
- Use the process of *significant event analysis* (SEA; see below) to implement change in order to reduce the likelihood of similar adverse events.

Significant event analysis (SEA)

An SEA is an investigation of individual events that have been identified by a member or members of the health-care team and are considered to be 'significant'. This approach has been proposed as one way to assist individual practitioners and health-care teams to improve the quality and safety of patient care by encouraging reflective learning and, where necessary, the implementation of change to minimise any recurrence of the events in question. So, significant event analysis and evaluation is about learning from events rather than finding out who is to blame.

A 'root cause' is that which, if removed, changed, or controlled, would prevent the event from happening or minimise the consequences should it occur again. However, significant adverse events are always multifactorial in cause.

There are seven steps to an SEA:

1. Identify and record significant adverse events.
2. Collect and collate as much factual information as possible about the event. This includes the thoughts and opinions of the people directly and indirectly involved in the event.
3. Convene a meeting to discuss and analyse the event in an open, fair, honest, and non-threatening atmosphere.
4. Analyse the event:
   - What happened?
   - Why did it happen?
   - What have we learned?
   - What needs to be changed?
5. Monitor the progress of the changes.
6. Write up the event.
7. Seek educational feedback on the standard of the analysis undertaken.

Specific issues in the United Kingdom
Clinical governance

In the United Kingdom, where the NHS provides state-funded health care, clinical governance is the framework used to safeguard the provision of high-quality care. The aim is to create an environment in which the principles of good clinical practice can be shared and spread throughout NHS organisations. It is most commonly defined as:

A framework through which NHS organisations are accountable for continually improving the quality of their services and safeguarding high standards of care by creating an environment in which excellence in clinical care will flourish.

The following elements are key to effective clinical governance:

- Education and training.
- Clinical audit.
- Clinical effectiveness.
- Research and development.
- Openness.
- Risk management.
- Information management

Most of the areas are covered in either this chapter or Chapter 2. The next short section considers the importance of continuing medical education, which is not discussed elsewhere.

Continuing medical education (also known as continuing professional development)

This refers to the process by which health-care professionals maintain their competence and also learn about new developments in their field. This may be by reading relevant medical literature, attending meetings, online learning, and so on. It is expected that all clinicians will meet the requirements specified by the professional organisations in respect of continuing medical education.

There is an onus on the health-care professional to ensure that any limitations and gaps in their knowledge are identified and addressed within a suitable time frame. Where practical skills are concerned, it is important to be able to demonstrate maintenance of competency by performing a reasonable number of procedures. The use of a log diary will support this.

Readers are referred to their professional organisations and to national guidance documents for further information.

Continuing professional development (CPD) should reflect the educational requirements identified in an individual's annual professional development plan (PDP). The principle behind the goals identified for a PDP is that they should be SMART: Specific, Measurable, Attainable, Relevant, and Time-bound. Within the UK, there are also specific annual CPD requirements for certain surgical roles.

The Care Quality Commission

In England, the Care Quality Commission (CQC) is responsible for ensuring that providers of health and social care are meeting government standards. To date, there has been an emphasis on the inspection of hospitals and care homes, but from April 2013 the providers of primary medical services, including GP practices, will need to register as providers of health care and meet government standards appropriate to the range of services they provide. This will be of importance to GPs providing minor surgery on their premises, who will be required to be familiar with and meet the standards required by the CQC.

Summary

Complaints can be difficult and distressing. Prevention is always better than cure, and the key to avoiding complaints lies in good communication skills and professionalism, two of the key elements of good medical practice. Mistakes do, however, occur, and care may sometimes not reach acceptable standards. In addition, complaints may arise where patients perceive their care to be of an unacceptable standard.

Clinicians therefore need to equip themselves with the skills and tools to successfully manage complaints, prevent their escalation, and mount a robust defence in the event of legal medical negligence claims or investigations into fitness to practice. To facilitate this, membership of an MDO, with access to the MDO's medicolegal expertise and financial indemnity insurance, is mandatory. Ensuring high-quality care, and thereby reducing the number of complaints, is facilitated by using a framework of clinical governance, something which is required for health-care professionals working in the NHS in the United Kingdom.

HEALTH AND SAFETY AT WORK

It is common sense to protect the health, safety, and welfare of workers in and people entering a workplace, such as patients entering a hospital or surgery. This is the principle of 'health and safety', and in many countries employers have formal legal obligations to ensure a safe and healthy workplace. Consequently, employees have legal rights, but they also have responsibilities for their own well-being and that of their colleagues.

In the United Kingdom, it is the Health and Safety Executive that identifies areas relevant to health-care workers and creates the necessary regulations to protect people in the workplace. In reality, looking after health and safety in the workplace is a real-world practical approach to looking after ourselves and our patients as we deliver a service to help others.

> **DON'T FORGET** ▶▶
> 'Health and Safety' is about protecting both patients and staff

Risk assessment and its importance

The key to ensuring a safe workplace for staff and patients is to consider the risks that might be encountered in the clinical setting by undertaking a risk assessment. This is a systematic approach that identifies risk and develops practical solutions to it. By implementing simple risk management principles, it is possible to manage the risks that may compromise staff and patient safety. The process offers an opportunity for all members of the health-care team—doctors, managers, nurses, receptionists, and therapists—to work together, talk openly, and develop practical solutions that promote safer practice. An example of this and the steps required might be as follows:

- Identify the hazard, for example scalpel blades or needles.
- Recognise who might be harmed—for example, patients and health-care professionals—and how.
- Evaluate the risks, for example blood-borne infections.
- Decide on the necessary precautions that need to be taken, such as 'sharps' bins and a needle-stick injury policy.
- Record the findings of the risk assessment and implement any necessary recommendations.
- Review and update the assessment as necessary.

Below is a description of some of the important health and safety 'risks' that relate to minor surgery, with suggested systems that need to be in place to manage these risks and reduce the likelihood of injuries to other staff and patients.

Important health and safety issues in minor surgery

Sharps and infection control

In most organisations where minor surgery is performed, there will be clearly documented policies relating to the following:

- The safe use and disposal of medical sharps.
- Infection control.

Staff need to be familiar with these policies, which should be regularly reviewed, and should comply with their recommendations (see Chapter 3 for more information about this). It is important that staff only use equipment and devices supplied for the purpose they are intended for. Equipment should also be regularly checked and maintained.

Substances hazardous to health

Some of the substances recommended in this book, such as phenol or liquid nitrogen, can be hazardous to health. In the United Kingdom, there is specific guidance about the handling of these substances (Control of Substances Hazardous to Health [COSHH]). All health-care professionals handling these substances should be aware of the dangers and any special safety requirements.

Personal protective equipment

Staff involved in minor surgical procedures need to be aware of, and use, the protective equipment that is appropriate to their role. This is discussed in Chapter 3. For example:

- Disposable plastic aprons—single-use.
- Eye protection, where appropriate (Figure 4.1).
- Disposable face visors (where necessary)—single-use.
- Non-sterile examination gloves.
- Sterile surgical gloves.

Management of surgical instruments and clinical waste

Clinical and surgical equipment should be appropriately decontaminated and sterilised (see Chapter 3). Systems should be in place for labelling, tracking, packing, and returning used (contaminated) reusable instruments.

Correct flooring

Correct flooring is necessary on two health and safety counts, first to reduce the likelihood of slips and trips, and second as an infection control measure:

- All floor coverings should be smooth, slip-proof, impervious, and washable. It should be appropriately hard-wearing and must be able to withstand cleaning with disinfectants, particularly chlorine-releasing products up to 10,000 ppm. The most common material is vinyl.
- The flooring should be turned up at the walls in an integral covered skirting that is continuous with the floor and flush with all walls and structures. The coving between the floor and the wall prevents the accumulation of dust and dirt in corners and crevices (see Figure 1.4).

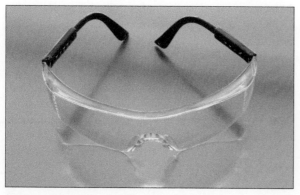

Figure 4.1 Protective goggles.

Latex sensitivity

It is estimated that between 1% and 6% of the general population in the United Kingdom are sensitised to natural latex rubber (NLR), and up to 17% of health-care workers are at risk of reactions to it. These reactions fall into type IV and type I hypersensitivity reactions, with deaths from anaphylaxis reported from the latter. The type IV delayed hypersensitivity reactions are due to the chemicals used to convert NLR during manufacture, and the type I immediate reactions are to the natural proteins in NLR.

How and why has this come about?

NLR products have been used for decades, although the first report of a type I reaction appeared in 1979. The introduction of guidance requiring health-care workers to wear gloves to protect themselves from blood-borne pathogens led to a huge jump in the demand for latex gloves (Figure 4.2). This in turn led to manufacturing changes resulting in high-protein examination gloves entering general medical use.

These proteins have sensitised workers and subsequently caused hypersensitivity reactions through either direct skin contact or inhalation of the airborne allergen carried by the cornstarch powder in powdered gloves. The routine use of gloves in health care also increases exposure to NLR in both the givers and the recipients of medical care. The risk is therefore to both the sensitised health-care provider and also the sensitised patient.

Why do we continue to use latex gloves?

Their continued use is because of their qualities of tactility and dexterity, which are unmatched by the alternatives on the market (vinyl, nitrile; Figure 4.3). In addition, despite the prevalence rate of sensitisation in the general population, not all of these individuals develop symptoms and therefore it can be argued that the majority of the population is not at clinical risk from use of NLR. The importance of risk assessment is to make an informed decision on whether an alternative is effective for the task. Where latex gloves are used, they must be low protein (less than 50 µg/g) and powder-free.

Musculoskeletal disorders

Several studies have shown that surgeons are prone to developing backache and other musculoskeletal problems. The following are sound recommendations for improving working posture and equipment design:

- *Change posture.* Alternate between sitting and standing. This will both produce a variety of postures and avoid postural (static muscle) fatigue.
- *Use support.* When sitting or standing, avoid leaning forward or stooping for prolonged periods unless supported. Maintain a good, upright posture when sitting, and if necessary use a footrest. When standing for prolonged periods, ensure you have something to lean on.

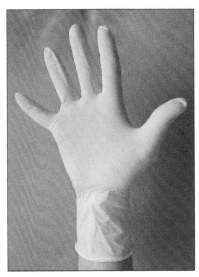

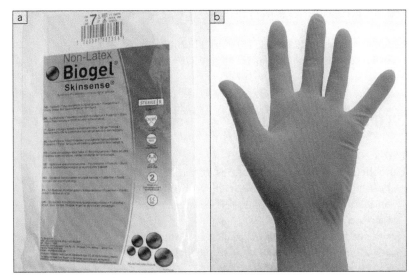

Figure 4.2 Latex surgical glove.

Figure 4.3 Example of latex-free gloves.

- *Safe reaching.* Keep equipment within easy reach. Items used frequently should be no further than about 50 cm from where your hands are operating, and your operating assistant should be trained to keep such equipment within reach.
- *Normal arm posture.* Avoid holding the upper arms away from the body while operating, and try to keep the wrists in a neutral position. Keeping the upper limbs free of tension and unnatural positions will minimise muscle, tendon, joint, and nerve problems.
- *Use comfortable equipment.* Equipment that is not too heavy and is ergonomically designed will help to avoid injury, especially to the upper limbs and back.
- *Manage time.* Avoid series of long appointments if possible—it is better to have numerous short surgical sessions with a change of position and posture in between. Therefore try to avoid multiple procedures on one patient in one appointment.

Stress

Unfortunately, stress is common in surgeons.

Evidence

The responses from a postal questionnaire sent to a sample of 1000 members of the Association of Surgeons of Great Britain and Ireland (Green *et al.*, 2005) revealed that surgeons showed mean scores significantly higher than those of the general population on two subscales of the mental health index (free-floating anxiety and hysterical anxiety). Although stress had both positive and negative effects, undue levels of stress impaired judgement, decision-making, and communication.

Strategies

Although stress poses significant risks, coping strategies are not taught explicitly during surgical training. Those used by the surgeons in a study on the effects of stress on surgical performance have the key elements of recognition of stress as a risk factor and of problems when they arise; and control over self and the situation:

- *Early recognition* of internal signs as indicators of stress.
- *Stop and stand back.* The cycle of anxiety and time pressure is broken by standing back mentally and regaining self-control, reassessing the situation and then making a decision, and finally preparing for the next stage.
- *Control of self.* The return to an appropriate physical, cognitive, and emotional state through physical relaxation methods, distancing techniques, and self-talk.
- *Control of the situation.* Surgeons follow the stages of reassessment, decision-making, intraoperative planning, preparing and leading the team, and solving the problem.

Methods for the primary prevention of stress should be offered to individuals through training, career counselling, and educating about error. It is essential to accept that tackling stress among health-care professionals is an important part of ensuring patient safety.

REFERENCE

Green A, Duthie HL, Young HL, Peters TJ (2005) Stress in surgeons. *British Journal of Surgery* 77: 1154–8.

FURTHER READING

Latex

Bandolier. Latex allergy: Implications for patients and health care workers. Available from: www.medicine.ox.ac.uk/bandolier/bandopubs/NHSSlatex.html (accessed July 2012).

Health and Safety Executive. Latex allergies. Available from: www.hse.gov.uk/skin/employ/latex.htm (accessed July 2012).

Musculoskeletal disorders

British Medical Association (2003) Specification for a directed enhanced service. Minor surgery (revised 2004). Available from: www.bma.org.uk/employmentandcontracts/independent_contractors/enhanced_services/DESsurgery.jsp (accessed October 2011).

Hedge A (2009) Back care for dentists and surgeons. Available from: www.spineuniverse.com/wellness/ergonomics/back-care-dentists-surgeons (accessed July 2012).

Humphreys H, Coai JE, Stacey A, *et al.* (2012) Guidelines on the facilities required for minor surgical procedures and minimal access interventions. *Journal of Hospital Infection* 80: 103–9.

Stress

Firth-Cozens J (2003) Doctors, their wellbeing, and their stress. *British Medical Journal* 326: 670–1.

Wetzel CM, Kneebone RL, Woloshynowych M, *et al.* (2006) The effects of stress on surgical performance. *American Journal of Surgery* 191: 5–10.

Chapter 5

Patient assessment

INTRODUCTION

This chapter is about assessing your patient prior to minor surgery. A careful assessment of the patient prior to commencing a surgical procedure is essential to reduce the likelihood of complications during surgery and after. If you are operating on a patient you have not met before, it is even more important to be sure that a proper assessment of the patient was made prior to surgery. A checklist is a useful way of ensuring that this is the case. The following section considers important issues that should have been discussed as part of the patient assessment.

ASSESSMENT OF PATIENT EXPECTATIONS

It is essential to familiarise yourself with the clinical record before the patient enters the operating room so that you are aware of the reason for the proposed surgery. You should confirm the following:

- What is the patient expecting and/or hoping you can do? In particular, what procedure are they expecting will be performed?
- What information about the procedure has the patient already been given?
- Has the patient had minor surgery before, and if so, what was the outcome? Were there any complications?
- Does the patient have significant illnesses and are they taking any medications?
- Does the patient have any problems with anaesthetics or needles?
- Are there any factors that may be relevant to wound healing or aftercare (e.g., travel, occupation, heavy lifting, etc.)?

As part of the process of obtaining informed consent (see Chapter 2), you need to be sure that different treatment options have been discussed. Do not rely upon this having already taken place. Remember the following:

- You should provide options for treatment, one of which may be to do nothing.
- You should be able to discuss the benefits and risks of those options.

Some patients have unrealistic expectations; for example, an excellent surgical scar may be described by the patient as poor. It is always worth inspecting any old scars the patient has, in order to gain information about the patient's healing tendencies and expectations.

YOUNG PATIENTS

There will be specific needs when operating on children and young adults. In the United Kingdom, there are very specific requirements relating to the care of children that are documented in the *National Service Framework for Children, Young People and Maternity Services* (Department of Health, 2004). This specifies the need for appropriately trained staff to be available during the procedure. In addition, remember the following:

- Parent(s) or guardian(s) should be available and involved in the consent process.
- Topical anaesthetics (and time for them to work), along with dilute or buffered injectable anaesthetic via very fine needles, may be helpful.
- The procedure may sometimes need to be performed under general anaesthesia.

ELDERLY PATIENTS

With elderly patients, there may be concerns about whether they have sufficient understanding to give informed consent. There may be a range of co-morbidities that may interfere with healing, such as diabetes, and this may complicate the postoperative period. This is particularly true for patients taking regular immuno-suppressive agents, such as prednisolone. There may be increased bleeding secondary to hypertension, varicose veins, and venous hypertension, and the skin may have reduced elasticity. This group is also more likely to be taking a range of medications.

MEDICAL HISTORY

A good medical history will identify most potential problems. Key aspects include medication, cardiovascular disease, allergies, problems likely to delay wound healing, haemorrhagic tendencies, and infectious diseases.

Regular medication

The most obvious relevant medications are those which interfere with bleeding, aspirin, clopidogrel, dipyridamole, and warfarin being the most common, but novel oral anticoagulants (NOACs) should also be considered.

Warfarin

For patients fully anticoagulated with warfarin, it is important to know what their International Normalised Ratio (INR) is on or around the day of surgery in order to assess the level of anticoagulation. Most patients will carry a record of their anticoagulation medication and INR. Studies have shown that, for minor surgery, an INR of between 1.5 and 3 is unlikely to cause excessive bleeding, and simple procedures can usually be performed without too much trouble.

Patients are usually taking warfarin for very specific medical reasons and they should, wherever possible, remain on their anticoagulant therapy as the risks of discontinuing treatment may well be significant. Care is particularly needed in patients with replacement artificial heart valves, and it may be advisable to obtain a cardiologist's opinion if it is considered necessary to discontinue anticoagulation, including NOACs, prior to surgery. In addition, haematologists report an increased thrombotic risk if warfarin is stopped suddenly.

If surgery is undertaken with an INR of greater than 3.5, not only is perioperative bleeding likely to be excessive, but also the risk of postoperative bleeding is increased. The use of pressure bandaging, rest, and, in the case of legs, elevation after surgery becomes more important than ever.

Antiplatelet medication

Even in low doses, aspirin can have prolonged (<10 days) effects on bleeding, and as it is available without prescription, it might not be noted in the medical records. Clopidogrel interferes with platelet action for up to 7 days. Dipyridamole has effects similar to those of aspirin.

The risk of stopping these medications needs to be weighed against the risk of bleeding with surgery. If the medication is being taken to protect a cardiac stent, the risk of stopping antiplatelet medication may be too great. Although current advice suggests aspirin is not a contraindication to minor surgery, more extensive surgical procedures may be complicated by the increased bleeding that can occur. If there is no contraindication to stopping antiplatelet medication, it should be discontinued at least 5 and ideally 7 days before planned surgery, especially where more complex procedures are anticipated.

Drug interactions

Other drugs exhibit interactions with anaesthetic agents or adrenaline (epinephrine). In practice, such interactions are unlikely to be significant as long as small doses of anaesthetic are used.

Lidocaine interaction

Beta-blockers (which can interact to produce hypertension and bradycardia), amiodarone, dipyridamole, and the histamine H2 antagonist cimetidine all tend to elevate lidocaine levels.

Adrenaline interaction

Tricyclic antidepressants can interact with adrenaline to cause hypertension, tachycardia, and even ventricular arrhythmia. With these drugs avoid large doses of local anaesthetic with adrenaline.

Cardiovascular conditions

Several potential problems can arise in people with cardiovascular disease. These include cardiac pacemakers, the risk of bacterial endocarditis, heart failure with resultant oedematous and poorly healing legs, and bleeding from varicose veins.

Pacemakers

There is some evidence that cardiac pacemakers can be affected by the use of unipolar and other forms of diathermy (including the hyfrecator), and particular care should be taken if a pacemaker is fitted. Potential problems depend on the type and age of the pacemaker, so the safest option is probably to use a conventional electrocautery machine in patients who have a pacemaker fitted.

Endocarditis

Although there is a theoretical risk of bacterial endocarditis occurring in patients with valvular disease, artificial heart valves, and valves previously damaged by endocarditis, current UK guidelines do not require the use of prophylactic antibiotics for most minor surgical procedures, such as excision of skin lesions. There is a theoretical small risk in those with pacemakers and angioplasty stents. Clinicians are advised to be up to date with current guidelines in this area. For example, the *Guidelines for the Prevention of Endocarditis: Report of the Working Party of the British Society for Antimicrobial Chemotherapy* (Gould *et al.*, 2006) makes the following statement:

'Procedures involving non-infected skin incision but no mucosal breach, for example, cardiac catheterisation or cosmetic piercing of nipple or pinna, do not require prophylaxis but adequate skin disinfection should be carried out prior to the procedure'.

A useful statement has also been published by the British Association of Dermatologists (BAD) and the British Society for Dermatological Surgery (BSDS) (BAD Therapy Guidelines and Audit Subcommittee, undated), which includes the following summary points:

- Antibiotic prophylaxis is effective in reducing bacteraemia, but there are no prospective data to confirm that it prevents endocarditis.
- There have been only four reported cases of endocarditis associated with skin surgery.
- The incidence of bacteraemia during skin surgery is comparable to the 2.1% incidence of random bacteraemia detected in normal volunteers.
- The commonest isolate present on preoperative surgical sites is coagulase negative staphylococcus which would require cover by vancomycin given intravenously.

As a result of the above, the BAD and BSDS, in agreement with the British Society for Antimicrobial Chemotherapy, state:

'Antibiotic prophylaxis for endocarditis is not required for routine dermatological surgery procedures, even in the presence of a pre-existing heart lesion'.

If any doubt exists, it is suggested that the clinician seek the advice of a microbiologist, consult a cardiologist or cardiothoracic surgeon, and/or refer to national guidance, which will be updated as appropriate. Endocarditis prophylaxis is most important where the area to be operated is infected or has a traumatised surface, and expert advice should be sought about the dosage, frequency, and type of antibiotic prophylaxis that is indicated.

In the United Kingdom, the *British National Formulary* is a useful source of up-to-date advice on this issue; see also National Institute for Health and Clinical Excellence (2008).

Allergies

The patient should be questioned about allergies to the following:

- *Latex*. Type I latex allergy is a well-recognised problem. Patients will describe anything from itchy blotches (urticaria) to angioedema and anaphylaxis. The use of latex-free gloves prevents this problem.
- *Skin cleansers*. Historically, iodine-containing products caused occasional allergies. Iodine is now rarely used as a skin cleanser. Sensitivity to common skin cleansers is unlikely but has been reported for chlorhexidine.
- *Local anaesthetics*. True allergy to the common local anaesthetics is rare. Many patients describing a reaction to a local anaesthetic may, on further questioning, be indicated to have had a vasovagal episode. Type I reactions can occur rarely to lidocaine, and if this is confirmed on prick-testing and/or radioallergosorbent (RAST) testing, an alternative should be used; prilocaine is often suitable.
- *Wound dressings*. Always check whether the patient is allergic to Elastoplast®, and choose the dressing appropriately.

Problems that may lead to delayed wound healing

Wound healing is a particular problem in the following situations:

- Individuals with diabetes tend to have problems with healing, especially if the wound is situated on the lower legs. This is likely to be related to microvascular compromise.
- Prolonged courses of oral steroids will result in not only delayed healing, but also skin atrophy and friable skin that may be difficult to repair.
- Patients with swollen legs resulting from cardiovascular or renal disease are likely to encounter difficulties with healing.

Haemorrhagic tendencies

Individuals with haemophilia pose a significant risk. Patients with thrombocytopenia may also be at risk. In addition to idiopathic causes, leukaemias and chemotherapy may cause significant problems due to low platelet counts. If there is any history of spontaneous bruising or excessive bleeding, arrange a clotting screen and blood film before operating.

Infectious diseases

The risk here is both with blood-borne diseases (hepatitis and HIV being the most obvious) and also acute infectious conditions. In general, and unless the procedure is part of investigating an ill patient, minor surgery should be avoided in any patient with a raised temperature or an active skin infection close to the surgical site.

ASSESSMENT CHECKLIST

The World Health Organization's Surgical Safety Checklist is a process to ensure that important factors are not overlooked prior to and after surgery. Although the steps (Sign in, Time Out, Sign Out) are not all relevant to minor surgery, the process remains relevant. It is advisable to consider the use of a checklist prior to minor surgery. Questions for the checklist that can be considered are listed below:

- Full name and date of birth.
- Any known allergies: to medicines, to plasters, to latex?
- On any medications (especially aspirin or warfarin)?
- Any problems with local anaesthetics?
- Any problems with healing?
- Tendency to faint?
- Pacemaker?
- Anything loose in the mouth (risk of choking if patient faints)?

- Able to comply with postoperative advice (travel, holidays, need for wound to be kept dry/sutures to be removed)?
- Consent obtained?
- Operation site confirmed and marked?

This is discussed in Chapter 2, where a sample form is provided.

REFERENCES

British Association of Dermatologists Therapy Guidelines and Audit Sub-Committee (undated) Antibiotic prophylaxis for endocarditis in dermatological surgery. A joint statement from the Therapy Guidelines and Audit Sub-Committee (TGASC) of the British Association of Dermatologists and the British Society for Dermatological Surgery. Available from: www.bad.org.uk/Portals/_Bad/Guidelines/Position%20Statements%20&%20Other%20Documents/Antiobiotic%20prophylaxis%20for%20endocarditis%20in%20dermatological%20surgery.pdf (accessed July 2012).

Department of Health (2004) *National Service Framework for Children, Young People and Maternity Services*. London: Department of Health.

Gould FK, Elliott TS, Foweraker J, *et al.* (2006) Guidelines for the prevention of endocarditis: Report of the Working Party of the British Society for Antimicrobial Chemotherapy. *Journal of Antimicrobial Chemotherapy* 57: 1035–42.

National Institute for Health and Clinical Excellence (2008) Antimicrobial prophylaxis against infective endocarditis in adults and children undergoing interventional procedures. http://www.nice.org.uk/nicemedia/pdf/CG64NICEguidance.pdf (accessed July 2012).

Chapter 6

Anatomical hazards and pitfalls

INTRODUCTION

The predictable anatomical complications awaiting the surgeon relate not only to the area being operated on, but also to what lies below it. This chapter considers first the areas of anatomical concern below the surface, followed by the forces that affect the healing of the skin itself, the areas of the body prone to poor healing, and finally the potential impact on haemostasis.

ANATOMICAL HAZARDS

A good knowledge of surface anatomy is essential for safe minor surgery, and a clear, illustrated textbook of surface anatomy is a sensible inclusion in the surgeon's library. We will look at the areas of concern starting from the head down.

The head

The objects of particular concern are:

- Nerves:
  - Facial nerve.
- Arteries:
  - Temporal artery.
- Other structures:
  - Parotid duct.
  - Lacrimal apparatus at the medial canthus.
  - Superficial lymph nodes.

These will be considered in turn.

The facial nerve

The two branches at greatest risk of damage during surgery are the marginal mandibular branch and the temporal branch (Figure 6.1). In addition, the posterior auricular branch is superficial enough to be damaged as it crosses the mastoid process.

Marginal mandibular branch

The nerve emerges 1 cm in front of or below the angle of the mandible, deep to the platysma muscle. This muscle may, however, have a minimal number of fibres, and the nerve may be exposed beneath the mandible as the head is extended. Damage results in drooping of the corner of the mouth and dribbling.

Temporal branch

The nerve crosses the zygomatic arch, anywhere over half the length of its inferior border. The nerve is particularly vulnerable to damage over the zygomatic arch and to a lesser extent in the lateral brow, especially if a large, infiltrating tumour is excised from the lateral forehead. Damage results in loss of innervation to the frontalis muscle, leading to loss of forehead wrinkles and inability to raise the eyebrow.

Posterior auricular branch

This rises close to the stylomastoid foramen and runs upward in front of the mastoid process.

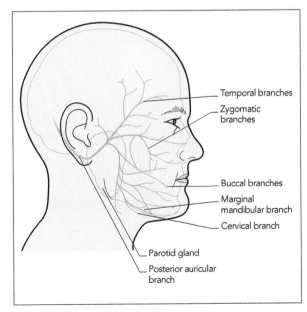

Figure 6.1 Branches of the facial nerve.

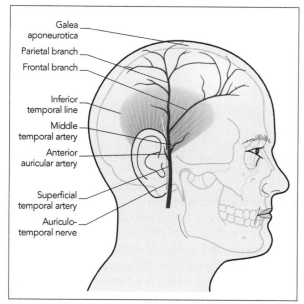

Figure 6.2 Temporal artery.

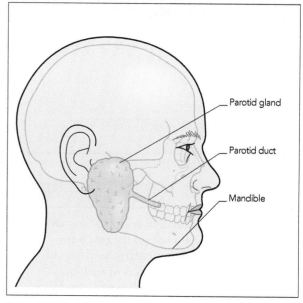

Figure 6.3 Parotid duct.

Temporal artery

The superficial temporal artery begins in the substance of the parotid gland, behind the neck of the mandible, and passes upwards to divide into two branches, the frontal and the parietal, both of which are superficial enough to be encountered (Figure 6.2). The temporal artery is very small (1.5–2 mm in diameter) and will go into spasm with trauma. Unless the damage is rectified, a reactive haemorrhage can be expected as the artery comes out of spasm.

The *frontal branch* runs tortuously upwards and forwards to the forehead, and the *parietal branch* is larger than the frontal, and curves upwards and backward on the side of the head, lying superficial to the temporal fascia.

Parotid duct

The location of the parotid duct, or Stensen duct, is shown in Figure 6.3. The duct lies superficial enough to be in danger from removal of deeply located lesions such as epidermoid cysts. Damage to the duct is characterised by a salivary fistula producing clear fluid days after the surgical procedure.

Lacrimal apparatus

The *lacrimal ducts,* one in each eyelid, open at minute orifices, termed *puncta lacrimalia* or lacrimal puncta (Figure 6.4). The *superior duct*, the smaller and shorter of the two, at first ascends and then bends at an acute angle, passing medially and downward to the lacrimal sac. The *inferior duct* at first descends, and then runs almost horizontally to the lacrimal sac. At the acute angles of the ducts, they are dilated into *ampullae*. This is an area fraught with complications, and surgery here should be entrusted to an ophthalmic expert.

Superficial lymph nodes

Postauricular lymph nodes in particular may be encountered or misdiagnosed as cysts in this area. Therefore it is advisable to be familiar with the lymph node chains around the head and neck.

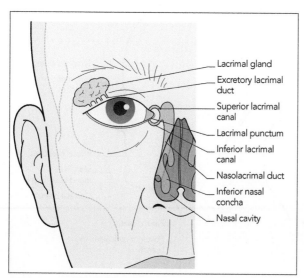

Figure 6.4 Lacrimal apparatus.

Neck

Those areas of particular concern include the anterior and posterior triangles and the supraclavicular fossae. The structures at particular danger include the:

- Spinal accessory nerve.
- External jugular vein.
- Pleura in the supraclavicular fossa.
- Thoracic duct on the left.

Spinal accessory nerve

The nerve (XIth cranial nerve) emerges beneath the posterior border of the sternomastoid at the junction of its upper and middle thirds (Erb's point; Figure 6.5). The nerve runs very superficially as it crosses from the posterior border of the sternomastoid almost vertically down to the anterior aspect of the trapezius. It is one of the most commonly damaged structures, resulting in shoulder drop from loss of innervation to the trapezius muscle.

External jugular vein

The external jugular vein drains most of the blood from the face and scalp. It begins in the region of the parotid gland, running backward and downward, and then across the surface of the sternomastoid (Figure 6.6). At this point, it pierces the deep fascia and enters, in the majority of cases, the jugulo-subclavian confluence. With the patient lying down, the location of the vein is usually easily seen, marked, and avoided.

Supraclavicular fossa

This is the area above the clavicle, and the unique danger here is the apex of the thoracic cavity and the outer, parietal pleura. The pleura is dome-shaped with its apex approximately 3 cm superior to the middle third of the clavicle. Covering the pleura is the suprapleural membrane, a strong fascial connective tissue layer.

Thoracic duct

This lies on the left side of the neck. It drains into the subclavian vein at the junction with the internal jugular vein.

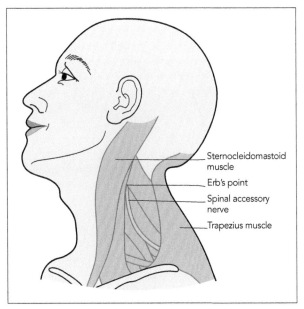

Figure 6.5 Spinal accessory nerve.

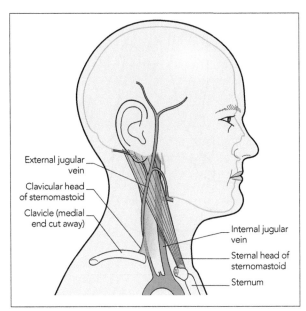

Figure 6.6 External jugular vein.

> **GOLDEN RULE** ❋
> Before you ever operate on skin, recall what lies underneath. If you can't recall, look it up!

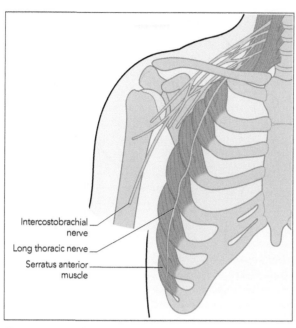

Figure 6.7 Long thoracic nerve.

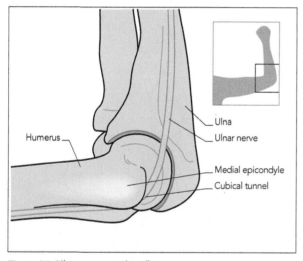

Figure 6.8 Ulnar nerve at the elbow.

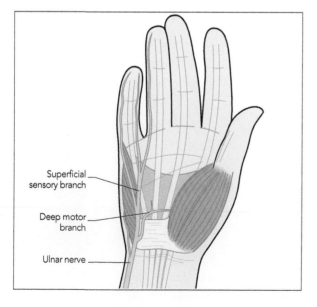

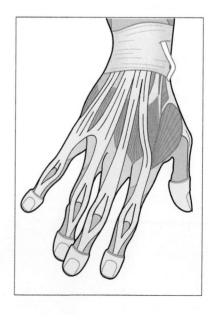

Upper limb

The main areas of concern are the axilla, elbow, wrist, hand, and fingers.

Axilla

The axilla contains the axillary vessels and the brachial plexus of nerves, with their branches, some branches of the intercostal nerves, and a large number of lymph glands, together with a quantity of fat and loose areolar tissue. It is best avoided entirely. The structures that are most superficial include:

- The long thoracic nerve, descending on the surface of the serratus anterior muscle, which it innervates (Figure 6.7).
- The intercostobrachial nerve, perforating the upper and anterior part of the axillary wall, and passing across the axilla to the medial side of the arm. This nerve runs superficially under the hair-bearing skin of the axilla. Even though it runs deep to the fat layer, there is little fat in this location. Damage leads to a winged scapula.

The ulnar nerve at the elbow and wrist

The concern here is the ulnar nerve as it travels around the medial epicondyle, where it is very superficial and easily damaged (Figure 6.8).

Similarly, in the distal part of the forearm, the ulnar nerve becomes relatively superficial, covered only by fascia and skin. Near the pisiform bone of the wrist, it passes superficial to the flexor retinaculum and ends by dividing into superficial and deep branches (Figure 6.9). The muscles innervated by the ulnar nerve are mainly concerned with fine movements of the hand, including adduction and abduction of the fingers (interossei), adduction of the thumb (adductor pollicis), and flexion and adduction at the wrist (interossei). Damage to this nerve will therefore have major implications for movement of the muscles of the hand.

Figure 6.9 (Left) Ulnar nerve at the wrist.

Figure 6.10 (Right) Extensor tendons of the hand.

Hand and wrist

Extensor tendons

These run just under the thin skin on the dorsum of the fingers and hand. They are therefore at risk from both the scalpel and cryosurgery (Figure 6.10).

Palm

Not only are the flexor tendons close to the skin, but there is no slack at all in the palm of the hand. Never excise a lesion from the palm since the wound may prove impossible to close; instead, leave this to a suitably trained specialist hand surgeon.

Groin and lower limb

The femoral vessels and femoral nerve can be damaged within the groin. Lower down, the common peroneal nerve is open to damage as it passes over the neck of the fibula, and the sural nerve as it passes over the posterior calf. The long saphenous nerve runs superficially over the medial side of the leg, and any dilated superficial veins over the lower legs are at particular risk of damage from skin surgery. The short saphenous vein lies within the popliteal fossa.

Common peroneal nerve (lateral popliteal nerve)

This nerve travels laterally just behind the biceps femoris and distally down just lateral to the fibular head (Figure 6.11). This nerve is very superficial near the knee. It is, therefore, easily injured, especially where it passes lateral to the fibular head, just as the fibular head tapers. It is, however, a large (4–5 mm diameter) nerve so can be easily identified using a careful technique. This nerve can also be traumatised by continued pressure over this area. Damage leads to foot drop.

Sural nerve

The sural nerve is a very small nerve and easily missed. It is particularly superficial as it runs from the centre of the posterior calf to the tendo achilles, close to the small saphenous vein (Figure 6.12). Damage results in numbness of the lateral border of the foot.

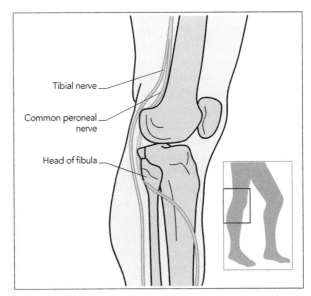

Figure 6.11 Common peroneal nerve.

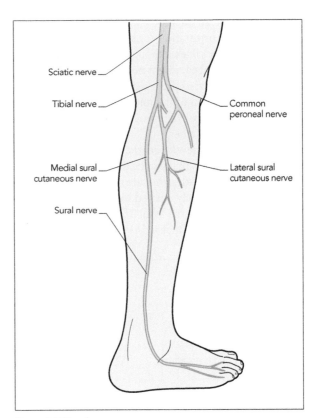

Figure 6.12 Sural nerve.

Anatomical hazards

LINES OF SKIN TENSION: OPTIMISING YOUR INCISION

When operating on skin, it is important to be familiar with Langer's lines, although today we are more likely to think in terms of relaxed skin tension lines (RSTLs; Figure 6.13) when deciding how to locate an incision to optimise healing and minimise scarring.

Langer was an anatomy professor in Vienna. In order to study the way skin reacts when incised, he mapped out the effect of stabbing a round-tipped awl into hundreds of fresh cadavers. He found that the puncture wounds made in fresh cadavers assumed a slit or oval configuration, the long axis corresponding to the greatest static tension of the skin. Langer constructed his lines to follow these long axes, but he was an anatomist and not a surgeon. It was Kocher who later recognised the surgical importance of the Langer tension lines and advised that surgical incisions should follow them.

However, not all surgeons found Langer's lines to provide the best orientation for scar healing, and it was felt that the Langer's lines, although relevant to the cadavers that Langer studied, might not have been correct for use in the living. Kraissl preferred lines oriented perpendicularly to the action of the underlying muscle, finding that the contraction of the muscles tended to bring the edges of a wound together.

In 1962, Borges developed the idea of RSTLs. The RSTLs follow furrows that can be formed when the skin is relaxed. Unlike wrinkles, they are not visible features of the skin; they are merely derived from the furrows produced by pinching on the skin. The RSTLs correspond to the directional pull that exists in relaxed skin. This pull is determined by the protrusion of the underlying bone, cartilage, and tissue bulk, not only the bulk that the skin covers, but also nearby tissue bulk (e.g., the breast). Although the RSTLs are not caused by the underlying musculature, they frequently run perpendicular to them (as described by Kraissl). The RSTLs exert a constant tension even during sleep, and are only temporarily altered by muscle contraction. It is for this reason that incisions made parallel to tension lines heal better than those made in other orientations.

In general, the best cosmetic results may be achieved by following Borges' lines on the face (i.e., RSTLs) and Kraissl's lines on the body (i.e., perpendicular to the underlying muscle).

Putting theory into practice

A skilled surgeon observes the skin tensions and plans an excision to produce the least skin tension, but the reality of translating the theory of using RSTLs into practice is not always straightforward. The first of the next two sections provides useful tips on how to identify the RSTLs and use them to make the correct incisions in different parts of the body. There will, however, be occasional exceptions to the rule of using the RSTLs, either when the orientation of the lesion is completely wrong (i.e., when following the RSTL will result in a huge scar as opposed to a small one) or when the excision will damage or distort neighbouring structures (e.g., the lips, the forehead leading to a browlift, or the lower eyelid resulting in an ectropion). The second section therefore describes situations when using RSTLs may not be the best approach, explains why, and suggests alternative approaches to deciding the optimal surgical incision in areas where healing and scarring can be a problem.

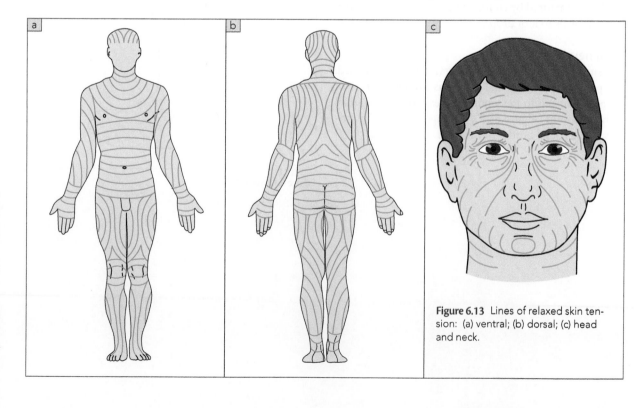

Figure 6.13 Lines of relaxed skin tension: (a) ventral; (b) dorsal; (c) head and neck.

Using RSTLs

Prior to cutting out a lesion, the surgeon can ascertain the RSTLs and the effects of the underlying muscles using the following approaches.

Head and neck
- For the *forehead and temple*, it is a good idea to ask the patient to raise their eyebrows and then to frown.
- On the *cheek or close to the lips*, ask them to alternately pout their lips and bare their teeth.
- On the *neck*, ask the patient to flex, extend, and then rotate the neck.

Torso
- Over the *upper back*. Get the patient to arch the shoulders back and then hunch them forward. Then observe the effect of abducting the adjacent arm.
- Overlying the *vertebrae* of the back. Here, the orientation of excision may depend upon the patient's flexibility. On a very rigid back, the least tension may be in the horizontal plane (across the vertebral column), whereas in a young, flexible back, a vertical excision may be best (although in theory it will be subject to more tension when erect as the wound edges are 'brought together' in flexion).
- *Anterior chest*. The female breast is a particular challenge due to both the potential for poor scarring and the effect that posture can have (see below).

Limbs
Prior to an excision near to a joint, examine the area in full extension, flexion, and, if relevant, rotation (Figure 6.14).

Tips for when you can't work it out
If there are still concerns about the correct orientation, the surgeon has two options:
- Mark the skin and then observe what happens to the ellipse when the skin is moved as above. It may be necessary to mark out several potential ellipses and observe which is affected least by movement.
- Cut out the lesion as a circle. The skin will then stretch along the lines demonstrated by Langer, and extending the circular wound to the shape of an ellipse will then allow closure. This is a useful technique when closing a punch biopsy wound.

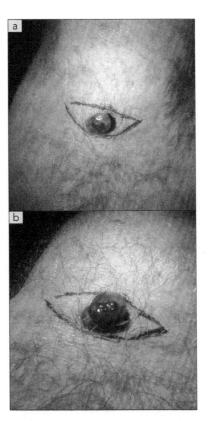

Figure 6.14 Knee (a) extended and (b) flexed.

Modified use of RSTLs in areas prone to poor healing and scarring

Working down from the head, there are various areas of the body where changing the traditional approach of using RSTLs to create an elliptical excision can have advantages, and it is important to recognise these situations.

Head
Central forehead
The centre of the forehead presents challenges (Figure 6.15). The natural skin creases often have a curved appearance, and a standard ellipse here can produce an unnatural straight line. Crescentic excisions tend to produce a distortion to other skin lines. Excising a large vertically orientated lesion above the eyebrow with a horizontal ellipse can lead to 'browlift'. There are two alternatives:

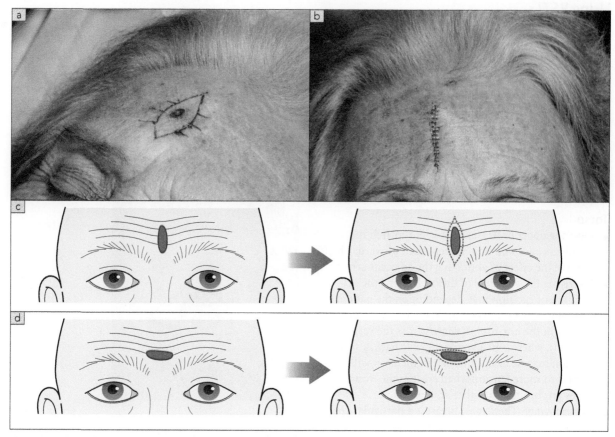

Figure 6.15 Examples on the central forehead: vertical (a, b, c) and horizontal (d). (a) The lesion has been marked out with a vertical excision; skin creases marked prior to anaesthesia. (b) The wound after closure.

- An ellipse can be created in which both ends are inverted to produce a very natural-looking scar (Figure 6.15d).
- If the lesion is large or orientated vertically, the only option may be to undertake a vertical elliptical incision. When this is undertaken, it is essential to ensure that skin creases line up after removal. As the anaesthetic will tend to relax all the skin creases, it is essential that they are marked with a fine skin marker prior to anaesthetising (Figures 6.15a, c). The marks are then brought together during suturing (Figure 6.15b).

Lateral forehead

Lateral to the eye lie RSTLs running perpendicularly to each other. The classic 'crow's feet' lines radiate out from the lateral canthus, and perpendicular to these are the forehead lines. If the lesion to be excised is orientated in a particular direction, the excision will be reduced in size by following that orientation (Figure 6.16). If it is not, however, the patient should be asked to undertake several facial expressions in order to assess the correct orientation for the incision:

- First, 'Raise your eyebrows as high as possible.' This will demonstrate the forehead lines.
- Second, 'Screw your eyes up tight.' This will demonstrate the 'crow's feet' (Figure 6.16a).

If there is any doubt over the best orientation, the surgeon should, with the surrounding skin relaxed, mark out the excision lines for both 'frown lines' and 'crow's feet' excisions. Figure 6.16b demonstrates a number of options. Figures 6.16c and 6.16d demonstrate an excision along the 'crow's feet' to avoid interfering with the eye.

Ear

Skin lesions commonly occur over the edge of the pinna. Although simple ellipse excision following the line of the ear may appear attractive, this may lead to distortion of the curve of the pinna, with a noticeable defect (Figure 6.17a). It is preferable instead to mark the excision of the lesion as a 'wedge' excision, an ellipse with one apex anteriorly and the other posteriorly, and then the lesion can be excised with the minimum of scarring (Figures 6.17b–d). If the lesion is one of chondrodermatitis nodularis helicis, the underlying affected cartilage will also require shaving (see Chapter 9).

Once the ellipse has been excised, the skin overlying the pinna to each side will need undermining. The resultant scar will be minimal. The size of the pinna may have been minimally reduced, but this will not normally be detectable.

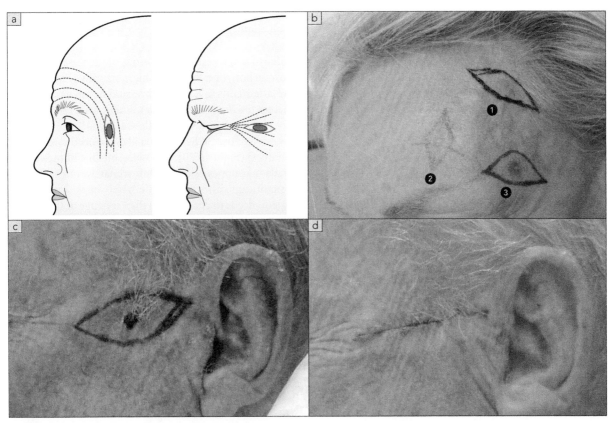

Figure 6.16 Examples on the lateral forehead. (a) Minimising the excision size by following the lesion orientation. (b) 1: Semi-crescentic, distant enough not to affect the eyebrow; 2: Vertical orientation to avoid eyebrow lift; 3: Crescentic excision lateral to the eyebrow. (c, d) Excision following the 'crow's feet'.

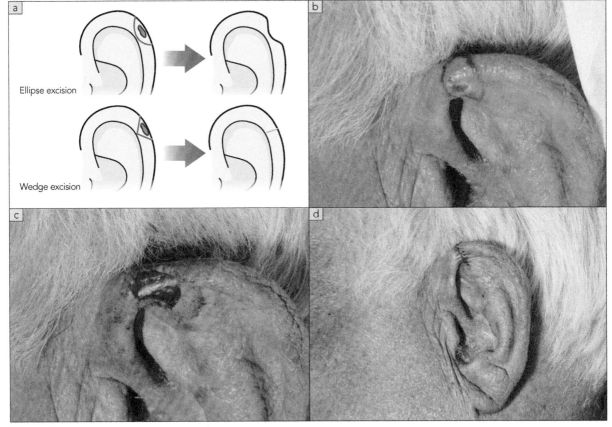

Figure 6.17 Incisions on the curve of the pinna, demonstrating the advantage of a wedge excision versus an ellipse.

Anterior cheek

The area below the eye presents a specific problem (Figure 6.18). The RSTLs radiate around under the eye and then curve down around the cheek. It is tempting to try to follow these curved relaxed tension lines under the eye excision (Figure 16.18a[1]), but the loss of skin may, on closure, cause excessive traction on the lower eyelid. The result may be the development of an ectropion and a permanently watering and irritated eye.

Eyelid tension can be assessed by pulling the lower lid down, away from the eye. If it 'snaps' back into place, the lower lid will probably withstand a small ellipse. If, however, the lid returns to normal very slowly, the risk of ectropion will be great. In these circumstances, it may be preferable to take an ellipse out vertically (Figure 6.18a [2]). Care needs to be taken to align the skin lines for closure. The effect of this direction of excision is that it will actually tend to lift the lower lid as the two curved edges of the wound are brought together and straightened. The scar may be less than ideal, but lid function will be preserved (Figures 6.18b–d).

Nose

Small elliptical excisions on the nose can be undertaken so that they have little if any effect on the shape and profile of the nose. Over the bridge of the nose, it is better to excise horizontally rather than vertically (Figure 6.19). The latter tends to leave a depression in the nasal profile, whereas the former tends to minimally raise the tip of the nose and produce a very subtle scar.

Lesions close to the nasal ala likewise need careful consideration (Figure 6.20). Following the line of the edge of the ala may appear simple. Unfortunately, this will result in significant distortion of the nasal shape. Instead, the surgeon needs to cut down to the very edge of the nostril. It is essential to obtain perfect apposition of the edges to produce a good cosmetic result. The ellipse will often curve around almost into the nostril.

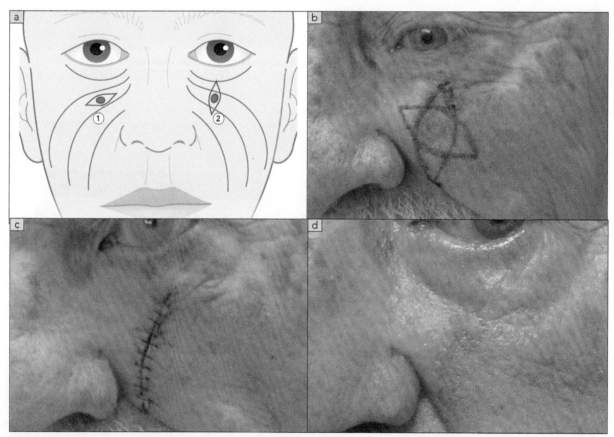

Figure 6.18 Examples (a) on the anterior cheek showing the options between RSTL orientation [1] and vertical orientation [2], and (b–d) below the eye (preoperatively, after excision, and 3 weeks postoperatively).

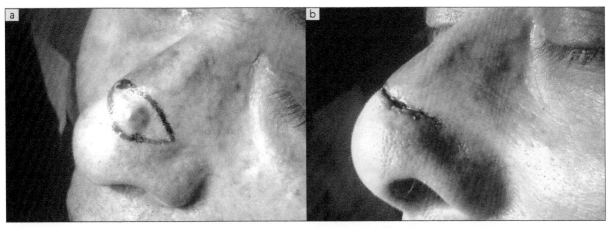

Figure 6.19 (a) Excision across the bridge of the nose avoids a depressed scar. (b) Closed prior to skin sutures.

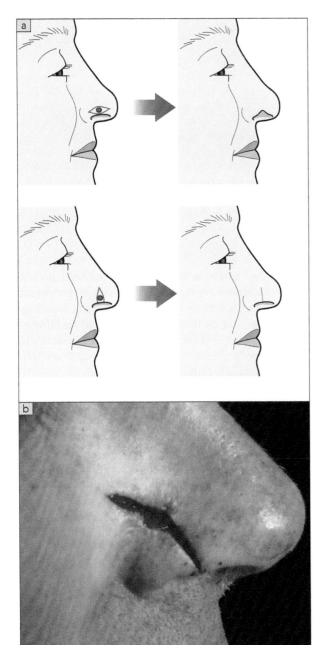

Figure 6.20 Nasal ala excisions: (a) orientation options; (b) correct (vertical) excision prior to skin sutures.

Lips

Excisions near the vermilion border are some of the most cosmetically visible. When considering surgery involving the lips, it is advisable to know the anatomy and terminology:

- The upper lip extends from the base of the nose superiorly to the nasolabial folds laterally, and to the free edge of the vermilion border inferiorly (Figure 6.21a).
- The lower lip extends from the superior free vermilion edge superiorly, to the commissures laterally, and to the mandible inferiorly.
- Around the border between the vermilion and the skin, a fine line of pale skin accentuates the colour difference between the vermilion border and the normal skin.
- Along the upper border between the vermilion and the skin, two paramedian elevations of the vermilion form the Cupid's bow: between two raised vertical columns of tissue lies a midline depression called the philtrum.
- The philtrum is located between the paramedian elevations of the vermilion border and the columella above.
- The labiomental crease passes horizontally in an inverted U-shape across the lower lip, which intraorally corresponds to the depth of the gingivolabial sulcus.

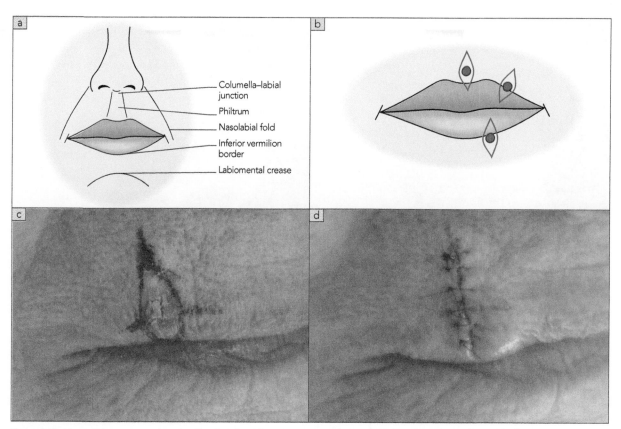

Figure 6.21 Lip excisions across the vermilion border: (a) correct nomenclature, (b) orientation, (c) marking, (d) after closure.

Labels in (a): Columella–labial junction; Philtrum; Nasolabial fold; Inferior vermilion border; Labiomental crease

When excising a lesion close to or on the vermilion border (Figure 6.21), the exact orientation of the elliptical excision can be assessed by asking the patient to purse the lips, thereby accentuating the RSTLs. The edge of the vermilion border should be very carefully marked with a fine skin-marking pen on each side of the ellipse. After anaesthetic with adrenaline (epinephrine) has been injected, the vermilion border may not be so easily visualised, but the skin markings will allow exact closure. By using anaesthetic volume, the surface of the lip may be expanded slightly. This facilitates a very clean cut through the epidermis. Suturing is achieved with fine 6-0 monofilament suture. Some surgeons advocate the use of absorbable sutures on the lips, but as the skin sutures will require removal, there is little advantage to this.

A lesion located centrally over the philtrum can also be excised in the same manner, but care needs to be exercised to avoid changing the shape of the lips and the paramedian elevations. If the lesion occurs at the commissures or over the paramedian elevations, standard elliptical excisions may either be impossible to achieve or result in anatomical distortion. In these circumstances, the excision can be achieved by the use of a simple 'M-plasty' excision (see Chapter 25).

Back

Experienced surgeons know just how difficult it is to achieve good cosmetic results over the back. Hypertrophic and keloid scars are more common toward the shoulders. The dermis is at its thickest over the back, resulting in much increased skin tension during wound closure. In addition, body movements ensure that wounds are subjected to significant stretching (Figure 6.22).

Lateral to the midline, the best orientation is usually to follow the line of the ribs, which usually corresponds to the RSTLs. Lesions over the midline, or very close to it, are, however, different. There are two possibilities here.

- **The vertical incision:** Cutting across the RSTLs and down the line of the vertebrae results in excision margins that are brought together as the back flexes. This orientation works well if the skin is not too tight, and this is best judged on an individual basis.
- **The horizontal excision:** By cutting across the line of the vertebrae, the surgeon follows the RSTLs. This may make the wound easier to close and reduce suture tension. As the back flexes forward, however, the wound will be subjected to significant stretching. Patient advice during healing is essential.

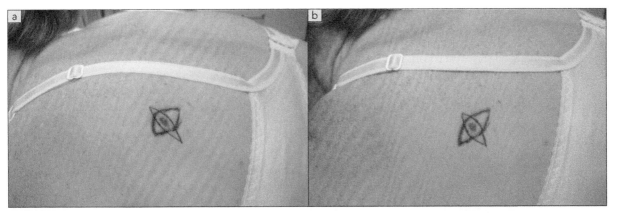

Figure 6.22 Back marking altered by the arm being (a) adducted and (b) abducted.

Female breast

Surgery to the skin over the breast is difficult, and decisions about orientation are dependent upon the size of the breast, the age of the skin, and the size and exact location of the lesion. In order to correctly assess skin tension, it is advisable to undertake skin marking with the patient sitting up and the breast unsupported by clothing—this will be the most natural orientation for the skin. If the orientation is determined and the skin marked with the patient lying down, the resultant scar is likely to be sub-optimal. The orientation of the incision also depends upon where around the breast the lesion is located (Figure 6.23).

Upper section

Skin tension lines tend to align to the areola, and the optimum orientation is to follow these lines. A more horizontal line avoids a scar running across the edge of clothing, but such a scar will require extra support to avoid stretching. Encouraging the patient to wear a supportive bra day and night for several weeks will help to avoid the wound stretching.

In Figure 6.23b, the right breast has been marked with what would be assumed to be a cosmetically sensitive excision—and with the ipsilateral arm raised (Figure 6.23c), the incision looks good. However, skin tension will produce a very poor scar. In Figure 6.23b the left

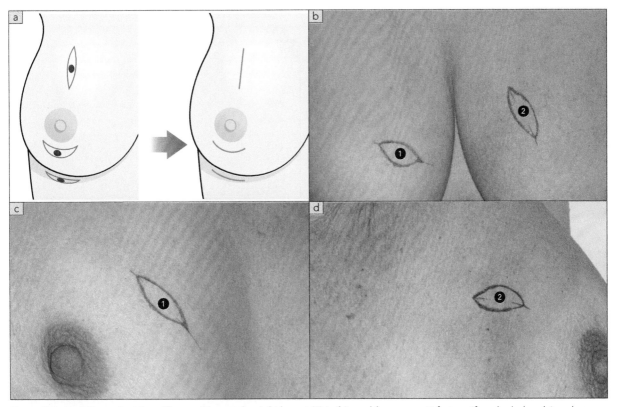

Figure 6.23 (a–d) Breast incisions. The marking on the right breast (1) in (b) would appear satisfactory, if marked when lying down and the arm abducted as in (c). Conversely, the marking on the left breast (2) in (b) is correct, but would not be chosen with the patient lying with the arm abducted, as in (d).

breast has been marked with the patient erect, the breast unsupported. This will produce the best healing, but the orientation would not be chosen with the patient supine and the arm abducted (Figure 6.23d).

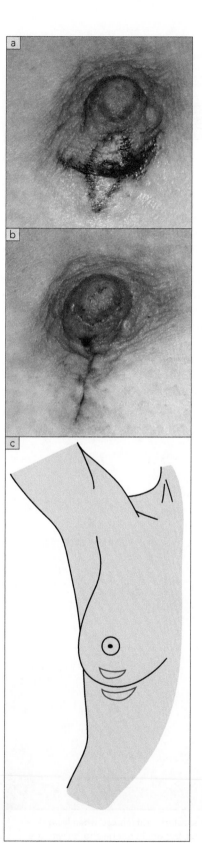

Figure 6.24
(a, b) Marking and excision across the areolar border. (c) Breast, lower section: crescentic incisions.

Peri-areolar

Two main options are possible here. The first is to excise an ellipse across the edge of the areola (Figure 6.24a, b). It is essential that the edge of the areola is marked prior to anaesthetising. With wound closure, there must be perfect apposition of the areola edge to avoid distortion. Under the areola, it may be possible to excise more of a crescentic scar (Figure 6.23a). The short side of the crescent can be curved to follow the areolar edge.

Lower section

Here the weight of the breast tissue tends to compress the skin, so crescentic excisions work well (Figure 6.24c). These can be aligned to follow the lower curve of the breast edge. Excising in a line radially to the areola (as recommended for the upper section of the breast) will result in a scar that is distorted by the breast when the patient is upright.

Shoulder

The RSTLs tend to run from the neck down toward the shoulder and arm, and for the majority of simple excisions following these lines is appropriate (Figure 6.25). However, the resultant wound/scar will run across the line of straps on clothing and cause irritation. In these situations, orientating the scar more vertically going from anterior to posterior shoulder may have advantages as long as shoulder movements do not put the skin under undue tension.

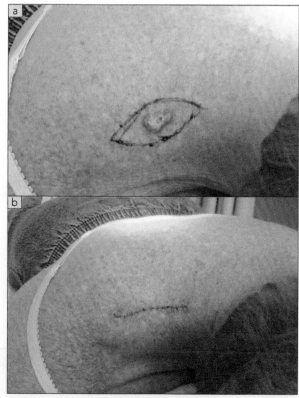

Figure 6.25 (a) Upper back incision and (b) closure along the line of the shoulder.

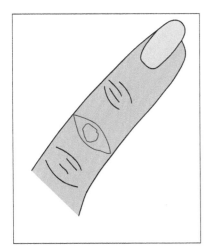

Figure 6.26
Incision on the finger.

ANATOMICAL FACTORS AND HAEMOSTASIS

Bleeding during surgical procedures is affected by anatomical factors, some of which are considered in this section.

Scalp

The scalp has a particularly extensive blood supply that runs predominantly radially but with extensive anastomoses. It is not uncommon for surgical wounds on the scalp to bleed profusely. Because of the anastomoses, it may be necessary to apply pressure circumferentially around the wound to establish haemostasis.

Underlying blood vessels

Although the list is not exhaustive, the following vessels may cause problems:

- Temporal artery.
- External jugular vein.
- Axillary artery and vein.
- Veins around the antecubital fossa.
- Femoral vessels in the groin.
- Short saphenous vein in the popliteal fossa.
- Any underlying varicose veins or other areas of venous hypertension.

The temporal artery can be a particular problem as injuring the artery causes it to spasm, thereby reducing or even halting bleeding. When the artery comes out of spasm, which can occur after surgery has been completed, there may occur brisk bleeding unless the artery has been ligated or repaired.

Sites of increased skin tension

Bleeding is more likely to occur if the skin is under increased tension. Examples of this are as follows:

- On the digit as there is little laxity of the skin on the fingers and toes.
- Where a large lesion is being removed and it is difficult to oppose the edges of the wound easily.
- Over or close to the extensor surfaces of joints.
- In the pretibial region.

Areas of poor healing

In addition to poor healing, distal parts of the lower limb are prone to venous oozing and leakage of interstitial fluid. This is particularly a problem in individuals with diabetes or arteriopathy, and those with marked lower limb oedema, as there may be difficulty in achieving closure because of thin, easily damaged skin.

Digits

Fingers and toes present particular problems. Not only does the skin lie in close proximity to the joints, but there also tends to be very little redundant tissue. The trick is to excise in a circumferential and not in a longitudinal direction (Figure 6.26).

Anterior shin

This is a difficult location for skin closure, especially in the elderly whose skin will be fragile and thin. Extensive undermining, mattress sutures, and an assistant helping to bring the edges together may all be required. Warn the patient in advance that the wound may need to heal slowly by secondary intention.

Palms of the hands and soles of the feet

The skin here is particularly difficult to excise and close without skin tension, so avoid surgery in these locations if at all possible. The orientation of any scar should be made viewing the function of the limb as paramount. Deep sutures are usually impossible to use as there is no depth to the dermis. In addition, although the epidermis may be very tough, especially on the sole of the foot, the skin is actually torn very easily by a tightly pulled suture. Particular care needs to be taken to avoid undue skin tension, perhaps with the use of mattress sutures. Sutures tend to need to be left in for longer to ensure adequate healing, and this makes stitch marks more likely.

FURTHER READING

Borges A (1984) Relaxed skin tension lines (RSTL) versus other skin lines. *Plastic and Reconstructive Surgery* 73: 144–50.

Wilhelmi BJ, Blackwell SJ, Phillips LG (1999) Langer's lines: to use or not to use. *Plastic and Reconstructive Surgery* 104: 208–14.

Chapter 7

Local and regional anaesthetic agents

INTRODUCTION

Most minor surgical procedures require local anaesthesia, with the injection of a local anaesthetic agent into the skin, where local anaesthesia is defined as any technique that is used to cause a loss of sensation in a particular part of the body. Successful local anaesthesia in the context of minor surgery ensures that the patient does not experience any pain during the surgical procedure, even if they are aware of other sensations.

The procedures in this book will usually be performed using local or regional anaesthesia, thereby avoiding the need for general anaesthesia. *Local anaesthesia* usually relates to anaesthesia of a small area of the body such as a tooth or an area of skin, whereas *regional anaesthesia* implies the anaesthetising of a larger part of the body, for example a digit or a limb. Using appropriate local or regional anaesthetics *any* minor operation should be performed *completely painlessly*, and effective anaesthesia is essential to the success of minor surgical procedures.

This chapter provides essential information about available anaesthetic agents and their usage, safety, and potential side effects. Chapter 15 describes techniques for topical, local and regional anaesthesia.

COMMON LOCAL ANAESTHETIC AGENTS AND THEIR PROPERTIES

Local anaesthetics cause reversible interruption of the conduction of impulses in peripheral nerves by a local decrease in depolarisation of the nerve membrane so that the threshold potential for transmission is not reached and no electrical impulse travels down the nerve. These effects are due to a blockade of sodium channels, which impairs sodium ion flux across the membrane.

There are two groups of local anaesthetic agents— esters and amides—with amides being the most commonly used. *Esters* (e.g., procaine and amethocaine) are relatively unstable and short-acting, and are rapidly broken down into para-aminobenzoic acid (PABA), which can produce hypersensitivity reactions. *Amides* (e.g., lidocaine, prilocaine, and bupivacaine) are more stable and longer lasting, being metabolised in the liver, and these rarely produce hypersensitivity reactions (fewer than 1% of cases). The clearance rate is fastest with prilocaine, followed by lidocaine, and slowest with bupivacaine. Lidocaine and prilocaine have a moderate duration of action (70–140 minutes), with bupivacaine having the longest action (about 200 minutes).

In solution, amides are acidic and need relatively alkaline tissues in which to work. The reason local anaesthetics are relatively inactive when injected into inflamed tissues is that these have an acid pH, and the lack of alkali reduces the release of the free, active base.

LOCAL ANAESTHETIC PREPARATIONS

Topical or surface local anaesthetics

Mucous membranes absorb local anaesthetics very rapidly, efficiently, and painlessly. Thus, the cornea and conjunctiva can be readily anaesthetised with local anaesthetic drops, of which there are several varieties including lidocaine, oxybuprocaine hydrochloride 0.4%, or amethocaine hydrochloride 0.5%. Onset of anaesthesia is rapid and lasts for up to 1 hour. Repeated small applications produce more effective anaesthesia than a single application of large volume.

The lining of the nose, buccal mucosa, larynx, pharynx, oesophagus, trachea, tympanic membrane, vagina, glans penis, and urethra may all be anaesthetised using topical anaesthetic preparations such as lidocaine aerosol spray. The maximum safe dose of topical or surface anaesthetic, which can be given to any particular patient for specific sites, should be known and not exceeded. These may differ for different agents, and if in doubt the clinician is advised to refer to the manufacturer's data sheet.

Topical anaesthetic creams

Absorption of conventional local anaesthetic agents through the skin is slow, poor, and unreliable. Newer eutectic mixtures of local anaesthetic agents can provide useful surface anaesthesia that is particularly helpful in paediatric practice.

There are two commonly available products: Emla® cream, which contains 25 mg lidocaine and 25 mg prilocaine per gram, and Ametop™, which is 4% amethocaine gel. Both need to be applied under an occlusive dressing for up to an hour to optimise absorption and create satisfactory surface analgesia for needle puncture (e.g., 2 g Emla® under occlusion). Some surgeons use Emla® cream for superficial cautery or split-skin grafting, for which it is recommended that 2 g per 10 cm² is applied as a thick layer under occlusion for at least 120 minutes.

Topical anaesthetic creams should not be applied to open wounds or mucous membranes, or on patients with atopic dermatitis. Prolonged exposure can produce erythema and skin irritation. The most useful application is in children before needle puncture, enabling infiltration anaesthesia to be accomplished painlessly.

Local anaesthetic for infiltration

Lidocaine

Lidocaine is the most widely used local anaesthetic for infiltration anaesthesia in minor surgery. It is an effective and safe drug provided the surgeon understands its limitations.

Preparations

Lidocaine solution is available in three strengths: 0.5%, 1%, and 2%. For most purposes, 1% lidocaine is adequate. A 1% solution contains 100 mg lidocaine in 10 ml. Each strength of lidocaine is also available with adrenaline (epinephrine; see below). Lidocaine solution is supplied in single-dose vials and multidose bottles. Although single-dose vials are slightly more expensive than multidose bottles, they are preferable because their use minimises the risk of contamination.

For *children*, it is possible to mix 1% lidocaine 50:50 with normal saline. This is isotonic, produces minimal sting, and, if suturing a laceration, can be injected through the cut sides painlessly. Such weak solutions have a short duration of action so should be followed with usual anaesthetic concentrations.

Dosages

Although there are widely quoted safe dosages for lidocaine in the literature, every patient should be assessed as an individual since the effect of a local anaesthetic depends on a number of factors, for example the size of the patient, tissue perfusion, the presence of infection, cardiac output, and drug distribution and metabolism. In principle, lower doses should be used in the elderly and in children.

As a rule of thumb, 3 mg/kg is widely used to calculate the maximum safe dose. So for an average 70 kg man, 210 mg lidocaine could theoretically be used. The widely quoted 'maximum adult dose' of 200 mg corresponds to:

- 40 ml of 0.5% lidocaine solution *or*
- 20 ml of 1% lidocaine solution *or*
- 10 ml of 2% lidocaine solution.

In practice, for the types of procedure described in this book, you will not usually approach these maximum doses. But be careful if you are treating multiple lesions at the same time, as the effects of each injection are cumulative.

> ## GOLDEN RULES ❋
> - The correct dose of local anaesthesia is the smallest dose required to produce the desired anaesthesia.
> - You should be aware of the signs of overdosage and act quickly if they occur.

Symptoms of overdosage

The early symptoms and signs of lidocaine overdosage are circumoral tingling, tinnitus, and slight confusion or oddness of speech. The patient will sometimes complain of a metallic taste. By talking to the patient, you will notice these signs immediately and stop giving further anaesthetic. If overdosage continues, the patient may develop nystagmus, dysphasia, or muscular fasciculation. In later stages, loss of consciousness supervenes, with fits, cardiac arrhythmias, and respiratory and cardiac arrest.

Addition of adrenaline to lidocaine

Most local anaesthetic agents produce some vasodilatation, and this enhances their absorption. Adrenaline is added to anaesthetic agents to produce vasoconstriction, thereby:

- Reducing bleeding from the operation site.
- Prolonging the action of the anaesthetic agent.
- Decreasing peak plasma local anaesthetic levels by slowing absorption.

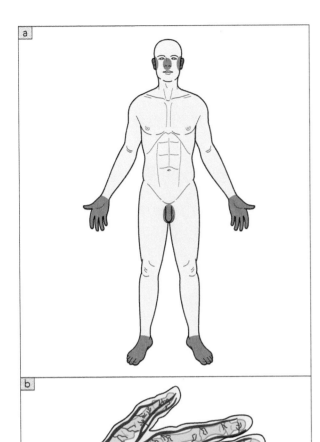

Figure 7.1 (a) Location of end-arteries (pink shading). (b) End-arteries of the hand.

In addition, the safety of lidocaine is said to increase 3.5-fold by the addition of adrenaline, theoretically allowing much larger quantities of lidocaine to be used.

However, the vasoconstriction can also be a disadvantage: adrenaline in an end-artery (Figure 7.1) causes intense vasospasm and may completely cut off the blood flow. If the collateral circulation is inadequate, the territory of the affected artery will become ischaemic, with disastrous consequences. The ear and nose are unlikely to be affected unless very large volumes are injected all around their base, as they have good collateral blood supplies. However, the digital arteries respond with prolonged vasoconstriction and subsequent ischaemia, necrosis, and loss of the appendage. There is no effective treatment for this. Small volumes injected very locally intradermally are unlikely to produce this devastating complication.

> **GOLDEN RULE** ✳
> Never use local anaesthetic containing adrenaline when anaesthetising any part of the body supplied by an end-artery (e.g., a digit, the penis, or the tip of the nose).

For the most part, plain lidocaine is adequate for almost all the procedures we describe. If you avoid stocking solutions containing adrenaline, there will be no possibility of confusion. Many surgeons do, however, use adrenaline, and provided you are aware of the possible hazards, it is perfectly safe and reduces bleeding.

Adrenaline: safety issues

When using adrenaline-containing solutions, it is wise not to exceed a total dose of 100 µg. This dose is contained in:

- 1 ml of a 1:10,000 solution (100 µg/ml).
- 10 ml of a 1:100,000 solution (10 µg/ml).
- 20 ml of a 1:200,000 solution (5 µg/ml).
- 40 ml of a 1:400,000 solution (2.5 µg/ml).

Commonly used lidocaine and adrenaline products contain a 1:200,000 solution of adrenaline. Dental cartridges contain the higher concentration of 1:80,000. This results in more profound vasoconstriction and a greater chance of adrenaline side effects (anxiety, tremor, tachycardia, sweating, etc.).

Buffered lidocaine with adrenaline

Lidocaine has a pH of 6.36 but this reduces to 3.82 with the addition of 1:200,000 adrenaline. This low pH increases the stability and shelf-life of the anaesthetic, but it makes it painful when injected. The addition of 8.4% sodium bicarbonate can be used to raise the pH, thereby making the solution much less painful on injection (Younis and Bhutiani, 2004).

For 20 ml of 1% lidocaine with 1:200,000 adrenaline, 2 ml of 8.4% sodium bicarbonate should be added. For 2% lidocaine and 1:200,000 adrenaline, this should be doubled to 4 ml per 20 ml. The mixed solution should be date labelled and used within 24 hours of preparation.

REFERENCE

Younis I, Bhutiani RP (2004) Taking the 'ouch' out— effect of buffering commercial xylocaine on infiltration and procedure pain. *Annals of the Royal College of Surgeons of England* 86: 213–17.

Chapter 8

Postoperative management

Madeleine Flanagan

INTRODUCTION

Postoperative care is very important and aims to optimise healing, reduce unsatisfactory scarring, and, in particular, diminish the likelihood of surgical site infection (SSI). Patients can expect to receive clear, sensible advice about likely postoperative problems and what they can do to prevent them. This chapter aims to provide enough information for clinicians to provide evidence-based postoperative care and also to support the development of resources for patients in order to enable them to care for their surgical wound appropriately.

PRE- AND PERIOPERATIVE FACTORS

Reducing the risk of SSI is particularly important. Good infection control measures perioperatively are important to reduce the risk of SSI, and these are discussed in Chapter 3. Chapter 5 emphasises the importance of patient assessment, which will make the surgeon aware of important risk factors that may predispose to SSI and poor healing. Special care is required pre-, peri-, and postoperatively for the following groups of surgical procedures, in order to reduce postoperative complications:

- Procedures below the waist.
- More advanced dermatological procedures such as skin plasties, wedge excisions, and skin grafts, and surgery on the ears or lips, or in the groin.
- Prolonged procedures, lasting for more than 24 minutes.
- Patients who are taking immunosuppressant drugs, such as transplant recipients, and those taking corticosteroids.
- Patients who smoke: this should be discussed with the patient and, if possible, abstinence encouraged, as smoking cessation can influence epidermal healing and reduce risk.
- Diabetes: patients must be encouraged to keep their blood sugars at an optimum level to reduce this risk.
- Lesions that have ulcerated and patients taking anti-hypertensive medication are further risk factors.

The following list highlights the important perioperative factors that matter for optimising healing and reducing postoperative complications:
- Clean surgical technique.
- Effective handwashing (World Health Organization guidance).
- Good surgical technique including early haemostasis, apposition and eversion of the skin edges, and tension-free closure.
- The use of subcutaneous sutures after an ellipse excision, to reduce tension on the skin edges.

IMMEDIATE POSTOPERATIVE WOUND CARE AND ADVICE

Pain management

Simple analgesia is usually all that is required after minor surgery. Some procedures can be painful when the local anaesthetic effect has worn off. This is particularly the case for surgery on the nail bed (e.g., wedge resection). Here, postoperative pain can be reduced by mixing a long-acting local anaesthetic (e.g., bupivacaine) with rapid-acting lidocaine at the time of local anaesthesia.

Patients should be advised to avoid aspirin-containing analgesics immediately postoperatively (in order to reduce the risk of bleeding) and, where pain may be predicted, to take simple analgesia such as paracetamol before its onset.

Dressings and wound care

The aim of surgical wound care is to facilitate the body's capacity to heal and replace injured tissue with regenerated tissue in the most favourable conditions in an optimal environment. The surgeon should choose an appropriate dressing for the surgical wound and provide the patient with information on how best to care for the wound. Remember that, in young, fit, healthy patients, most wounds will heal readily without the need for expensive dressings.

There is extensive literature from the early 1960s that moist wound healing has the following beneficial effects:

- Reduction in inflammatory response.
- Increase in leucocyte activity.
- Reduced infection rates.
- Reduced fibrosis.
- Increase in healing rates.

As long ago as the early 1960s, the important features of a good surgical dressing were identified as follows:

- High permeability to moisture vapour.
- Sterile.
- Non-adherent to wound/good adhesion to the surrounding skin.
- Absorbent.
- External protection.
- Hypoallergenic.
- Conformable.
- Cost-effective.

A Cochrane Review in 2004 (Vermeulen *et al.*, 2004) compared different dressings for wounds healing by secondary intention and found no convincing evidence of superiority for any dressing. The weight of evidence therefore supports the following:

- An appropriate dressing should be applied postoperatively.
- Leaving the dressing in place, or replacing it with a new one as required, is a good idea as a moist environment optimises wound healing.
- It is not necessary to use expensive special dressings for minor surgery wounds.
- Hypoallergenic waterproof dressings are preferable.

Suggested dressings are as follows:

- A wound contact dressing held in place by a vapour permeable film, *or*
- Composite wound contact and film dressing.

Should the surgical wound be kept dry?

Patients are given varied and sometimes conflicting advice on whether or not their wound should be kept dry. There is very good evidence from a randomised controlled study (Heal *et al.*, 2006) that no increased risk of infection is seen in skin wounds washed within the first 48 hours of surgery. There is also good evidence that there is no difference between cleaning surgical wounds with saline or tap water. It therefore seems reasonable to reassure patients that there is no requirement to keep the wound dry after the first 24 hours after surgery.

The role of prophylactic antibiotics

There is no evidence to support the widespread use of prophylactic antibiotics to prevent SSI, other than in high-risk patients. A study from Australia in 2009 (Heal *et al.*, 2009) suggested that a single application of chloramphenicol ointment to the wound immediately postoperatively may reduce the risk of wound infection in high-risk sutured wounds. There is no evidence to support the routine use of antimicrobial dressings.

Reducing the likelihood of wound dehiscence

It is important to remember that wounds take about 2 months to achieve full strength and even then have only about 60% of the tensile strength of normal skin (Figures 8.1 and 8.2). Wound strength is often reduced about 3 weeks after surgery. Understanding this is important, and both the surgeon and the patient can help to prevent wound dehiscence.

What the surgeon can do: perioperative tips

- Always consider using buried absorbable sutures to maintain wound support where possible. These sutures take 4–6 weeks or more to dissolve and will improve the tensile strength of the healing wound after the skin stitches have been removed.

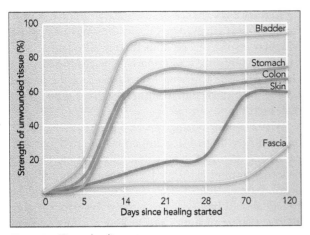

Figure 8.1 Tissue healing rates.

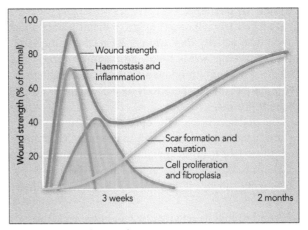

Figure 8.2 Wound strength over time.

- Although deep buried absorbable sutures allow for the use of finer calibre skin sutures (or no skin sutures), it is still important to have an adequate calibre of skin sutures when they are used, in order to avoid wound dehiscence.
- Avoid the use of rapidly dissolving deep sutures.
- Ensure there are sufficient sutures of sufficient calibre to avoid the sutures breaking or the skin tearing.
- There is a balance between having too many sutures too close together and too few too far apart. In general, space sutures according to the size of the 'bite' (Figure 8.3).
- Consider the use of deep interrupted absorbable sutures with extended tensile strength (such as Ethilon PDS™ II) where wound stretching is likely. You can use the same suture as a continuous subcuticular suture (especially suitable for the back) and/or supplement with adhesive skin tapes. These sutures will retain tensile strength until the wound has achieved strength (Figure 8.4).

Preventing wound dehiscence: removing skin sutures

Try to remove the skin sutures only after the wound has developed sufficient tensile strength. If there is any doubt about this, consider:

- Supporting the wound after the sutures have been removed with adhesive skin tape.
- Removing every other suture initially, and leaving the remaining sutures to support the wound for a little longer.
- Delaying suture removal (remembering that scars will form around the puncture marks after 7–10 days).

Recommended times for skin suture removal
Head and neck: 5–7 days.
Torso and upper limbs: 7–10 days.*
Lower limbs: 10–14 days.*
* These are likely to leave permanent suture marks.

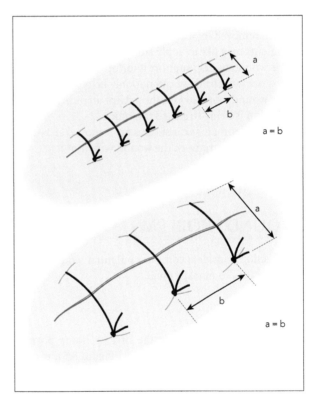

Figure 8.3 Ratio of suture width to spacing.

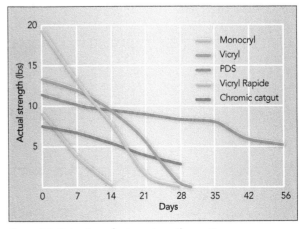

Figure 8.4 Retention of suture strength over time.

Immediate postoperative wound care and advice

Advice for patients

It is particularly important to give patients advice about how much activity they can expect to do immediately after and in the weeks following a surgical procedure. The need to avoid strenuous activity should be discussed with the patient preoperatively as part of the informed consent process.

- The patient will leave the operating room with the area anaesthetised and needs to be reminded of this and advised to avoid any undue exertion immediately postoperatively because there will be no way of patients knowing if they are causing damage to their wound.
- Avoid strenuous activity *as a minimum* while the sutures are in place.
- In areas of particular tension and stress, such as the back or shoulders, it is sensible to avoid strenuous activity for a further 2 weeks after the sutures have been removed in order to avoid stretching of the scar.
- Patients may like to apply adhesive skin tapes across the wound to help support it for up to 2 months postoperatively: these can not only help to support the wound, but also give the patient an indication if the skin is being stretched too much.
- Remember that if skin sutures are removed at 1–2 weeks postoperatively, the wound will be at its weakest at 3 weeks.

WOUND PROBLEMS

This section considers common potential wound problems and how to manage them.

Bleeding

Bleeding may occur during the first 48 hours postoperatively (reactionary haemorrhage; Figure 8.5), usually because a thrombus has been displaced or a ligature has slipped. Alternatively, it tends to occur 8–14 days later (secondary haemorrhage) when the wound has become infected and eroded a vessel, usually quite a small one but sometimes a larger one.

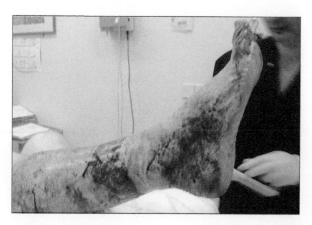

To reduce the chance of reactionary bleeding, ensure haemostasis is achieved before any dressings are applied. This may involve the use of diathermy, adequate sutures, or simple pressure. It is important that sufficient time elapses between achieving haemostasis and the patient leaving the surgical unit to ensure that there is no immediate bleeding.

Where venous oozing can be anticipated (especially on the lower limbs), it is important to apply pressure bandaging on top of the usual wound dressing. This can be in the form of elasticated crêpe bandage or adhesive dressing over a folded swab or a cotton fibre roll. The patient should be advised to remove the extra dressing after a number of hours and to look out for overtight bandaging causing swelling. Advice about elevating the limb as much as possible is also important. In other areas, pressure dressings using one or two dental rolls held in place with tape can be useful. Use of an alginate dressing under pressure can be helpful for wounds where venous oozing is anticipated; it is left in place for 48 hours and then soaked off with normal saline.

Advice for patients

Patients should receive simple, straightforward advice about what to do if their wound starts to bleed. It is recommended that the following be included:

- The importance of applying firm, constant pressure to the bleeding wound.
- Elevation of the lower leg above the waist if the wound is located on the lower limb.
- What to do if the bleeding does not stop: for example, visit the GP surgery or the place where the procedure was performed, or attend the local hospital accident and emergency department (the latter if the bleeding is pulsatile or spurting).

Wound dehiscence

Dehiscence occurs either because undue tension has been applied to the healing wound, wound support is inadequate (Figure 8.6) (either in the quality or length of time of support), or the wound becomes infected. Management of wound dehiscence is as follows:

- In the immediate postoperative period (the first 48 hours), the wound can usually be cleaned, anaesthetised, and re-sutured.
- After the first 48 hours, the risk of introducing infection is greater, and it is usually advocated that the wound be left to heal by secondary intention.

Each case will need to be considered carefully; there are no hard and fast rules. The surgeon needs to balance the risk of unacceptable secondary intention scarring against the risk of wound infection or inevitable dehiscence (if the wound has already started to granulate).

Figure 8.5 Early bleeding after punch biopsy.

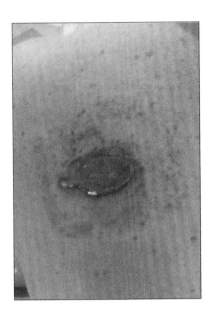

Figure 8.6 Dehiscent wound on the back through lack of buried sutures.

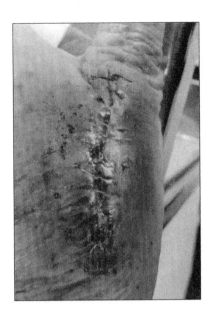

Figure 8.7 Infected thumb wound related to the use of braided skin sutures.

Surgical site infection (SSI)

Diagnosing postoperative wound infection is sometimes difficult, and some amount of postoperative inflammation and discomfort is to be expected. True infection rates should be relatively low, and practitioners should regularly audit these. Expected SSI rates for skin surgery are around 5%, although some centres report 1–2%. Wherever possible, operating on infected skin should be avoided. If this is unavoidable, you should ensure that wound closure allows any pus, if it forms, to escape. For example, avoid the use of continuous subcuticular sutures and heavy, occlusive dressings, and ensure that the wound is assessed 48 hours postoperatively. Try to avoid braided skin sutures (Figure 8.7).

Management of surgical site infection

Where infection is suspected, the following management is recommended:

- Take a swab for bacteriology.
- Consider removing some, if not all, of the sutures (especially important with continuous subcuticular sutures). The wound may dehisce (Figure 8.6), but it is better to allow a significant infection to drain, and the wound to granulate and heal by secondary intention, than to risk developing a deep-seated abscess.
- Make arrangements to inspect the wound regularly.
- Start oral antibiotics if the clinical diagnosis of infection is not in doubt (Figure 8.7), and modify the choice of antibiotic depending on the microbiology results. The usual first-line choice of antibiotic is co-amoxiclav in patients not allergic to penicillin, and a cephalosporin or erythromycin in patients with a history of penicillin allergy.
- Consider the use of a topical antibacterial agent such as fusidic acid if the infection looks low grade and localised—you can always add in an oral antibiotic at a later date.

- Be particularly attentive toward any sign of ascending infection (lymphangitis, temperature, or pain) or of catastrophic complications such as necrotising fasciitis.

It is important to make the patient aware of the signs and symptoms of wound infection and advise them to seek help without delay. Increasing pain and discomfort is one of the most reliable indicators of wound infection and should not be ignored.

Scarring
Managing expectations

Chapter 2 describes in detail the process of informed consent and the need for patients to be absolutely clear about the risks and benefits of any surgical procedure, in particular the likely scar. It is essential that patients are given detailed and realistic details of the likely cosmetic outcome and potential risks of a surgical procedure, including infection and bleeding. There are several key points to emphasise to patients:

- Skin incisions always leave a scar of some sort, and it is impossible to accurately predict the exact appearance of the likely scar.
- It may take a year or even longer for their scar to mature and hopefully fade (scars can gradually fade over decades).
- A scar resulting from the removal of a skin cancer is usually easily justified, whereas a scar resulting from the excision of a lesion that does not medically need to be excised is less easily justified.
- Always try to be sure that the scar from the surgery you perform will look better than the lesion you are removing. This is particularly true when removing benign lesions.

Tips to improve scar results

- Always try to follow the relaxed skin tension lines when operating (see Chapter 6).
- Wherever possible, avoid stretching the wound. This can be achieved by the use of buried, slowly absorbed sutures, closing the wound in layers, and using adhesive skin-closure strips. Advise the patient to avoid strenuous activity, which will stretch the wound or put it under tension during healing.
- Remember that wounds in most young, fit, healthy individuals will heal well, and it is important not to interfere with the wound as this may impair the healing process.
- Covering a wound and newly formed scar with a simple dressing may improve the final cosmetic appearance. The use of microporous tape to support a healed incision can also be effective.
- Where poor scar formation might be expected (e.g., shoulder tip, anterior chest, sternum, or breast), prophylactic use of occlusive silicone dressings applied for 2 months postoperatively can be tried, although there is limited evidence that this influences healing.

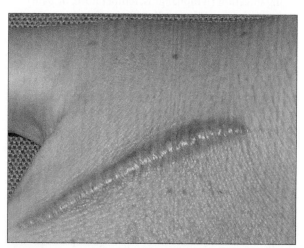

Figure 8.8 Hypertrophic scar. (© DermNetNZ.org. With permission.)

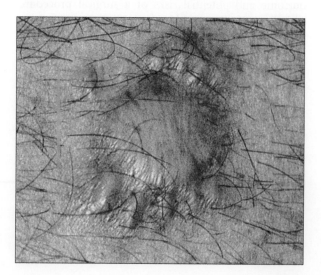

Hypertrophic scars and keloids

Hypertrophic scars (Figure 8.8) and keloid scars (Figure 8.9) represent an abnormal wound reaction to surgery, usually occurring in predisposed individuals. The clinical and histological features of these two types of abnormal scar differ, as does their natural history and prognosis. Wolfram *et al.* (2009) have published a very useful review of this topic, and the differences between the scars are summarised in Table 8.1, reproduced from that article.

Prevention of hypertrophic scars and keloids

It is very important to avoid unnecessary surgery in patients prone to developing keloids. Many of the tips to improve scar results are relevant for avoiding hypertrophic scars. These include:

- Closing wounds with minimal tension.
- Avoiding incisions across joint spaces.
- Following skin creases.
- Efficient haemostasis.
- Everting the wound edge at the time of closure.
- Avoiding subcutaneous sutures on the face unless absolutely necessary.

Management of hypertrophic scars and keloids

A range of therapeutic options are available for the management of hypertrophic scars and keloids, including the following:

- In those who have previously formed hypertrophic scars or keloids, there is limited evidence that silicone dressings and/or the application of pressure to the wound will act prophylactically.
- Local corticosteroids can be of value. These include steroid-impregnated tape (Haelan® tape), cut to the size of the scar and changed daily for 4–6 weeks, or intralesional triamcinolone (5 or 10 mg/ml). This is infiltrated into the scar, which is difficult as the tissue will be dense and fibrous. A 1 ml diabetic needle and syringe should be used (to avoid a separate needle 'blowing off'), or alternatively a Dermojet® unit can be employed (Figure 8.10).

Figure 8.9 Keloid scar.

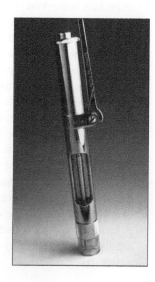

Figure 8.10 Dermojet® unit.

Table 8.1 Summary of the differences between hypertrophic and keloid scars	
Hypertrophic scars	**Keloids**
Develop soon after surgery	May develop months after the trauma
Usually improve with time	Rarely improve with time
Remain within the confines of the wound	Spread outside the boundary of the initial lesion
Occur when scars cross joints or skin creases at a right angle	Occur predominantly on the ear lobe, shoulders, sternal notch; rarely develop across joints
Improve with appropriate surgery	Are often worsened by surgery
Are of frequent incidence	Are of rare incidence
Have no association with skin colour	Are associated with dark skin colour

Caution needs to be taken with intralesional steroids because of the following problems:

- Injected intradermally they can cause significant fat atrophy.
- Depigmentation may occur on dark skins.
- For *hypertrophic scars only*, surgery may be indicated, but it is usually *contraindicated for keloids*.
- Surgical excision followed by low-dose radiotherapy to the wound in certain areas is used rarely in specialist centres.

Figure 8.11, adapted from Wolfram *et al.* (2009), summarises the different treatment options available.

Figure 8.11 Therapeutic recommendations for hypertrophic scars and keloids. (Adapted from Wolfram, D. *et al.*, 2009, Hypertrophic Scars and Keloids—A Review of Their Pathophysiology, Risk Factors, and Therapeutic Management, *Dermatologic Surgery*, 35(2): 171–181, John Wiley and Sons.)

Wound problems

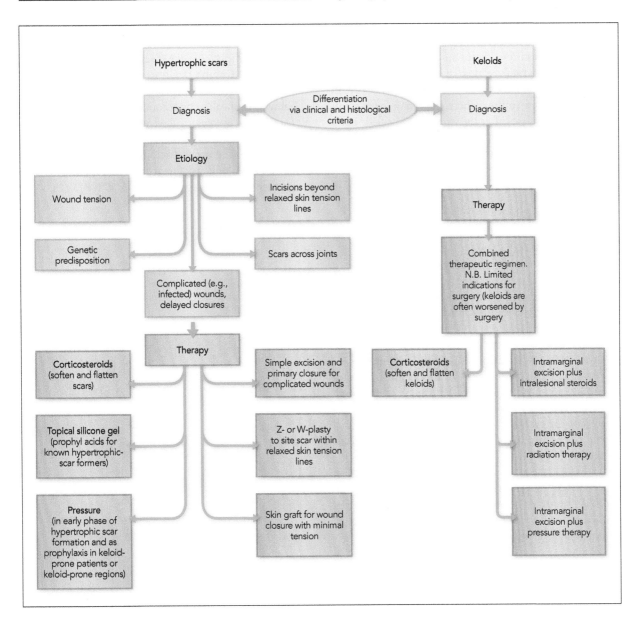

Suture problems

It is very important that the information the patient takes away from the operating session includes written details of when any stitches need to be removed and the number to be removed. Tips on sutures include the following:

- Avoid cutting stitches so short that they cannot be found, especially against the hair of the scalp.
- Avoid sutures being too tight—they will tend to become buried in the healing skin and prove very difficult to see when you want to remove them.
- Avoid long lengths of continuous subcuticular suture that need to be removed as they may well break in the process.
- Where buried sutures are trimmed, ensure the trimming is done under tension so that the cut end retracts under the surface of the skin.
- Warn patients about the length of time some absorbable stitches may take to be fully absorbed. This can be anywhere between a few weeks and several months.

One of the arguments against braided, absorbable sutures is that they can encourage infection more easily than monofilament sutures. Except in a few areas (mucous membranes, children's scalps, and genital areas) they should always be avoided as skin closure and usually avoided as buried sutures where they may form small, sterile stitch abscesses after the wound has healed. These are not a serious problem as long as the patient has been forewarned. Simple removal of the stitch remnant with a 21 G needle and fine Adson forceps is usually painless.

Nerve damage

Nerve damage is unusual but does occur in specific predictable situations as follows:

- Deep incisions over areas of high risk (see Chapter 6) can result in nerve damage. Minor damage to very superficial nerves may cause an area of anaesthesia to persist. Patients should be advised that any area of persisting anaesthesia around the wound should be expected to improve gradually over many months.
- Local anaesthesia may produce temporary muscle paralysis, particularly when the anaesthetic is injected into the forehead, where it may produce a temporary paralysis of the frontalis muscle with the inability to raise the eyebrow and a loss of forehead creases. Although alarming, this is usually a temporary anaesthetic effect.

If the surgeon is concerned about damage to a superficial but important nerve, the patient should be referred immediately to a plastic surgical unit for the wound to be explored and the nerve repaired.

Follow-up arrangements

The need to review a patient following a surgical procedure will depend on the nature of the procedure, and advice for specific situations is given in the relevant 'knowledge' chapters in Part 2 of the book. When a lesion has been removed, follow-up will depend on the nature of the lesion. For vasectomy patients, follow-up will include arrangements to check that the procedure has been successful.

REFERENCES

Heal C, Buettner P, Raasch B, *et al.* (2006) Can sutures get wet? Prospective randomised controlled trial of wound management in general practice. *British Medical Journal* 332: 1053–6.

Heal CF, Buettner PG, Cruickshank R, *et al.* (2009) Does single application of topical chloramphenicol to high risk sutured wounds reduce incidence of wound infection after minor surgery? Prospective randomised placebo controlled double blind trial. *British Medical Journal* 338: a2812.

Vermeulen H, Ubbink D, Goossens A, de Vos R, Legemate D (2004) Dressings and topical agents for surgical wounds healing by secondary intention. *Cochrane Database of Systematic Reviews* (2): CD003554.

Wolfram D, Tzankov A, Pülzl P, Piza-Katzer H (2009) Hypertrophic scars and keloids—A review of their pathophysiology, risk factors and therapeutic management. *Dermatologic Surgery* 35: 171–81.

PART 2

Knowledge: diagnosis and management

Chapter 9

Skin lesions

INTRODUCTION

This chapter includes the following topics:
- **Basic information about the clinical features and natural history of common skin lesions.**
- **Advice on the management of common skin lesions.**
- **Tips about how to manage a skin lesion when you do not know what it is.**
- **Guidance on how to manage the histology report.**

Specific dermatological techniques are discussed in Chapter 19.

OVERVIEW

This is a very important chapter for all surgeons excising skin lesions. It provides an overview of the common skin lesions surgeons should be familiar with in order to ensure that:
- The management of the skin lesion is *appropriate*.
- The decision to perform a surgical procedure at all is *appropriate*.
- The *appropriate* surgical technique is used.

This is necessarily a long chapter, as not all skin lesions require surgical removal and it is important that those performing skin surgery are aware of the full range of management options for particular skin lesions. The aim of the chapter is to help clinicians:
- Make sensible management decisions about patients.
- Deal with lesions themselves wherever possible.
- Identify when referral to specialist colleagues is recommended, particularly where there are doubts about what to do or how to do it.

There is mention of specific management techniques such as cryotherapy, curettage and cautery, and shave excision, but these are described in more detail in Chapter 19.

The chapter is divided into three key sections covering the following areas:
- Basic dermatological knowledge of common skin lesions.
- Management: basic principles and common clinical confusions, including tips on how to manage a patient when you do not know the diagnosis.
- Interpretation and management of the histology report.

A confident clinical diagnosis and a knowledge of the natural history of skin lesions are both vital when deciding whether surgical management of a particular lesion is appropriate. Where there is uncertainty about the diagnosis, it is better to avoid surgery. A patient with a poor cosmetic outcome is likely to be very dissatisfied if it becomes clear that the procedure was unnecessary, inappropriate, or both.

The emphasis here is on the common skin lesions that are most likely to be seen in day-to-day clinical practice, and readers are referred to dermatological texts for detail of the rarer skin lesions.

Important clinical principles

GOLDEN RULES ✳
- Before removing a lesion you *must* try and make a diagnosis.
- If you remove any tissue from a patient you *must* send it for histological examination.

- *Before removing a lesion you* **must** *try to make a diagnosis*. Without a diagnosis you have no basis for deciding the best treatment. It is unsatisfactory to *remove* a lesion out of curiosity without first committing yourself to a provisional diagnosis.
- *If you remove any tissue from a patient you* **must** *send it for histological examination*. Only by doing this will you find out whether your clinical diagnosis was correct. If it should prove to be wrong, you will need guidance on further management. This is provided in the section on managing the histology report, below.

- *If in doubt, refer.* Work within your limitations and only carry out procedures you feel confident about. Never be too proud to refer a patient to someone else. Sometimes you may be sure that a lesion is harmless and you will be able to reassure your patient that no treatment is required. At other times, you may think that a lesion needs to be removed but not feel happy to do this yourself—the lesion may be unsuitable, it may be in a difficult site, or you may simply not have confidence in your skills or your facilities. It is therefore essential to develop close links with local specialists.

BASIC DERMATOLOGY

Introduction

This section provides basic information about the clinical features and natural history of skin lesions. Benign conditions are described first, followed by premalignant and malignant lesions. Particular attention is paid to the more common lesions, although some of the more unusual ones are included for completeness. Common things occur commonly. If you see a lesion you cannot identify, it is much more likely to be an unfamiliar variant of a common condition than a rarity. Because this is a practical book, it is not exhaustive; conditions that you would expect to see only once in a lifetime have been deliberately omitted. Entries include a photograph of a typical lesion, some with a simple line drawing showing the part of the skin from which it arises. There follows a brief account of the lesion, with up-to-date information about management.

Classification of skin lesions

When examining a skin lesion and trying to make a diagnosis, it is helpful to consider the part of the skin from which the lesion is derived. This is illustrated in Figure 9.1.

Lesions can arise from various parts of the skin as follows:

- From *melanocytes* (Figure 9.2): for example, freckle, lentigo, junctional melanocytic naevus, compound melanocytic naevus, intradermal melanocytic naevus, halo naevus, atypical melanocytic naevus, and malignant melanoma. Melanocytes produce pigmentation, so many of these lesions, but not all, will be pigmented.

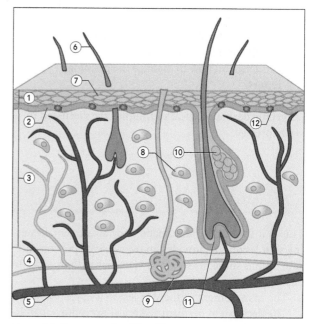

Figure 9.1 Components of the skin:

1. Epidermis	5. Blood vessel	9. Sweat gland
2. Basal layer	6. Hair	10. Sebaceous gland
3. Dermis	7. Keratinocyte	11. Hair follicle
4. Fat	8. Fibroblast	12. Melanocyte

Figure 9.2 Types of melanocytic lesions.

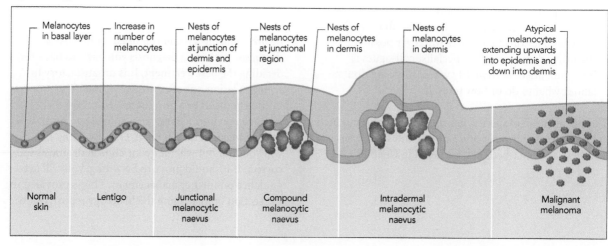

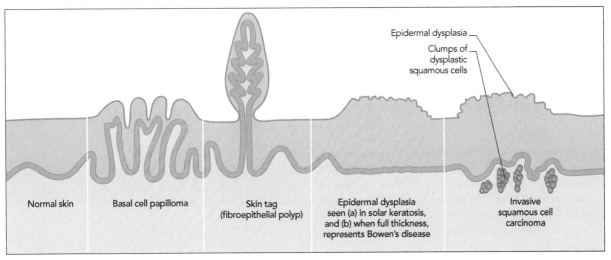

Figure 9.3 Types of epidermal lesion.

- From the *basal layer*: for example, basal cell skin cancers. These immature cells bulge up onto the surface (producing the rolled edge), easily ulcerate (rodent ulcer), and may carry pigment from the basal layer (pigmented basal cell carcinoma [BCC]), spread along the basal layer (superficial or multinodular), or infiltrate the deeper tissues (infiltrative or morphoeic).

- From the *epidermis* (Figure 9.3): for example, basal cell papilloma (also known as seborrhoeic wart or seborrhoeic keratosis), solar keratosis, Bowen's disease, and squamous cell carcinoma (SCC). These arise from the upper part of the skin, so have a very superficial appearance.

- From *hair follicles* (Figure 9.4): for example, epidermoid cysts (also known as pilar cysts). These are often incorrectly described as sebaceous cysts.

- From *fibroblasts* in the dermis (Figure 9.5): for example, dermatofibroma (sometimes known as histiocytoma).

- From *blood vessels* in the dermis: for example, spider naevi, Campbell de Morgan spots, and pyogenic granuloma.

Figure 9.4 Lesion arising from pilo-sebaceous unit: epidermoid/pilar cysts.

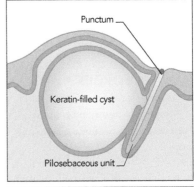

Figure 9.5 Lesion arising from fibroblasts, e.g. dermato-fibroma.

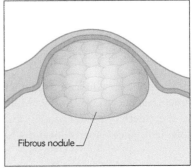

Table 9.1 Skin lesions most commonly removed in general practice	
Lesion	Frequency (%)
Melanocytic naevus	29
Basal cell papilloma (seborrhoeic keratosis)	24
Epidermoid cyst	16
Fibroepithelial polyp (skin tag)	12
Dermatofibroma	5
Malignant lesions	2
Other, e.g., pyogenic granuloma	12

What is common?

Table 9.1 shows the skin lesions most commonly removed in general practice. These data were obtained from histopathology reports of all lesions excised by general practitioners in South West Hertfordshire in a year.

Benign skin lesions
Pigmented melanocytic lesions

Melanocytes are present in the basal layer of the epidermis (see Figure 9.1). The melanosomes in melanocytes produce the pigment melanin, responsible for skin pigmentation. The melanocytes of darker skin types produce more melanin than the melanocytes of fairer skin types.

Freckles (ephelides)

Freckles are pigmented macules that are usually 1–3 mm in diameter (Figure 9.6). Typically, they start to appear in childhood. They do not occur as a result of an increase in melanocytes. Rather, the melanosomes in the melanocytes of the freckle produce melanin much more readily in response to sunlight than the melanosomes in the surrounding skin.

Management

Most people with freckles have them in large numbers. Although some consider them a cosmetic nuisance, treatment is inappropriate.

> **DON'T FORGET ▶▶**
> Axillary freckling and café-au-lait patches are markers of neurofibromatosis.

Lentigo

A lentigo is also a small pigmented macule (usually 1–3 mm), but here the increase in pigmentation is due to an increase in the number of melanocytes in the basal layer (Figure 9.7). Unlike freckles these may be solitary, and they do not darken as much after sun exposure (Figure 9.8).

It may be very difficult to distinguish a lentigo from a junctional naevus (see below). Multiple lentigines occur in the elderly on sun-exposed skin, these being called solar lentigines (Figures 9.9 and 9.10).

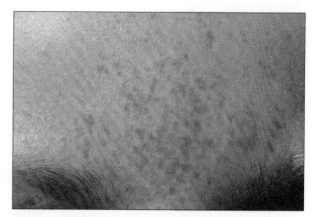

Figure 9.6 Freckles.

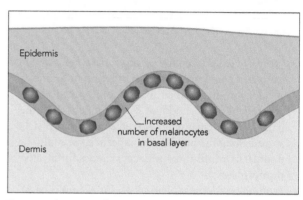

Figure 9.7 Lentigo: schematic representation.

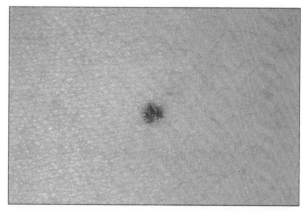

Figure 9.8 Lentigo.

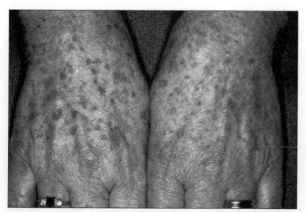

Figure 9.9 Solar lentigines.

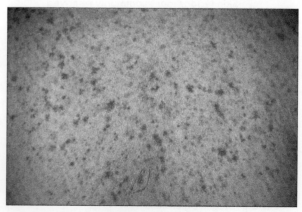

Figure 9.10 Solar lentigines.

Management

These lesions are usually very small and best left alone. Excision of a small lentigo leaves a scar much bigger than the original lesion. Larger lesions (5–10 mm) occurring on the sun-damaged skin of the elderly may look worrying. In this group, you may wish to arrange referral for a dermatological opinion for diagnostic confirmation. In the case of a lentigo on the face (Figure 9.11), it is important to consider the possible diagnosis of Hutchinson's freckle, which is also known as lentigo maligna. This premalignant melanocytic lesion is discussed in more detail later in the chapter.

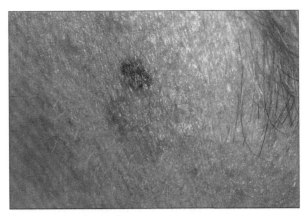

Figure 9.11 Lentigo maligna.

DON'T FORGET ▶▶
Multiple lentigines presenting in childhood can be a cutaneous marker of systemic abnormalities, for example Peutz–Jeghers syndrome.

Benign melanocytic naevi

The term 'mole', if used, should be reserved for this group of lesions. The term 'melanoma' is best avoided when describing benign melanocytic naevi as it may cause confusion with malignant melanoma. Seborrhoeic keratoses (basal cell papillomas) and solar keratoses are better referred to as keratoses rather than moles.

Benign melanocytic naevi are common, usually appearing in childhood and puberty. They disappear in later life, and it is rare to see melanocytic naevi in the elderly. Seborrhoeic keratoses (basal cell papillomas; see below) are much more frequent in this age group.

It is quite common to find 30–40 naevi, usually occurring on light-exposed skin. The fair-skinned, those with a family history of moles, and those with a history of increased sun exposure in childhood are more likely to have large numbers.

A melanocytic naevus usually evolves through three stages: from a new junctional naevus to a compound naevus, and finally to a mature intradermal naevus. The clinical features of these three lesions are different. Complete evolution through the stages does not always occur, and some people have many melanocytic naevi of different types. A melanocytic naevus will sometimes develop a halo of depigmentation and then disappear (halo naevus; see below).

Junctional melanocytic naevus

These occur as a result of melanocytic proliferation at the junction of the dermis and epidermis, hence the term 'junctional' (Figure 9.12).

Clinical features

A junctional naevus is typically flat and brown (Figure 9.13). It may be irregularly pigmented. It is sometimes difficult to tell a new junctional naevus from a malignant melanoma.

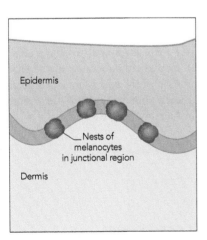

Figure 9.12 Junctional melanocytic naevus: schematic representation.

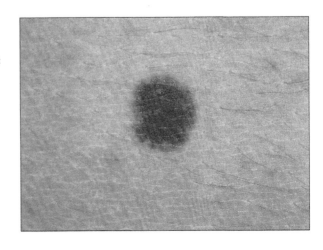

Figure 9.13 Junctional melanocytic naevus.

Management

If you are confident of the diagnosis, there is no need to excise junctional naevi. If the patient is keen to have the lesion removed, this is best done by ellipse excision with a 2 mm margin (see below). If there is the slightest possibility of malignant melanoma, you should refer the patient urgently for a dermatological opinion.

> **DON'T FORGET** ▶▶
> Be careful about making a diagnosis of a junctional naevus if the lesion has appeared for the first time in a patient over the age of 40, if it is growing rapidly, or if it has an irregular border or is variably pigmented. With any of these features, the diagnosis could be malignant melanoma.

Compound melanocytic naevus

In this lesion, many of the proliferating naevus cells (nests of melanocytes) have dropped into the dermis. This pushes up the overlying epidermis, resulting in a raised lesion (Figure 9.14). As melanocytic proliferation at the dermo–epidermal junction continues, the lesion remains pigmented.

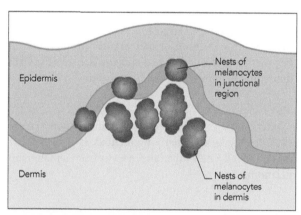

Figure 9.14 Compound melanocytic naevus: schematic representation.

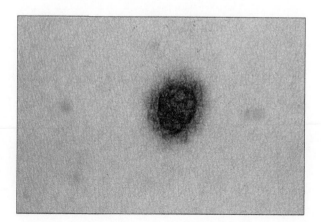

Clinical features

This type of naevus is raised and is usually pigmented (Figure 9.15). Because it is easily caught or knocked, causing bleeding, excision is often requested.

Management

Shave excision with or without cautery avoids suturing and usually gives a good cosmetic result (see Chapter 19). However, patients should be warned that pigmentation of the scar is not uncommon, that occasionally the naevus recurs and that if there were any hairs on the lesion, these may regrow at the site of the scar.

Ellipse excision inevitably leaves a linear scar and should be avoided if possible. Before proceeding with ellipse excision, be sure that the cosmetic result will be acceptable to the patient.

Again, if there is the slightest concern about malignant melanoma, you should refer the patient to a dermatologist.

> **DON'T FORGET** ▶▶
> Shave excision biopsy is the wrong procedure if the lesion is subsequently shown to be a malignant melanoma. Similarly, a large diagnostic ellipse excision is unacceptable if a shave excision would have sufficed.

Intradermal melanocytic naevus

In this lesion, the junctional activity is no longer present and the naevus is located predominantly in the dermis. These lesions are therefore raised. Because of the lack of junctional activity, there is often no pigment (Figure 9.16).

Clinical features

These are common, particularly on the face of women. Raised and typically non-pigmented, they may have hairs growing out of them (Figure 9.17). They are usually stable and unchanging but are often considered a cosmetic nuisance. In men, lesions found on the face may catch and bleed during shaving.

Management

Intradermal naevi lend themselves well to shave excision (see Chapter 19). In particular, because of the lack of pigment, repigmentation of the scar is not a problem. However, you should warn your patient that the lesion may recur and that the hairs may regrow.

Figure 9.15 Compound melanocytic naevus.

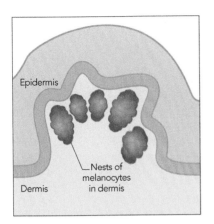

Figure 9.16
Intradermal melanocytic naevus: schematic representation

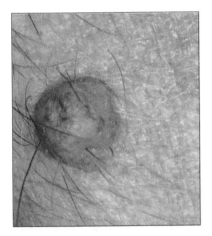

Figure 9.17 Intradermal melanocytic naevus.

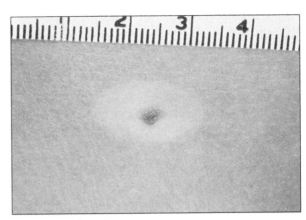

Figure 9.18 Halo melanocytic naevus.

Clinical confusion

The pale, rather cystic appearance on the face sometimes suggests a BCC. However, an intradermal naevus will usually have been present unchanged for a long time, making the diagnosis of BCC unlikely. Since shave excision is the wrong treatment for a BCC, you should refer if the diagnosis is in doubt.

Halo naevus (Sutton's naevus)

Halo naevi usually occur in young adults and are often a source of considerable anxiety to patients and doctors alike. They arise as a result of a localised immunological response to the pigment cells in and around the melanocytic naevus.

Clinical features

The pigmented lesion suddenly develops a halo of depigmentation (Figure 9.18). The central naevus gradually becomes smaller and eventually disappears. The remaining small area of hypopigmentation usually, but not always, slowly repigments over the next few months.

Management

The presence of the halo alone should not cause concern. Reassure the patient and explain the likely outcome. Review the patient every 6–8 weeks to reassure both yourself and the patient that the lesion is behaving as expected.

There is no need to remove the pigmented lesion at the centre of the halo unless it behaves suspiciously. Should the naevus in the centre change in size, shape or colour, it should be treated like any other suspicious pigmented lesion.

Atypical melanocytic naevi

At least 5% of the population have one or two atypical melanocytic naevi, previously known as 'dysplastic naevi'. This term is no longer used because many clinicians associate dysplasia with inevitable malignant transformation and there is no convincing evidence that dysplastic naevi are premalignant.

Clinical features

Atypical naevi are large (usually larger than 5 mm in diameter) with an irregular border, are often variably pigmented, and sometimes have a pinkish inflammatory appearance (Figure 9.19). They are most common on the trunk but also occur on the limbs.

> **DON'T FORGET ▶▶**
> The differential diagnosis of atypical naevi is malignant melanoma.

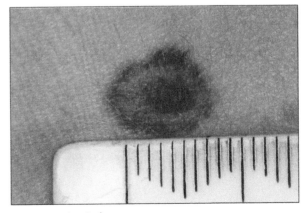

Figure 9.19 Atypical naevus.

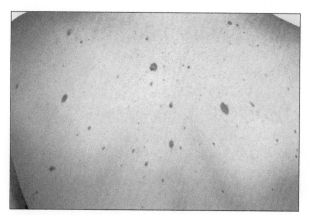

Figure 9.20 Multiple atypical melanocytic naevi.

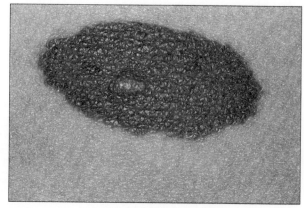

Figure 9.21 Small congenital melanocytic naevus.

Management

The confident diagnosis of an atypical naevus is some-times difficult. A useful tip is the so-called 'fried egg' sign. This is where the lesion has a darker centre (yolk) and an obvious, paler peripheral area (the white around the yolk). Atypical naevi showing this feature are more likely to be innocent. Simple management advice is as follows:

- *Solitary atypical melanocytic naevus*: The history is very important. If the atypical naevus has been present and unchanging for years, it is unlikely to be a malignant melanoma. If the lesion is new or you are concerned about it, refer the patient for a derma-tological opinion. It can sometimes be very difficult to distinguish an atypical melanocytic naevus clini-cally from an in-situ melanoma.

- *Multiple atypical melanocytic naevi*: A patient with many atypical naevi, particularly on unusual sites such as the scalp, buttocks, or dorsum of the feet, should definitely see a dermatologist. The patient may have atypical mole syndrome (Figure 9.20), which is associated with an increased incidence of malignant melanoma. It is most important to give this group of patients advice on sun avoidance and information about checking their moles for changes in size, shape, or colour.

Congenital melanocytic naevus

These are melanocytic naevi which by definition are present at birth or appear within the first 12 months of life. They are typically dark brown and may be raised, often having mammillary projections. Hair is often, but not always, present in varying amounts. Size is variable, but these naevi can be divided broadly into two groups:

- Small congenital melanocytic naevi (Figure 9.21), which are relatively common and occur on any part of the body. There is very little evidence of increased risk of malignant change in these lesions.

Figure 9.22
'Bathing trunk' congenital melanocytic naevus.

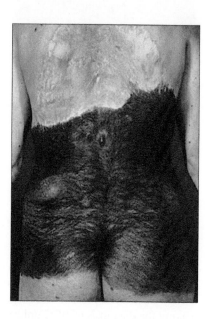

- Very extensive lesions covering large areas of the skin, such as the so-called 'bathing trunk' or 'garment' naevi (Figure 9.22). Fortunately, these are relatively rare. There is a definite increase in malignant trans-formation in these lesions.

Management

Patients with extensive congenital naevi should have long-term follow-up looking for malignant change. Babies born with extensive bathing trunk naevi should be referred for specialist assessment as neural melano-sis may need to be excluded. Those with small congeni-tal naevi should be advised to check them regularly for changes in size, shape, or colour. Any such changes are an indication for referral.

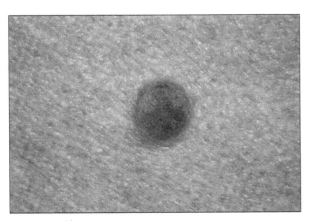

Figure 9.23 Blue naevus.

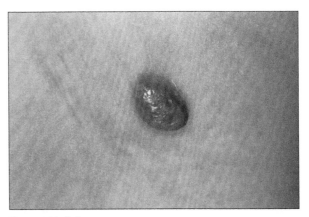

Figure 9.24 Spitz naevus.

Blue naevus

This melanocytic lesion is less common than those already described.

Clinical features

A blue naevus typically appears in childhood or early adult life, most commonly on the extremities. It is usually solitary, less than 1 cm in diameter, slightly raised, and has a distinctive dark blue/slate grey colour (Figure 9.23). Although the appearance is usually typical, it can sometimes resemble a malignant melanoma.

Management

If the clinical diagnosis is not in doubt and the lesion is unchanging, there is no need to remove it. If the diagnosis is in doubt or the lesion is changing, refer the patient to a specialist.

These lesions can be unsightly, and patients may request excision for cosmetic reasons. Ellipse excision with a 2 mm margin is the best treatment, provided that the site is suitable.

Spitz naevus

A Spitz naevus is a rare benign melanocytic lesion. The histological features may resemble malignant melanoma, hence the alternative term 'juvenile melanoma', which is sometimes used by histopathologists.

Clinical features

Spitz naevi occur most commonly in young children but may be seen in young adults. The most common site is the cheeks. The lesion typically presents as a rapidly enlarging red or reddish-brown nodule up to 1–2 cm in diameter (Figure 9.24). The differential diagnosis includes pyogenic granuloma and, in young adults, malignant melanoma.

Management

If you suspect this diagnosis, refer the patient for a specialist to confirm the diagnosis and arrange management. It will usually be necessary to excise the lesion for histological assessment. In the case of a young child, this may require general anaesthesia. If the pathologist has any doubts about the histological diagnosis, wider excision may be necessary.

If you receive a histology report suggesting the diagnosis of a Spitz naevus or juvenile melanoma, particularly when the patient is an adult, you should discuss the case with the histopathologist or dermatologist.

Seborrhoeic keratosis

Clinicians sometimes have difficulty with the terminology of these lesions. Seborrhoeic keratosis describes the clinical appearance of the lesion, and basal cell papilloma the histological appearance (Figure 9.25). Both are acceptable terms and can be used synonymously. Other terms, such as senile keratosis, seborrhoeic wart, and senile wart, are best avoided. Many patients find the term 'senile' derogatory, while 'wart' suggests a viral aetiology, which may lead to the inappropriate use of antiviral wart preparations.

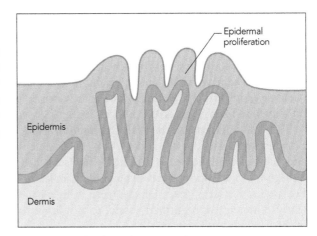

Figure 9.25 Seborrhoeic keratosis: schematic representation.

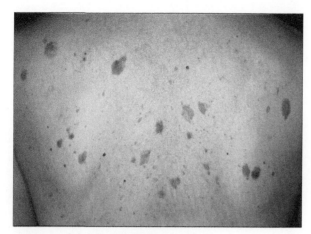

Figure 9.26 Seborrhoeic keratoses.

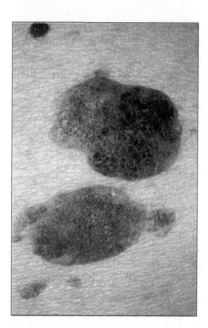

Figure 9.27
Seborrhoeic
keratoses.

Clinical features

These pigmented lesions usually start to appear in the fifth decade of life. They occur equally in men and women. They continue appearing in predisposed people for many years and do not resolve spontaneously. The lesions are commonly multiple and occur particularly on the upper trunk and face. They are much more common in those who are fair skinned. Usually ovoid, they vary in size from a few millimetres to 2–3 cm.

The lesion typically consists of a keratotic, greasy (seborrhoeic) plaque, most of which is above the skin surface. It is adherent to the epidermis but looks as if it could be easily lifted off. The keratotic surface often falls off only to re-form (Figures 9.26 and 9.27).

The colour is variable but most commonly black. Brownish-yellow lesions also occur. They are often itchy and may become inflamed or 'irritated' when scratched. A diagnostic clue is the presence of plugged follicular orifices on the surface of the lesion, best seen using a hand lens. Dermoscopy is particularly useful to aid diagnosis of these lesions (see Chapter 10).

Malignant change in seborrhoeic keratoses is extremely rare, and it is often said that it never occurs. The differential diagnosis of seborrhoeic keratosis is that of any pigmented lesion and includes benign melanocytic naevi and malignant melanoma. Indeed, in many dermatology clinics, the most commonly referred pigmented lesions suspected of being malignant melanoma are, in fact, seborrhoeic keratoses.

Management

Explanation and reassurance are often all that is needed. Where the diagnosis is certain and the lesions are multiple, it is important to tell the patient that new lesions are likely to continue appearing. You should avoid removing them in large numbers.

Some patients can be very bothered by their appearance, and in such cases it is important to help the patient come to terms with the problem. Some patients request treatment, and it is not unreasonable to treat seborrhoeic keratoses that are symptomatic or disfiguring.

These lesions can be removed by curettage and cautery (see Chapter 19). Curettage leaves a flat surface that rapidly re-epithelialises. Ellipse excision is *not* appropriate as it leaves an unjustifiable scar. However confident your diagnosis, always send the curettings for histological examination. Alternatively, seborrhoeic keratoses can be treated with cryotherapy (see Chapter 19), but remember that this treatment does not provide any histological confirmation, so you must be completely confident of your diagnosis.

Skin tag (fibroepithelial polyp)
Clinical features

Skin tags are common and often occur in people with seborrhoeic keratoses. These small, fleshy, pedunculated lesions are usually seen on the neck, in the flexures, and around the eyes of the middle aged and elderly (Figure 9.28).

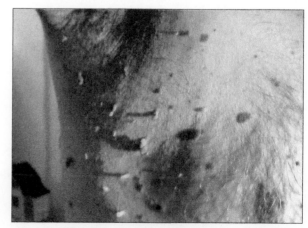

Figure 9.28 Skin tags.

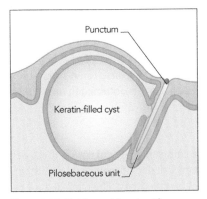

Figure 9.29 Epidermoid cyst, with punctum.

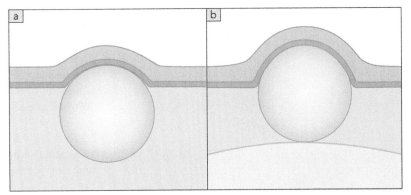

Figure 9.30 (a) Cyst pushing up overlying skin on the back (epidermoid cyst) and (b) on the scalp (pilar cyst).

Management

As with seborrhoeic keratoses, new tags often continue to appear in predisposed individuals. Skin tags are easy to remove by snip excision, with or without cautery, and some patients can be encouraged to snip them off themselves. Cotton can be tied round the base, but this can lead to swelling and an unpleasant inflammatory response and is not recommended.

Epidermoid and pilar cysts

These epithelial, keratinous, walled cysts are best considered as derived from the pilosebaceous unit.

Epidermoid cysts

Epidermoid cysts are often incorrectly referred to as 'sebaceous cysts'. True sebaceous cysts, which contain oily sebum, are actually very rare.

An epidermoid cyst is a very common skin lesion that arises from the traumatic entrapment of surface epithelium (epidermal inclusion cyst) or, more often, from aberrant healing of the infundibular epithelium during an episode of follicular inflammation or folliculitis. The lining of an epidermoid cyst looks like the epidermis. Often, but not always, these cysts connect to the surface of the skin by a punctum (Figure 9.29). Epidermoid cysts can be differentiated histologically from pilar cysts by the presence of a granular layer in the lining epithelium. The epidermoid cyst wall surrounds a core containing keratin and its breakdown products. The contents have a characteristic semi-solid cheesy appearance and often a foul odour.

Clinical features

Epidermoid cysts are common in young adults, but rare in childhood. Teenagers with significant acne vulgaris are particularly prone to them. The cysts are often asymptomatic but tend to enlarge slowly and sometimes become inflamed. The most common sites are the head, neck, chest, and back. They never occur on the palms or soles. Cysts may be single or multiple.

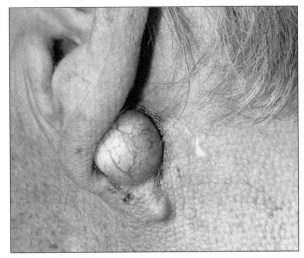

Figure 9.31 Epidermoid cyst.

The spherical cyst is situated in the dermis. The overlying epidermis is normal, and the cyst lifts this to a varying degree to give a domed appearance. In sites such as the back, where it has room to expand into the subcutaneous tissue, the cyst is less likely to be raised than where there is little subcutaneous tissue; a cyst on the scalp (pilar cyst, see next page) may be raised above the surrounding skin, causing the overlying epidermis to become taut (Figures 9.30 and 9.31). Epidermoid cysts usually have a keratin-filled punctum marking the point of attachment to the epidermis (and from which rancid contents may leak); these are absent in pilar cysts.

Management

Many patients elect to have epidermoid cysts excised. Excision of a non-inflamed epidermoid cyst is usually straightforward and is the type of procedure that is very suitable to undertake in general practice. The technique is described in Chapter 20.

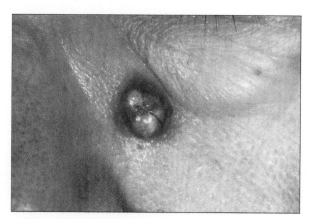

Figure 9.32 Calcified pilomatrixoma.

Pilar cysts

Pilar or trichilemmal cysts occur in 5–10% of the population, are more common in women than men, occur in middle age, and are often familial. Of patients with these cysts, 70% have several lesions and 10% have more than 10 lesions. They arise preferentially in areas of dense hair follicle concentrations; therefore, 90% of cases occur on the scalp.

Pilar and trichilemmal cysts are derived from the outer root sheath of the hair follicle. No punctum is present. These cysts also tend to be less attached to surrounding structures and are usually more easily enucleated than epidermoid cysts. These too contain a cheesy keratinaceous material.

Calcified pilomatrixoma

These less common lesions are also derived from the pilosebaceous unit. They are usually seen on the head, neck, or upper arms (Figure 9.32), typically in children. Full of dead and calcified epithelial cells, these have a characteristically rock-hard and lobulated feel owing to calcification, and are located from the deep dermal to the subcutaneous tissue.

Dermatofibroma (histiocytoma)

This can be considered to be a proliferation of fibroblasts in the dermis (Figure 9.33). There is debate about the derivation of these lesions, with some people believing they develop as an abnormal response to an insect bite, although a history of such a bite is obtained in only about 20% of those affected.

Clinical features

Dermatofibromas are common, particularly on the lower limbs of women. They usually present as a persistent, firm, hard nodule that is often itchy. The clinical appearance varies, depending upon the appearance of the overlying epidermis (Figure 9.34). Some are pigmented and may be confused with compound naevi. The universal finding is of a hard, rubbery-feeling nodule that can be pinched between the fingers.

Management

Where the clinical diagnosis is not in doubt, there is no medical indication to excise a dermatofibroma. Patients often request excision for cosmetic reasons, but you should select patients carefully because of the tendency of these lesions to occur on the lower limb. This is a bad area for healing, and the resulting scar may look worse than the nodule you removed. Be sure to discuss fully with the patient the likely cosmetic outcome and draw the excision lines out for the patient to see. Remember that, as much of the lesion occurs below the surface, your excision margin will need to reflect this.

If you decide to proceed, ellipse excision is the appropriate procedure. If the lesion is on the lower leg, it is recommended that the patient wears a support bandage in the immediate postoperative period and ideally, until the sutures are removed, as with all procedures on the lower limb (see Chapter 8).

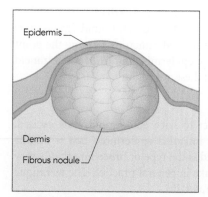

Figure 9.33 Dermatofibroma: schematic representation.

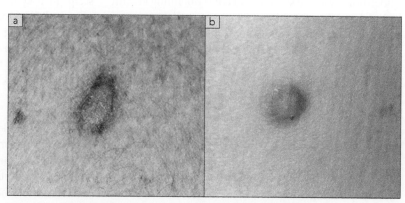

Figure 9.34 Dermatofibroma.

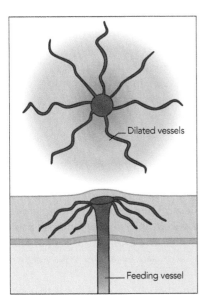

Figure 9.35
Spider naevus: schematic representation.

Dilated vessels

Feeding vessel

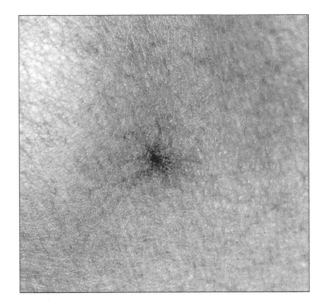

Figure 9.36
Spider naevus.

Angiomatous lesions

Spider naevi

These are small vascular malformations that usually occur on the face, neck, upper trunk, and arms. They are common in women, particularly during pregnancy and as a sign of photo-aging. Circulating oestrogens are thought to be relevant in the aetiology. A central dilated vessel is surrounded by numerous smaller vessels (Figures 9.35 and 9.36). A useful diagnostic test is to press on the spider naevus with a glass microscope slide, which makes the lesion disappear.

Management

Many spider naevi disappear spontaneously; in particular, those which develop during pregnancy usually resolve after delivery. Cold-point electrocautery and unipolar diathermy (hyfrecator) can be used to coagulate the central vessel. Local anaesthetic is not usually necessary and indeed, with adrenaline (epinephrine), can make them disappear (see Chapter 7). They may recur, and a suitable cosmetic laser provides definitive (but expensive) treatment. If you do not have the necessary equipment, you may choose to refer the patient to a cosmetic dermatologist for treatment.

> **DON'T FORGET** ▶ ▶
> Although multiple spider naevi can be a feature of chronic liver disease, solitary spider naevi unrelated to liver disease are much more common.

Campbell de Morgan spots

These are caused by a benign proliferation of blood vessels high in the dermis, with overlying hyperkeratosis.

Clinical features

Campbell de Morgan spots are very common, particularly in older people. They are small cherry-red spots, up to about 5 mm in diameter (Figure 9.37), and are usually multiple. They occur most commonly on the trunk. Excised lesions will be reported histologically as angiokeratomas.

Management

In view of the large numbers that may be present, these are best left untreated. Patients should be warned that they are likely to develop new ones from time to time. If they are treated, it should be with unipolar diathermy set at approximately 3–6 W (usually requiring a small bleb of local anaesthetic; the spots tend not to blanch with this).

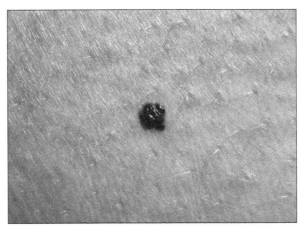

Figure 9.37 Campbell de Morgan spot.

Basic dermatology

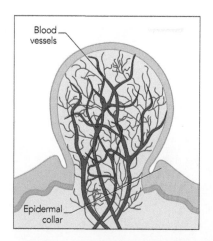

Figure 9.38
Pyogenic granuloma: schematic representation.

Figure 9.39
Pyogenic granuloma.

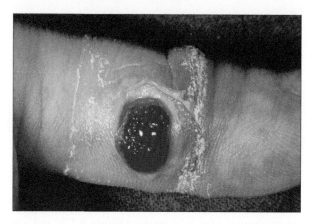

Pyogenic granuloma

A pyogenic granuloma is caused by a proliferation of blood vessels in the dermis (Figure 9.38). The name is a misnomer as they are neither pyogenic nor a granuloma, but an exuberant vascular response to injury.

Clinical features

Pyogenic granulomas occur equally in both sexes and at any age. They are not uncommon in childhood. The most common presentation is of a rapidly enlarging, juicy, non-pigmented lesion, usually on an extremity. They are usually bright red and may be up to 10 mm in diameter (Figure 9.39). They bleed easily and profusely. Some patients give a history of a minor penetrating injury a few weeks before the development of the lesion.

Management

Pyogenic granulomas lend themselves well to curettage and cautery (see Chapter 19), but be prepared for bleeding, which may be profuse. Although haemostasis can often be achieved by cautery, it may be necessary to suture the skin after the lesion has been removed. A combination of styptic (in the form of aluminium chloride) and unipolar diathermy is often successful.

Viral warts and molluscum contagiosum

Clinical features

Warts are very common, and management is often a problem for the clinician. They come in various shapes and sizes. Most are caused by infection with human papillomavirus (Figure 9.40). The exception is molluscum contagiosum, which is caused by a pox virus (Figure 9.41).

The most important message about warts is that the vast majority will resolve spontaneously without scarring when the patient has developed an adequate immunological response. This may take months or years, during which time the patient may become fed up because of the cosmetic appearance. In older patients (particularly over 35 years), it may take much longer for the immune response to kick in. People with viral warts often ask to have them removed, but the temptation to remove warts surgically should be resisted wherever possible for the following reasons:

- Warts commonly recur at the site of surgical removal.
- The resulting scar is unnecessary, since the wart will eventually resolve without intervention.
- Curettage of large plantar warts inevitably leaves a large wound on the sole of the foot: this may be painful to walk on, and the wart often recurs within the scar.
- Ellipse excision of warts leaves an inappropriate linear scar, and warts may develop within this scar (this phenomenon is known as koebnerisation).
- Most warts occur in children, in whom unnecessary surgery should be avoided.

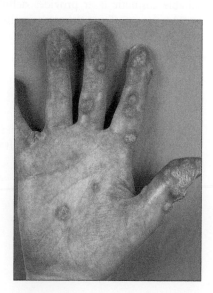

Figure 9.40 Viral warts.

- Molluscum contagiosum can be very extensive, particularly in children, but the lesions usually resolve spontaneously without scarring in 6–9 months.
- The only possible exception might be filiform warts: these have a very narrow base, and curettage, with or without cautery, will leave only a small scar (the wart may nevertheless recur!).

Accepted treatments

- *Time.* Most warts will resolve spontaneously in 3–6 months. The evaluation of any treatment method has to take this into account.
- *Keratolytic wart paints.* Many products are available, usually containing salicylic and lactic acids. These need to be used every night for up to 3 months. The patient should be instructed to soak the area in water. After drying, the hard skin should be pared down using a pumice stone or emery board. Finally, the preparation is applied. The newer gels avoid the need to protect the surrounding normal skin and to wear an occlusive dressing.
- *Liquid nitrogen cryotherapy.* Details of this procedure are to be found in Chapter 19. For cryotherapy to be effective, it must cause tissue destruction (as the wart virus is not destroyed by freezing). This is inevitably painful and should therefore be avoided in children. Adequate cryotherapy to plantar warts may leave the patient unable to walk for several days after the treatment. Overall, the evidence does not support the widespread use of liquid nitrogen as an effective treatment for viral warts.
- *Formaldehyde soaks.* This rather old-fashioned method is sometimes recommended as a treatment for mosaic plantar warts, although evidence of its efficacy is lacking. A litre of 3% formaldehyde is supplied to the patient. The affected foot is soaked in a bowl of the solution for 15 minutes each evening—warn the patient to use an old bowl. The solution is then poured back into the bottle (using a funnel) and can be reused. Because of evaporation, it is necessary to top up the bottle from time to time with water.
- *Occlusive tape.* There has been evidence from one small trial of tape (known as tank, gaffer, duck, or duct tape) applied to recalcitrant digital warts in children with good results, but this was not subsequently reproduced in further studies.

> **DON'T FORGET** ▶▶
> Viral warts can be particularly troublesome and recalcitrant in immunosuppressed patients, such as post-transplant patients, HIV-positive patients, or those taking long-term immunosuppressants (particularly azathioprine) for medical problems. Modification of the immunosuppressant therapy may occasionally be necessary.

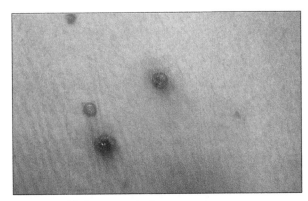

Figure 9.41 Molluscum contagiosum.

Chondrodermatitis nodularis helicis

Chondrodermatitis nodularis helicis is a benign condition involving inflammation of the cartilage of the pinna, with overlying dermal and epidermal inflammation. It is quite common, and the diagnosis is usually straightforward.

Clinical features

The condition usually occurs in older men, although women are also affected. Although other parts of the pinna can be involved, the patient typically presents with a very painful and exquisitely tender inflamed nodule (0.5–1.0 cm in diameter) at the upper pole of the helix (Figure 9.42). The condition usually occurs on the side on which the patient sleeps, and the severe pain often interferes with sleeping.

Management

Simple measures to relieve pressure on the helix may prevent the need for surgery. Corn plasters can be used, cutting out a central disc to the size of the nodule, and special pillows with a central hole are available and can be helpful. Surgical excision of the lesion, making sure to remove the inflamed underlying cartilage, with a margin of normal skin, is the treatment of choice if pressure-relieving measures fail. The affected cartilage is usually softer than the healthy cartilage. Care is needed to avoid leaving sharp edges on the remaining cartilage.

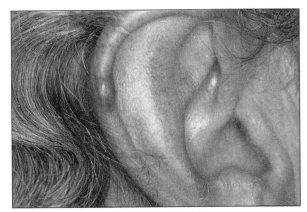

Figure 9.42 Chondrodermatitis nodularis helicis.

Although the extreme tenderness of the lesion usually makes the diagnosis straightforward, remember that SCC on the pinna can sometimes mimic chondrodermatitis nodularis helicis and vice versa.

Lipoma
Clinical features

Lipomas are slow-growing benign tumours of fatty tissue that form a lobulated soft mass enclosed by a thin fibrous capsule (Figure 9.43). They are the most common benign soft tissue tumour found in adults. Occurring usually in 40–60 year olds, and slightly more common in men, the incidence is probably between 1:100 and 1:1000 of the general population.

The lesions may be multiple and are usually painless and asymptomatic, with malignant sarcomatous transformation virtually never seen. Angiolipoma is a common variant that has a proliferation of small vessels scattered throughout the fat and, unlike common lipomas, these are usually painful when pressed.

The symptoms and signs will depend on location:

- Those arising from fatty tissue between the skin and deep fascia have the typical features of a soft fluctuant feel with lobulation, and the free mobility of overlying skin.
- Lipomas arising from fat in the intramuscular septa cause a diffuse palpable swelling, which is more prominent when the related muscle is contracted.
- A lipoma will sometimes produce a small protuberant swelling in the skin. The naked-eye appearance is the lipoma herniating out through the subcutaneous fat.
- Lipomas may arise from the subcutaneous tissues of the vulva. These usually become pedunculated and dependent.
- The breast is a common site for lipomas, although not as frequently as expected considering the amount of fat that is present.

Confirming the diagnosis

The clinical diagnosis is not usually in doubt, but imaging can sometimes provide confirmation. Because lipomas are radiolucent, soft tissue radiographs may be indicated when the diagnosis is in doubt. Other imaging studies include ultrasonography, computed tomography, and magnetic resonance imaging.

Management

Indications for the excision of a lipoma include the following:

- When there is doubt about the diagnosis, for example if there is any suspicion that the lesion might be a liposarcoma.
- If the lesion is symptomatic.
- If the lipoma is enlarging and has grown to bigger than 5 cm (because of the possibility of liposarcoma).
- If it is a cosmetic nuisance.

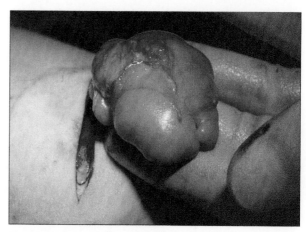

Figure 9.43 Lipoma after removal.

> **DON'T FORGET ▶▶**
> - Straightforward subcutaneous lipomas are usually not fixed to the underlying fascia.
> - Be wary of lipomas over the forehead. Although these may cause cosmetic concerns even when quite small, they may prove difficult to remove, are often located below the aponeurosis, and are more adherent than expected from palpation.

Digital myxoid cyst
Clinical features

Digital myxoid cysts (sometimes known as mucin cysts) typically occur in older people and are benign lesions. These lesions usually present as a cystic swelling around the distal interphalangeal joint of the fingers (Figure 9.44). They are often associated with adjacent nail dystrophy because of pressure on the nail plate. Patients will sometimes describe the lesions as discharging a thick gelatinous material from time to time. The lesions are often linked to the joint and are associated with osteoarthritis.

Management

There are a range of options for treatment, which include the following:

- Repeatedly extruding the contents using a sterile needle to perforate the cyst.
- Cryotherapy.
- Intralesional sclerosant injections.
- Curettage and cautery.
- Surgical excision.

Unfortunately, these lesions tend to recur so formal surgical excision is recommended if the lesion is particularly troublesome. Because the cyst is often connected to the joint space, it is recommended that this procedure is performed by an experienced hand surgeon (see page 245).

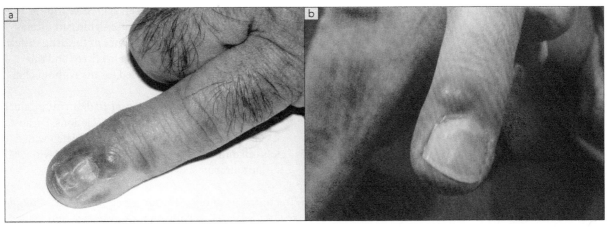

Figure 9.44 Digital myxoid cyst.

Premalignant skin lesions

This section considers solar keratoses, Bowen's disease, keratoacanthomas, and Hutchinson's freckle (lentigo maligna). Although not truly benign, these conditions are not quite malignant. It is important to try to make a firm clinical diagnosis of these lesions as simple excision is often not the most appropriate treatment.

Solar keratoses are common on the sun-damaged skin of the elderly. Their association with the development of SCC is not clear-cut, and spontaneous resolution of solar keratoses often occurs.

Bowen's disease and keratoacanthomas are relatively uncommon. Bowen's disease has the potential to progress to SCC. Keratoacanthomas demonstrate many of the clinical and histological features of malignancy, but they behave very differently.

Hutchinson's freckle (lentigo maligna) is becoming more common and if left may progress to invasive lentigo maligna melanoma. Many patients will have what is called 'field change' where the whole area of skin shows sun damage, with lentigines, solar elastosis, and solar keratoses.

Solar keratosis (actinic keratosis, senile keratosis)

Solar keratoses are common on the light-exposed skin of fair-skinned people who have had a large amount of cumulative sun exposure. The relationship between sunlight and the development of solar keratoses is well documented. There is debate about the likelihood of malignant change, but it is generally accepted that the risk of transformation is very small, except in patients on long-term immunosuppression, for whom this is a very real risk.

Remember that the presence of one or two of these lesions is evidence that the patient has had long periods of sun exposure and is at risk of developing further solar keratoses as well as other tumours associated with chronic sun exposure.

Clinical features

The characteristic appearance is that of a pink, scaly, warty, keratotic lesion on the face, scalp, ears, or back of the hand (Figure 9.45). A solar keratosis will sometimes present as a cutaneous horn (Figure 9.46). The diagnosis is often confirmed by gently feeling the surface. The solar keratosis produces a rough, catching surface.

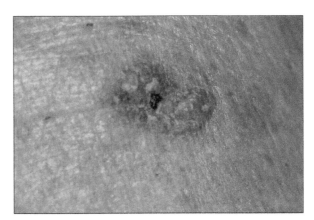

Figure 9.45 Solar keratosis.

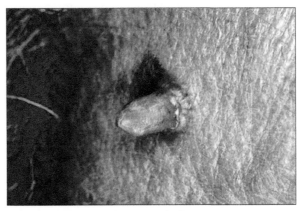

Figure 9.46 Cutaneous horn in a solar keratosis.

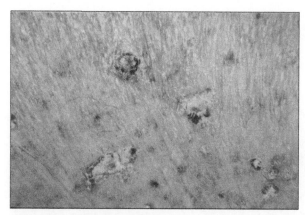

Figure 9.47 Multiple solar keratoses.

Lesions are often multiple (Figure 9.47) and are frequently more obvious in the summer. Patients will often report that keratoses regress spontaneously in the winter. Solar keratoses are often asymptomatic and are usually mostly a cosmetic nuisance.

Although malignant transformation is rare, it is suggested by induration at the base and an increase in the inflammatory change around the lesion. The appearance of a nodule within the lesion is also suspicious. Squamous cell carcinoma arising in a solar keratosis is usually, but not always, slowly growing (well differentiated), with little tendency to metastasise.

Management

Since these lesions regress when sunlight is avoided, a sunscreen and protective clothing (e.g., a hat) should be recommended for all patients presenting with solar keratoses. This may also prevent the development of new lesions. Medical management of these lesions is increasingly popular, and some of these approaches are included below; readers are referred to standard dermatology texts for more detailed information about these treatments.

For *solitary lesions*, the following are options:

- *No treatment.* If the lesion is asymptomatic and not troublesome, it is reasonable to offer no treatment other than to recommend sun protection/avoidance measures and topical emollients.
- *Cryotherapy.* If the patient is keen to have the solar keratosis removed, liquid nitrogen is an effective treatment, provided that the clinical diagnosis is not in doubt and histological confirmation is not required. The cosmetic result is usually good, but patients should be warned of the short-term effects of treatment and of the long-term possibility of developing a hypopigmented macule (see Chapter 19).
- *Curettage and cautery.* This is an effective treatment, with the additional benefit that the curettings can be sent for histological examination. However, this is even more likely than cryotherapy to leave superficial scarring, which may make the treatment unjustifiable (see Chapter 19).

- *5-Fluorouracil (5%).* This is an aggressive topical antimitotic agent that may cause significant ulceration during treatment. Experience of the drug's effect is required to use it safely and effectively, and this treatment is not recommended for use without clinical experience.
- *5-Fluorouracil 0.5%/salicylic acid 10.0%.* This product is applied with a brush to individual lesions. Because it contains less 5-fluorouracil, it is associated with less inflammation and ulceration compared with 5% 5-fluorouracil.

Treatment is more difficult when there are *multiple lesions*. Repeated cryotherapy or curettage and cautery should be avoided as unacceptable scarring may result. Other treatment options available include the following:

- *Diclofenac gel* applied twice daily for 3 months can be prescribed for multiple superficial lesions. This is usually reasonably well tolerated, although some patients complain of redness and irritation. The lesions often recur as soon as treatment stops, and it may be best reserved for patients with thin, less inflamed lesions.
- *Topical imiquimod* is a cutaneous immunomodulator and is effective when used in the treatment of solar keratoses. Side effects commonly include a significant inflammatory response, but this feature is often associated with higher efficacy of treatment.
- *Photodynamic therapy.* This treatment is available from specialist units and involves application to the lesions of a photosensitising cream followed, 3 hours later, by irradiation with light of a specific wavelength. The treatment is performed on one or two occasions a week apart.
- *Ingenol mebutate.* This is applied over an area of up to 25 cm^2 daily for 3 days; it may cause inflammation.

Patients who request treatment for widespread symptomatic multiple lesions, or in whom there is concern about malignant transformation, should be referred to a dermatologist.

> **DON'T FORGET ▶▶**
>
> Most people with solar keratoses can be managed conservatively. Remember, however, that in immunosuppressed patients, such as post-transplant patients or patients taking long-term immunosuppressants for medical problems (particularly azathioprine), malignant transformation is a real risk, and the treatment of solar keratoses should be more aggressive.

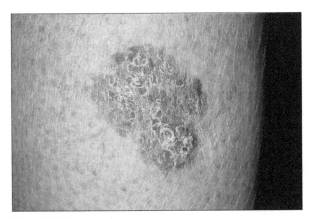

Figure 9.48 Bowen's disease.

Bowen's disease (intraepidermal squamous cell carcinoma)

Bowen's disease is less common than solar keratosis and represents a skin tumour that has progressed one stage closer to the development of SCC. Also known as intraepidermal carcinoma *in situ* (the equivalent of cervical intraepithelial neoplasia in cervical cytology), it has the capacity inevitably to transform to SCC, although this may take many years. Spontaneous resolution does not occur.

There is an association between cumulative sun exposure and Bowen's disease, although this is less clear-cut than with solar keratosis. Ingestion or topical application of arsenical preparations (e.g., tonics or Fowler's solution) is known to predispose to the development of this condition.

Clinical features

Bowen's disease presents as a persistent, well-demarcated, erythematous, scaly plaque on the lower limbs of the elderly. The plaque enlarges and may reach several centimetres in diameter (Figure 9.48).

Differential diagnosis

This includes inflammatory dermatoses such as psoriasis, tinea corporis, and discoid eczema. Treatment with topical steroids or antifungals is, however, ineffective. If ulceration or a nodule develops within the lesion, malignant change should be suspected.

Management

Since the tumour most commonly occurs on the lower limbs of the elderly, where healing after surgery is often poor, primary surgical excision is usually inappropriate, particularly if the lesion is large. Curettage and cautery for smaller lesions can be considered. Where Bowen's disease is strongly suspected clinically, and the patient is reluctant or too frail to be referred to hospital, histological confirmation of the diagnosis can be obtained by taking a small incision biopsy from the centre of the lesion.

Other treatment options include the following:
- *Liquid nitrogen cryotherapy.* If the lesion is large, it should be treated in stages, ensuring that healing has occurred before proceeding to the next part of the plaque. A reasonable interval between treatments is 4–6 weeks.
- *Medical treatments.* Topical 5-fluorouracil or imiquimod and photodynamic therapy can be used.
- *Radiotherapy.* This is now rarely used as the treatments listed above are more widely available, effective, and more straightforward.

The risk of progression to SCC should not be underestimated, and you should only embark on treating Bowen's disease if you fully understand the potential problems.

Keratoacanthoma

This is a spontaneously resolving tumour that is much less common than either solar keratosis or Bowen's disease. Keratoacanthoma occurs at about a third of the frequency of SCC, which is the most important clinical and histological differential diagnosis. It is often difficult to distinguish between the two conditions, particularly histologically. Again, there seems to be a link with sun exposure, since keratoacanthomas are most commonly seen on the head or upper limbs of older people.

Clinical features

A keratoacanthoma is usually a solitary lesion that enlarges rapidly over 4–12 weeks, often causing patients considerable alarm. The typical lesion is a neatly symmetrical pink nodule 10–20 mm in diameter that has a central crater filled with a keratin plug (Figures 9.49– 9.51).

The tumour may occasionally be as large as 50 mm in diameter. The surrounding skin is often normal, with a marked absence of the thickening and induration that occurs around a nodule of SCC. Left alone, spontaneous resolution is said to occur within about 3 months, often leaving a cribriform scar. The diagnostic clues suggesting keratoacanthoma are the short history and the tidy symmetrical appearance of the lesion.

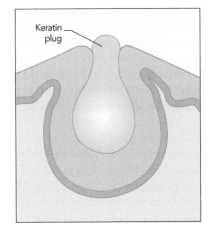

Figure 9.49 Keratoacanthoma; schematic representation.

Keratin plug

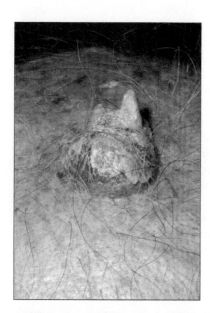

Figure 9.50
Keratoacanthoma.

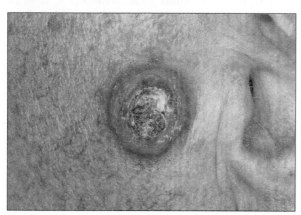

Figure 9.51
Keratoacanthoma.

Management

Despite the tendency to resolution, the treatment of choice is urgent excision. The important differential diagnosis is a rapidly enlarging SCC. It is therefore vital that the specimen is sent for careful histological examination and the histopathologist is given *all* the clinical details, in particular the history of the lesion.

The histopathology report itself may cause some difficulty. It will often state that the diagnosis of SCC cannot be excluded histologically, and that the history and clinical appearances of the lesion should be taken into consideration when deciding the definitive diagnosis and further management.

Shave excision or curettage is a simple way to treat small keratoacanthomas, particularly in the elderly, when the clinical diagnosis is not in doubt. However, removal by this method destroys the architecture of the lesion, making histopathological diagnosis more difficult. If this method of excision is chosen, it is important that a good wedge biopsy is taken from the lesion immediately prior to the curettage or shave excision. The wedge biopsy and curettage/shave specimen can be sent in the pot together and will help the histopathologist to make a diagnosis.

In view of the potential pitfalls, it may often be more appropriate to refer patients with lesions suggestive of keratoacanthoma to a dermatologist for assessment and surgery. The clinical appearance of the tumour is vital in making a correct diagnosis. Provided the tumour has been completely excised, the outcome is likely to be satisfactory (see Chapter 19). Always consider photographing a keratoacanthoma before treating it.

Lentigo maligna (Hutchinson's freckle, Stage 0 melanoma, in-situ melanoma)

This represents a proliferation of atypical melanocytes that are premalignant. The rate of malignant melanoma transformation is not predictable and varies. Although much less common than solar keratosis and Bowen's disease, lentigo maligna is not rare and is becoming more common as people live longer. Again, cumulative sun exposure is the important aetiological factor.

Clinical features

This is a slowly enlarging pigmented lesion that occurs on the face, upper cheek, temple, or forehead of an elderly person. It initially appears as a flat brown mark that then gradually enlarges and becomes darker, usually with variation in colour (Figure 9.52) and an irregular border. By the time the patient presents, the lesion may be quite large (more than 2 cm diameter). The changes may be so slow and subtle that presentation can be delayed.

The lesion with which lentigo maligna is most commonly confused is a seborrhoeic keratosis. The smoothness of the skin and absence of the typical warty texture of a basal cell papilloma can be useful clues to support the diagnosis of a lentigo maligna as can the appearance under dermoscopy (see Chapter 10). The uniform pigmentation of the seborrhoeic keratosis or solar lentigo contrasts sharply with the variable pigmentation of the lentigo maligna.

After slowly enlarging over a period of some years, a nodule may develop. This indicates transformation into an invasive lentigo maligna melanoma, which has a poor prognosis for survival.

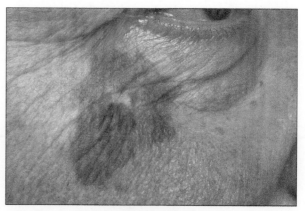

Figure 9.52 Lentigo maligna.

Management

A patient with a suspected lentigo maligna is best referred to a specialist. Unlike with other suspected melanomas (where incisional biopsies are to be avoided), the specialist may need to take multiple biopsies of suspicious areas to confirm the diagnosis as malignant change may be limited to only certain parts of the pigmented lesion.

Following histological confirmation, complete excision of the affected area is sometimes necessary, often with skin grafting. However, this decision needs to be taken after careful consideration of the patient's general medical condition as there is often a widespread field change of atypical melanocytes, and clearance of all the abnormal cells has the potential to lead to inappropriate and disfiguring surgery. Careful monitoring by specialists with a multidisciplinary approach is important.

Early studies suggest there may be a role for topical imiquimod treatment for some patients with this condition, but there is not yet enough evidence to support this as a safe option in all patients.

Malignant skin lesions

Malignant skin lesions are much less common than benign ones. The aim of this section is to describe the clinical features of the more common skin malignancies. In England and Wales, there is very clear national guidance about the management of all types of skin cancer, which all clinicians performing skin surgery should be aware of and cognisant with. Where such guidance is not in place, clinicians performing skin cancer surgery should think carefully before excising skin malignancies in general practice. Although these tumours are often fairly easy to remove, it is sometimes more difficult to make an accurate preoperative diagnosis unless you are seeing them often.

If you do decide to remove a lesion that may be malignant, you must have a clear management plan. In particular, you need to be aware of all the treatment options available so that you can offer the patient the same choices of management that would be available from a specialist service. You must have a clear idea of how you will proceed and what you will tell the patient when you receive the histology report. Remember that if you are uncertain about the clinical diagnosis, you should not perform the surgery yourself.

Table 9.2 Melanoma and non-melanoma skin cancer: the differences

Non-melanoma	Melanoma
Basal cell carcinoma, squamous cell carcinoma	Malignant melanoma
Common	Much less common
Older (50 years and upwards)	Younger (30–70 years, mean 51 years)
Sun-exposed sites, photodamaged skin	More common on the legs in women and the trunk in men
Slowly enlarging	More rapidly enlarging
Locally invasive. Metastases from basal cell carcinomas are virtually unheard of. Squamous cell carcinomas may metastasise, usually at a late stage	Metastasise early
Prognosis for survival is excellent. Second tumours are common	Prognosis for survival is excellent if diagnosed early, but remains poor if diagnosed late

Classification

Skin cancer can be divided into melanoma and non-melanoma skin cancer (Table 9.2). This is a very important distinction. Non-melanoma skin cancer is common, for the most part slowly growing, locally invasive, and usually easily treatable. Melanoma skin cancer is much less common, more aggressive, and will metastasise if not treated early. This distinction is important when counselling patients, many of whom think 'skin cancer, no hope'. This is because they have heard only about malignant melanoma, which was previously associated with a poor prognosis.

Non-melanoma skin cancer
Basal cell carcinoma (BCC, rodent ulcer)

A BCC, also known as a rodent ulcer, is the most common type of skin cancer seen on white skin. This tumour is much more common than any of the other malignant or premalignant tumours discussed in this chapter; indeed, it is the most common form of malignant disease. BCCs enlarge very slowly but can be highly invasive locally, especially when situated over areas of embryological differentiation. They are said not to metastasise.

The most common sites are the sun-damaged skin of the head and neck, especially in the elderly who have had long periods of sun exposure over many years. The growing popularity of recreational sun exposure has resulted in an increased incidence of these tumours in younger people.

Clinical features

Nodulo-cystic BCC. This is the most common type and usually appears on the face as a slowly enlarging nodule with a cystic, pearly appearance. It is often crossed by telangiectatic vessels (Figure 9.53). The nodule typically has a rolled edge, and the patient may present with a non-healing ulcer (Figure 9.54). Previously, these tumours caused extensive destruction of large areas of the face, hence the name rodent ulcer.

Other types listed below are variants of a typical BCC and are much less common:

- *Pigmented BCC.* Sometimes a BCC is pigmented (Figure 9.55), causing confusion with a melanoma.
- *Superficial BCC.* Unlike the other types, superficial BCCs are usually seen on the trunk. Cystic change is usually seen at the periphery of the lesion (Figure 9.56). The differential diagnosis includes Bowen's disease and inflammatory dermatoses such as eczema, psoriasis, and tinea corporis. As with Bowen's disease, treatment with topical steroids or antifungals will be ineffective.
- *Morphoeic BCC.* This is the least common type, which is fortunate since it is the most difficult to diagnose and treat (Figure 9.57). The affected area is often thickened and pale, and the typical cystic change with telangiectasia may be absent.

Differential diagnosis

To the inexperienced (and experienced!) eye, sebaceous gland hyperplasia (Figure 9.58) and non-pigmented intradermal naevi may be difficult to distinguish from BCC. If there is any doubt, the patient should be referred for a further opinion to avoid unnecessary surgery. Dermoscopy can help with the diagnosis (see Chapter 10).

Management

- *Nodulo-cystic BCC.* The treatment of choice is surgical excision. Radiotherapy is still sometimes appropriate although the cosmetic outcome is variable. Curettage and cautery has been advocated, and this technique works well for some patients, but it should only be performed by clinicians with a sound dermatological training and expertise in the diagnosis and management of skin tumours. Curettings should always be sent for histological examination, and the curettage and cautery repeated three times to ensure adequate clearance (with only the first curettings being sent for analysis). Diagnostic biopsy of BCCs is of little value if the patient is to be referred for definitive surgery anyway. This is particularly true of small BCCs that may appear to 'vanish' during healing after an incisional biopsy.

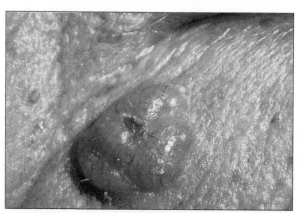

Figure 9.53 Basal cell carcinoma.

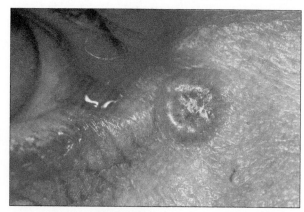

Figure 9.54 Basal cell carcinoma.

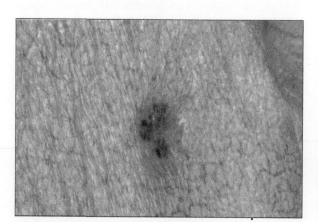

Figure 9.55 Pigmented basal cell carcinoma.

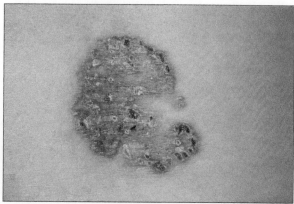

Figure 9.56 Superficial basal cell carcinoma.

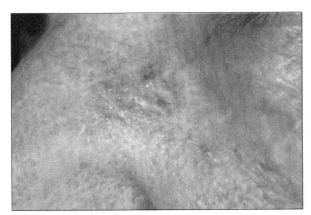

Figure 9.57 Morphoeic basal cell carcinoma.

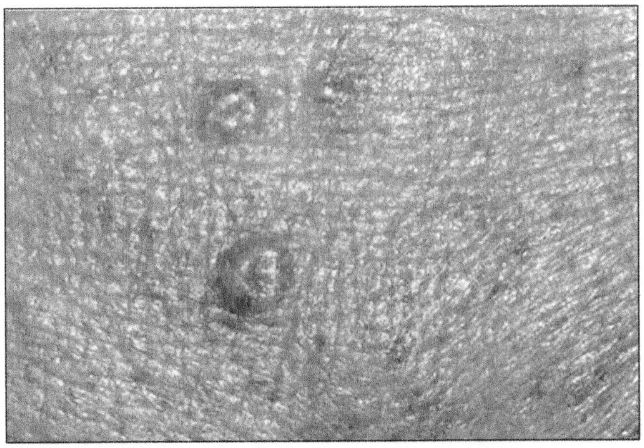

Figure 9.58 Sebaceous gland hyperplasia.

- *Morphoeic BCC.* Clinically, these tumours have a very poorly defined margin. They may require a procedure known as Mohs' micrographic surgery. This is usually performed by a dermatological surgeon in close collaboration with a histopathologist. A primary excision is performed and, with the patient still in the operating theatre, frozen sections of the specimen are examined to establish whether the tumour has been fully excised. Further excision can be performed as necessary and the process repeated until the tumour has been completely removed.
- *Superficial BCC.* A range of treatments are available for these lesions, including liquid nitrogen cryotherapy, topical imiquimod, curettage and cautery, photodynamic therapy, and radiotherapy. Small lesions can be excised by an elliptical excision, but for larger lesions other treatment modalities are preferable to optimise the cosmetic outcome.

Where a confident clinical diagnosis of BCC has been made in a frail, elderly patient, excision in the primary care physician's surgery may be a more convenient approach, but this needs to be performed in the context of any nationally agreed guidance for the management of skin cancer. Such guidance takes account of the need for specialist skills in the diagnosis and management of skin cancer, and is designed to ensure that the full range of skin cancer services is available to all patients.

Recurrence may take some years to develop, so the patient should be advised to return if the scar changes, even after a very long time. Second tumours are common, with up to 40% of patients developing a second BCC within 5 years. It is therefore important to check the remainder of a patient's skin if they present with a BCC. Further advice about follow-up is discussed in the section on managing the histology report (see below).

Squamous cell carcinoma

Squamous cell carcinoma (SCC) typically arises in the sun-damaged skin of the elderly. It is much less common than BCC. Since these tumours can be more aggressive, correct diagnosis and management are vital. The tumour can arise *de novo*, or there may be a history of a preceding long-standing solar keratosis or a patch of Bowen's disease.

Clinical features
The most common early clinical presentation is of an indurated, crusted keratotic plaque or nodule (Figures 9.59–9.61). Later, a non-healing ulcer may develop with an irregular raised border (Figure 9.62). The rate of enlargement is variable but is usually faster than that of a BCC and slower than that of a keratoacanthoma. Squamous cell carcinomas do metastasise, although tumours arising in solar keratoses are particularly slow to do so. Lesions on the lip spread earlier and have a worse prognosis. Usually, the faster growing the lesion, the less well differentiated it appears under the microscope (unlike a keratoacanthoma). Remember that SCCs are likely to behave more aggressively, and metastasise earlier, in patients on long-term immunosuppression, particularly transplant patients. UK guidelines suggest these patients should be reviewed annually by a dermatologist.

Differential diagnosis
Keratoacanthoma is the most difficult differential diagnosis. Even if the clinical diagnosis is keratoacanthoma, the histology report is often suggestive of an SCC. It may be necessary to arrange follow-up of these patients even if the lesion was completely removed (see above).

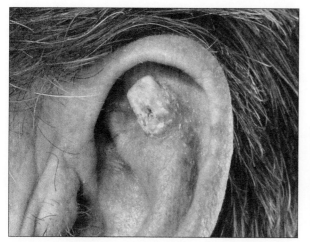

Figure 9.59 Squamous cell carcinoma.

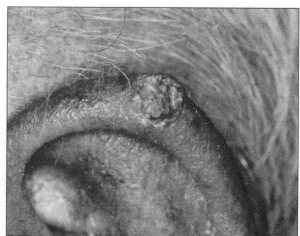

Figure 9.60 Squamous cell carcinoma.

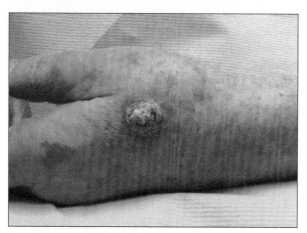

Figure 9.61 Squamous cell carcinoma.

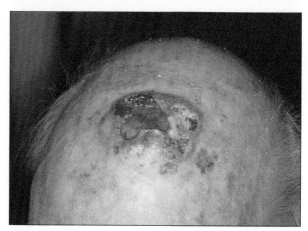

Figure 9.62 Squamous cell carcinoma.

Management

This depends on the clinical presentation, the site, and, most importantly, the histopathological features. If the diagnosis of SCC is suspected, it is advisable to seek a specialist opinion before proceeding, since the combined expertise of a dermatologist, plastic surgeon, and radiotherapist in the multidisciplinary team may be necessary. If an SCC is unexpectedly excised, you should refer the patient to a dermatologist for further assessment, histology review, and development of a management plan appropriate to the aggressiveness of the tumour.

Small tumours arising in actinic keratoses often do well with local excision alone, while larger, more aggressive tumours may require further wide local excision and occasionally radiotherapy. Radiotherapy alone is sometimes indicated.

DON'T FORGET ▶ ▶
- Squamous cell carcinoma is likely to be much more aggressive in immunosuppressed patients.
- Features of SCC and BCC may rarely be present within a single lesion—so-called baso-squamous lesions.

Malignant melanoma

Although the incidence of malignant melanoma has doubled in the last 10 years (and within the Western world, the incidence has been doubling every 10 years since the 1950s), this tumour is much less common than other types of skin cancer. The prognosis of a malignant melanoma is excellent if it is diagnosed and treated early, but remains poor if the tumour is diagnosed late.

Natural history

Malignant melanoma affects young adults, and females are affected more commonly than males. The tumour is more common in those who burn rather than tan in the sun. The history is of great importance since in many cases it forms the basis on which a decision to excise a pigmented lesion will be taken. Remember that in about 50% of cases, malignant melanoma presents as a new melanocytic naevus, and in the remainder it occurs in a pre-existing naevus. A new, enlarging pigmented lesion on the leg of a red-headed young lady should ring alarm bells even if it looks innocent at a first glance.

Retrospective studies of patients with malignant melanoma have shown that the three most important worrying clinical signs in a pigmented naevus are *change in size*, *in shape*, and *in colour*. These are the so-called major criteria (Table 9.3). Symptoms such as itching are much less important and are included in the minor criteria.

Clinical features

The most common type of malignant melanoma is the superficial spreading (80%). Invasive lentigo maligna melanoma is a condition of the elderly and is likely to become more common as people live longer. The other types (nodular, acral lentiginous, and subungual) are rare, and further information about them can be obtained from any standard dermatology text.

- *Superficial spreading malignant melanoma.* This is most common on the legs (women) and the trunk (men). It is a pigmented lesion, usually greater than 7 mm in diameter, and often with an irregular border (Figure 9.63). The pigmentation within the lesion is variable and in some parts may even be absent.
- *Lentigo maligna melanoma.* The development of a nodule in a long-standing Hutchinson's freckle (lentigo maligna) indicates the development of invasive lentigo maligna melanoma (Figure 9.64).

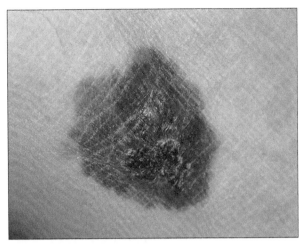

Figure 9.63 Malignant melanoma.

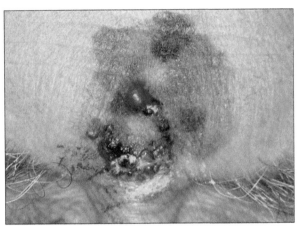

Figure 9.64 Lentigo maligna melanoma.

- *Amelanotic malignant melanoma.* Although this is a very rare type of malignant melanoma, it is worth mentioning briefly. An amelanotic malignant melanoma typically presents as a rapidly enlarging shiny red nodule that may resemble the much more common pyogenic granuloma (see Figure 9.39). The presence of a pre-existing pigmented lesion in which the nodule has developed is strongly suggestive of an amelanotic malignant melanoma. Because of the clinical similarity between the two lesions, all pyogenic granulomas should be excised urgently and the histology report checked carefully.

Table 9.3 Pigmented lesions: the major and minor criteria	
Major criteria	Minor criteria
Change in size	Inflammation
Change in shape	Crusting or bleeding
Change in colour	Sensory change
	Diameter greater than 7 mm

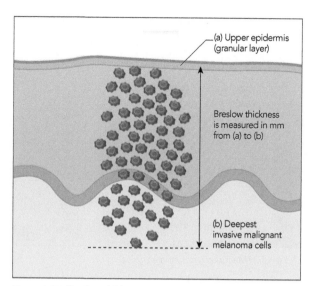

Figure 9.65 Breslow thickness.

Prognosis

The single most important prognostic factor in malignant melanoma is the thickness of the tumour, the so-called Breslow thickness (Figure 9.65). Excision of early lesions that are thin (less than 1.5 mm) is associated with 90% 5-year survival. If the tumour is 1.5–3.5 mm in thickness, 5-year survival is around 70%, and if it is greater than 3.5 mm this figure falls to only 40%.

Management

Treatment of malignant melanoma remains surgical since the tumour is unresponsive to either chemotherapy or radiotherapy. The extensive mutilating surgery previously performed is now felt to be inappropriate. Ideally, a malignant melanoma that is less than 2 mm in thickness should be excised with a 1 cm margin as a minimum.

All patients with malignant melanoma should be discussed by the multidisciplinary skin cancer team to agree the most appropriate excision margin for each individual patient. This is particularly relevant for patients with thicker, poorer prognosis tumours. Sentinel node biopsy (SNB), for patients with malignant melanoma, is available in many melanoma centres. This procedure has not to date been shown to be associated with improved survival; however, the results of SNB may indicate the appropriate use of immunotherapy agents, and the results of further studies are awaited.

Excision of melanoma in primary care

Whenever you examine a pigmented lesion you should ask yourself, 'Could this be a malignant melanoma?'

There are two possible scenarios. In the first, you suspect when you first see the patient that the lesion may be a malignant melanoma. In the second, you inadvertently excise a malignant melanoma, only finding out when you receive the histopathology report.

- *You suspect the lesion is a malignant melanoma.* Although you may have the technical expertise for primary surgical excision of a malignant melanoma, in the United Kingdom, you should *not* undertake this in general practice. National guidance in England and Wales requires that these patients are referred to specialist centres using the so-called '2-week wait' referral process. Because of the rarity of the tumour, you cannot be expected to have up-to-date knowledge about the management and prognosis of patients with malignant melanoma. When you receive the histopathology report, it is unlikely that you will be confident in counselling your patient and answering questions accurately. If a wider excision is required, the patient will need to be referred to a specialist anyway. All dermatologists should agree to see a patient urgently if the diagnosis is thought to be malignant melanoma. If this is the case, the subsequent treatment of malignant melanoma (wide local excision) will be determined by the histopathology of the initial lesion. All melanocytic naevi, and indeed most skin lesions, should be removed with a 2 mm margin so that if the lesion is subsequently reported as malignant, it will have been completely removed at the primary excision. *There is no place for performing a primary excision of a melanocytic lesion with a margin wider than 2 mm.* This is because it is the initial histology of the primary excision that determines the margin for wide local excision, and this may be 1–3 cm, depending on the Breslow thickness of the lesion.

- *It looked benign but the histopathologist reports it as a malignant melanoma.* Don't panic! Don't immediately phone the patient. Take advice. Discuss the histopathology report urgently with your local dermatologist or plastic surgeon. It is most helpful if you can read the histology report out verbatim. Having taken advice on how to proceed, contact the patient. Provided you act promptly, you will have done no harm to your patient; indeed, if you have removed a malignant melanoma that 'looked benign' you may well have improved your patient's life expectancy. Even if you have carried out an incomplete excision of a melanoma, this is no worse than an incision biopsy, as the patient will require further surgery anyway. However, shaving or curetting a malignant melanoma disrupts the architecture of the melanocytic lesions and removes the opportunity for the histopathologist to measure the Breslow thickness of the malignant melanoma. This is therefore to be avoided at all costs. The old wives' tale about 'interfering with moles making them go bad' is not true. In England and Wales, all patients with a malignant melanoma will be discussed by the local skin cancer multidisciplinary team, who will advise on further management.

APPROACH TO MANAGEMENT

This section provides a plan for the management of patients who present with a skin lesion, for although you should not *remove* a lesion without having made a diagnosis, you cannot refer every patient whose lesion you cannot identify. Managing uncertainty is an essential part of clinical practice. This section gives practical guidelines about dealing with uncertainty and using time as a diagnostic tool. It also highlights important conditions that are commonly confused.

Basic principles

It is not necessary to remove a lesion just because it is there. The right treatment for many lesions is to do nothing, and many patients only need reassurance.

The history usually gives you the answer to a diagnostic uncertainty. A lesion that has been present for a long time and is not changing is almost certainly benign. However, various points in the history may make you suspect malignant change. For example, malignant melanoma is suggested by a history of:

- Change in size, shape, or colour in a pre-existing melanocytic naevus.
- A new melanocytic lesion in a patient over the age of 30, particularly where it is rapidly enlarging, has an irregular outline, or is variable in colour.
- Development of a nodule in a pigmented patch on the face. This suggests development of invasive malignant melanoma in a Hutchinson's freckle.

Non-melanoma skin cancer is suggested by:

- A slowly enlarging, non-healing lesion on light-exposed skin (BCC).
- Thickening, ulceration, or nodule formation in a previously stable solar keratosis (SCC).
- A nodule arising on an erythematous plaque on the leg, which may be an SCC arising in a patch of Bowen's disease.
- Any new, enlarging lesion on the skin of the elderly (SCC, BCC).

Itching *alone* is not usually a symptom of malignancy. However, in combination with other symptoms, it should be taken more seriously. A personal history of previous skin cancer, or a family history (first-degree relative) of malignant melanoma, adds weight to the likelihood of a malignant lesion.

GOLDEN RULES ✳

- Take a careful history.
- Wherever possible, never remove a lesion without a diagnosis.
- In many cases, you will be able to make a confident clinical diagnosis.
- The earlier section in this chapter contains an outline of the different treatments that are available and recommendations on those most suitable for particular conditions.
- A patient will not infrequently present with a lesion you cannot identify; nevertheless, you can usually decide if it is benign or malignant.

If you can identify the lesion

If you can make a diagnosis, it is fairly straightforward to decide what to do next.

If obviously benign

Patients request removal of a lesion because it is a nuisance, it is unsightly, or they are worried that it might be something sinister.

Should you remove it?

Ask yourself whether there is any reason for the lesion to be removed. Many benign lesions are best treated with reassurance; tampering with these is unnecessary and meddlesome.

Can you remove it?

In the case of a benign lesion, you must decide whether your skill, experience, and facilities are adequate to deal with it. You should be certain that you can produce a result that will be better than the original lesion. You must set your standards high in respect of the likely outcome, and you need to weigh up the potential problems against your skills in dealing with them and decide each case on its merits. The site of a lesion, its size, and your own experience should all be considered.

There are a number of anatomical areas that should be avoided (see Chapter 6). In addition, you should steer clear of surgery in certain groups of patients such as young children, very anxious patients, and those whose expectations about the required cosmetic outcome are unrealistic. It goes without saying that you must send any lesion you remove for histological examination. You will sometimes get a surprise when the report comes back, and occasionally a nasty shock such as a completely unexpected malignancy. This scenario is covered later in this chapter.

If obviously malignant

Sometimes you will suspect strongly that a lesion is malignant.

Pigmented lesion

The worry is that it may be a malignant melanoma. This needs prompt action. *Do not remove the lesion yourself but refer the patient at once.* Telephone or fax your local consultant dermatologist and arrange for your patient to be seen within 1–2 weeks. In England, you will be expected to use the '2-week wait' referral process. If the patient prefers not to be referred, photograph the lesion and request the patient's permission to discuss their case with your local expert.

Non-pigmented lesion

You will usually suspect either a BCC or an SCC. Unless you have particular experience of treating patients with such lesions, they should all be referred to your local specialist dermatology service. The patient should preferably be seen at the dermatology clinic within 2–4 weeks. A suspected SCC needs to be seen sooner than a suspected BCC, and in England patients with a suspected SCC should be referred using the '2-week wait' referral process. If there is any diagnostic doubt at all, indicate this in the referral letter and ensure the patient is seen within 2 weeks.

If you cannot identify the lesion
If obviously benign

Even if you cannot make a definite diagnosis, you can often be sure that a lesion is harmless. Patients with such lesions do not have to be referred. If the lesion is stable, is unchanging, and has no sinister features, you may well feel able to reassure your patient that nothing further needs to be done. You should always provide a safety net, however, by telling your patient to see you again if they are at all concerned in the future.

Sometimes you may not be entirely happy with this approach. You may feel that there are features you are unsure about, or that your patient has not been fully reassured. In this case, arrange to review the patient after 6–12 weeks. There is little point in seeing them much sooner than 6 weeks as little will have changed.

It is useful to draw a diagram of the lesion and measure or photograph it in order to monitor any change in shape or size. You may ask the patient to photograph the lesion (if they have the equipment and skill) and for them to keep a digital record of it. If, when you review your patient, the lesion has not altered at all, you can provide strong reassurance. Nevertheless, you should always tell the patient to consult you in the future if the lesion changes or he or she is at all worried. If you are unhappy in any way, refer for a specialist opinion at this stage.

If possibly malignant

If you are not confident that the lesion is benign, you should refer the patient at this stage. Any change in the size, shape, or colour of a lesion is significant, and such a history should ring warning bells. Itching is a very unreliable sign, although patients are often alarmed by it. Obviously, you should have a low threshold for referring pigmented lesions, which can be very difficult to assess. *Always err on the side of caution.*

Rashes

There is an understandable temptation to biopsy rashes in order to spare the patient a visit to hospital. In general, you should resist the temptation as there are dangers, not least a dissatisfied patient!

- *Wrong site.* You may take the biopsy from the wrong site. The report you receive will show non-specific changes, and you are bound to refer the patient. The first biopsy will have resulted in a delay in diagnosis and treatment. If there is diagnostic doubt, a further biopsy may be necessary, and the patient may perceive the first one as having been inappropriate.
- *Incomprehensible report.* You may take a good biopsy from the correct site but receive an incomprehensible histopathology report. You will have to refer the patient anyway for the dermatologist to see the rash that goes with the report. The biopsy will have caused a delay in treatment, and the patient may have suffered undue anxiety.
- *Missed pathology.* In the worst scenario, the biopsy misses the pathological features completely, giving both patient and doctor false reassurance. The clinician at best misses a treatable condition and at worst misses a serious underlying disorder, for example cutaneous lymphoma.
- *Unnecessary biopsy.* Is a biopsy really necessary? Dermatologists look at lots of rashes and will often diagnose and start treatment without needing a biopsy at all.

Summary
Manage it yourself if:
- You are confident of a benign diagnosis.
- It needs no treatment.
- It needs treatment and you can do it yourself.
- It needs observation to reassure you and your patient.

Refer if:
- It is definitely malignant.
- It is suspicious.
- It is benign but needs treatment that is beyond your ability.
- It is an undiagnosed rash.
- You are in any doubt about the management.

Common clinical confusions

There will be situations when you are unsure about the diagnosis of a skin lesion. Where the lesions in the differential diagnosis are all benign and their management is *similar*, being unable to make a correct diagnosis is irritating to the doctor but causes no harm to the patient. There are situations, however, even with benign lesions, when making the wrong diagnosis may lead to serious errors in management.

Diagnosis wrong, lesion benign, acceptable procedure performed

A solar keratosis is sometimes thought to be a seborrhoeic keratosis and is treated by either cryotherapy or curettage and cautery. Provided that the patient was keen to have the lesion treated and the lesion was definitely benign, no harm has been done.

Epidermoid cysts and dermatofibromas may be confused. Here the correct diagnosis becomes clear during the surgical procedure, when a well-demarcated cyst rather than a fibrous dermal nodule is discovered, or vice versa. The outcome in both cases is a linear scar, and provided the patient has requested the excision no harm will have been done.

Diagnosis wrong, lesion benign, unacceptable procedure performed

By far the most common example of this is where a seborrhoeic keratosis is incorrectly diagnosed as a benign melanocytic naevus and is removed by ellipse excision, leaving a sutured linear scar. This procedure is inappropriate, and the patient will have reason to be dissatisfied with your management. The correct surgical procedure is curettage and cautery, which leads to a much better cosmetic result (see Chapter 19).

Diagnosis wrong, lesion malignant

This is the most worrying situation because an incorrect diagnosis can lead to inappropriate management and the patient's care may suffer as a consequence.

Examples of clinical confusion
Malignant melanoma versus seborrhoeic keratosis

These lesions are often mistaken for one another. Increase in size and change in colour, major criteria for the diagnosis of melanoma, are often the presenting features in both (see above). The lesion in Figure 9.66, despite its suspiciously variable pigmentation and central pinkish area, was confirmed histologically to be a seborrhoeic keratosis.

Management

If you think that the lesion might be a malignant melanoma, refer the patient for a specialist opinion. Curettage and cautery is inappropriate treatment for a melanoma. Ellipse excision may be necessary to confirm the diagnosis but, as this is an inappropriate procedure for a seborrhoeic keratosis, the decision to do this is best taken by a specialist. If you start to curette what was thought to be a pigmented seborrhoeic keratosis and it appears otherwise (black pigment seen, or the lesion is not curetting off with ease), either stop and refer the patient to hospital or, with the patient's consent, convert the process to an ellipse excision with a 2 mm margin.

Intradermal melanocytic naevus versus basal cell carcinoma

Basal cell carcinomas and benign intradermal melanocytic naevi are both most common on the face and both can have the typical nodular cystic appearance of BCC, with overlying telangiectasia (Figure 9.67).

Management

The best treatment for a benign melanocytic intradermal naevus is shave excision, whereas a BCC should be treated by ellipse excision. If you have any doubt about the diagnosis, refer the patient for a specialist opinion.

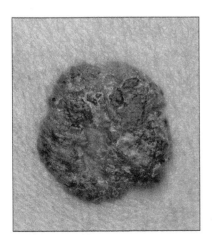

Figure 9.66 Suspicious-looking seborrhoeic keratosis.

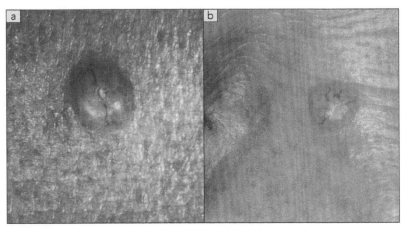

Figure 9.67 (a) Intradermal melanocytic naevus. (b) Basal cell carcinoma.

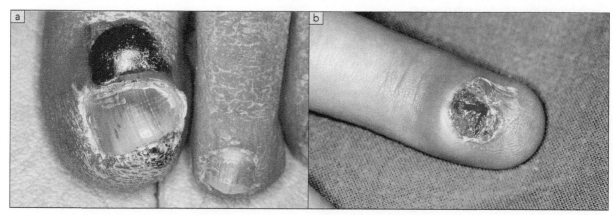

Figure 9.68 (a) Subungual haematoma. (b) Subungual melanoma.

Subungual haematoma versus subungual malignant melanoma

A brown tumour beneath the nail will often be mistaken for a subungual haematoma (Figure 9.68a). In the absence of a history of trauma to the nail, the diagnosis of a subungual haematoma can be very difficult to make. A longitudinal pigmented band in the nail suggests melanocytic proliferation. With time, a subungual malignant melanoma will lead to longitudinal splitting of the nail, oozing, paronychia, nail dystrophy, and finally destruction of the nail (Figure 9.68b).

The prognosis of subungual malignant melanoma is poor, and it is an important condition to diagnose early. It is therefore unacceptable to wait and see whether the nail grows out normally, as always happens when a subungual haematoma resolves. Most specialists have a very low threshold for performing a nail biopsy if there is any possibility that a subungual lesion is melanocytic.

Management

Refer the patient urgently to a specialist (to be seen within 1–2 weeks) with a view to an urgent nail biopsy.

Solar keratosis versus Bowen's disease versus squamous cell carcinoma

In patients with many solar keratoses, it is tempting to treat multiple lesions with cryotherapy. Although treating a patch of Bowen's disease with liquid nitrogen will cause no adverse effects, cryotherapy is the wrong treatment for SCC. Before treating the lesion, look carefully at any presumed solar keratosis for evidence of induration and infiltration of the surrounding skin, and question the patient about recent changes in the lesion (Figure 9.69). Lifting the crust may reveal a nodule or an ulcer if the lesion is an SCC.

Management

If you have any doubt about the diagnosis, you should refer the patient for a specialist opinion.

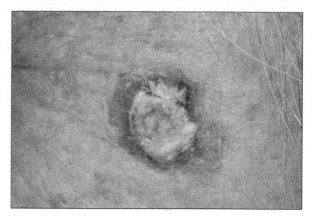

Figure 9.69 Early squamous cell carcinoma.

Cutaneous horn

A cutaneous horn represents an abnormal proliferation of keratin. It is a clinical and *not* a pathological diagnosis (Figure 9.70).

There are several possible underlying pathological processes that lead to the development of such a lesion. A viral wart is the most likely cause in a young patient, whereas a solar keratosis is most probable on light-exposed skin in an older patient. Squamous cell carcinoma is the most important differential diagnosis and should always be borne in mind.

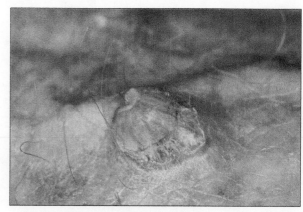

Figure 9.70 Cutaneous horn.

Management

It is most important to establish a histological diagnosis by examining the tissue at the *base* of the horn; examination of the keratin alone is of no value. Curettage and cautery or ellipse excision will provide the necessary information.

Beware cutaneous horns that have a cuff of red, raised skin at their base. This may well be an SCC, and diagnosis requires excision of this base. If the horn arises out of completely healthy skin at its base, the diagnosis is much more likely to be benign.

THE HISTOLOGY REPORT

This section discusses the interpretation of the histology report and what to do with unexpected results, for example an incompletely excised lesion, an unsuspected malignancy, or something completely baffling. Chapter 2 gives details of the information that you should include on the histopathology request form accompanying the specimen. Guidance based on numerous real scenarios is given here.

Principles

Should you send a specimen for histological examination even if you are absolutely certain what it is? The only safe answer is *yes, always*. This is for two reasons:

- No matter how certain you are of the clinical diagnosis, you may be wrong. All pathologists occasionally come across epidermoid cysts containing tumours, or seemingly benign lesions that turn out to be something rare and sinister.
- The patient from whom you have removed some simple benign lesion may subsequently develop a completely unconnected malignancy, often years later. Unless you have firm evidence that what you removed was benign, you may be unable to defend yourself against the charge that the original lesion was malignant and that you were negligent in missing the diagnosis.

The only safe policy is to submit everything you remove to the histology laboratory.

People often ask whether it is necessary to send skin tags, when large numbers are being removed. If they are tiny, it could be argued that the alternative treatment of cryotherapy would produce no histological specimens. A safe compromise is to send:

- At least one representative specimen.
- In addition, any unusual skin tags (unusually large or pigmented).
- Several specimens from one small area in one pot, provided this is clearly stated in the notes and on the request form (e.g., 'left axilla', 'right base of neck').

Pathology specimens

Throughout this section, the point is made that you should not remove a lesion without first making a clinical diagnosis. On the basis of that diagnosis, you will decide what procedure is most appropriate. You should provide the histopathologist with as much relevant information as possible and send the specimen properly fixed, identified, and orientated. It is very helpful to put in a marker suture on one side of the specimen. Although not strictly necessary with simple ellipse excisions, this is essential with non-orientated circular excisions, with a simple drawing on the request form showing the specimen's orientation. Remember also to record any previous cryosurgery since this may alter the histological appearance of the specimen.

Although curettings are disrupted tissue, they too should always be sent since they can provide satisfactory diagnostic information.

Interpreting the histology report

The histology report will usually be self-explanatory. Sometimes, however, it may be more difficult to interpret. It may be couched in unfamiliar technical terms, or you may be unsure of the clinical implications for managing your patient. The rest of this chapter is based on real examples and discusses what action to take in each case.

Pigmented lesions

Pigmented lesions form the largest group of lesions excised in general practice. The vast majority will be either benign melanocytic naevi (moles) or seborrhoeic keratoses. More rarely, a malignant melanoma is inadvertently removed.

Benign melanocytic naevi

The report will typically read:

- '... *dermal melanocytic naevus, completely excised.*'
- '... *compound melanocytic naevus, completely removed.*'
- '... *junctional melanocytic naevus, completely excised.*'

These histological descriptions correspond to the clinical descriptions elsewhere in the book. The distinction between compound, junctional, and intradermal is of no consequence with regard to managing the patient. Although the term 'benign' is often not included in the descriptive report of a melanocytic naevus, the examples above are all benign. Consequently, reports suggesting incomplete excision should cause no concern.

Dysplastic melanocytic naevi

To many clinicians, the term 'dysplasia' suggests premalignant change. Dysplasia is a term best avoided when describing the clinical appearance of melanocytic naevi as it suggests premalignancy. It is, however, a term widely used in the histological description of melanocytic lesions, and it is therefore very important to understand the use of this term in this context. It is important to know, first, the amount of dysplasia (i.e., mild, moderate, or severe), and second, whether the lesion was solitary or whether it was one of many other melanocytic lesions. The simple guidelines below will ensure safe practice.

'Junctional/compound melanocytic lesion with mild dysplasia'

- Whether the lesion has been completely or incompletely removed, this report should cause no alarm for you or the patient.
- Many solitary benign naevi show mild dysplasia.
- If the patient has many other melanocytic naevi, in particular odd-looking ones, you may wish to seek reassurance from a dermatologist that the patient does not have atypical mole syndrome (see above), which is associated with an increased incidence of malignant melanoma. Referral for a routine appointment is appropriate. While awaiting the hospital appointment, the patient should be advised to report whether any other pigmented lesion changes in size, shape, or colour.

'Junctional/compound melanocytic naevus with moderate dysplasia'

This report should not be ignored or inadvertently filed before careful assessment and appropriate action. Management depends on whether or not the lesion has been completely excised and whether or not the patient has multiple melanocytic naevi:

- The patient should be reassured that although the mole was active, it was not malignant.
- Because the diagnosis of malignant melanoma has implications for patients obtaining life insurance, it is important to stress to the patient that the diagnosis is *not* malignant melanoma.

Complete excision, very few other moles, and no atypical moles

- No further surgery is necessary provided the lesion is reported as completely removed.
- Advise the patient to return for review if new pigmentation develops within the scar.
- A recurrence at any time demands urgent referral to the dermatology department, where the initial histology can be reviewed and appropriate management instituted.

Complete excision, multiple moles, and/or several atypical-looking moles

- If the other moles look benign, refer for a routine dermatological opinion to consider the possibility of atypical mole syndrome.
- If any of the other moles look worrying, refer for an urgent dermatological opinion.
- Give simple advice about checking moles for changes in size, shape, and colour; expedite an outpatient appointment if any other moles change and cause concern. Make the patient aware of the harmful effects of sun exposure, and give advice about sunscreens and sun avoidance.

Incomplete excision, very few other moles, and no other worrying or unusual moles

- Take advice, preferably from your dermatologist, by telephone. The dermatologist will probably arrange to review the specimen with the histopathologist and then discuss management with you.
- If this is not practicable, refer urgently for excision of the scar.
- If you feel confident, arrange to excise the scar yourself. Meanwhile, either discuss the histology report with the dermatologist or refer the patient for a routine dermatology outpatient appointment.

Incomplete excision, multiple moles, and/or several other unusual moles

The guidelines in the previous section apply, but in addition:

- Ensure that the patient has a dermatological opinion in weeks rather than months.
- Give simple advice about checking moles for changes in size, shape, and colour; expedite an outpatient appointment if any other moles change and cause concern. Make sure the patient is 'sun aware'.

Melanocytic naevus with severe dysplasia

This is much more worrying, because the interpretation of severely dysplastic changes varies. Some histopathologists consider severe dysplasia to indicate in-situ melanoma (Stage 0 melanoma). In such cases, the histology should be reviewed by the dermatologist and histopathologist together to plan future management.

Severe dysplasia, complete excision

Although the time scale is not vital, request an urgent outpatient appointment for everyone's peace of mind. Include the histology reference number in your letter, so that the histology can be reviewed before the patient attends. If there is a high level of anxiety, telephone the dermatology department and ask for the histology to be reviewed at an early stage.

Severe dysplasia, incomplete excision

We would suggest urgent referral. Arrange an early out-patient appointment (within 1–2 weeks) by telephone, or, in England and Wales, use the '2-week wait' referral process.

This term often causes confusion. 'In-situ' indicates non-invasive, and, provided the lesion is completely removed, the prognosis is excellent. You should request an urgent appointment with the dermatologist so that the patient has the opportunity to discuss the diagnosis and management. It is, however, important to explain to the patient that this is not an invasive lesion, i.e. *not* a malignant melanoma. In-situ melanoma is also known as Stage 0 melanoma, lentigo maligna, and Hutchinson's freckle.

Malignant melanoma

Most pigmented lesions removed in general practice are benign. Most malignant melanomas are excised in hospital. Occasionally, however, a report will appear on your desk as follows:

> *'... skin with a superficial spreading malignant melanoma. The tumour depth is 0.9 mm. The mitotic rate is high and there is a marked lymphocytic reaction. Surface margin is 2.3 mm; deep margin 3.5 mm.'*

This is a real 'heart-sink' report that usually comes as a complete surprise, and often you cannot even put a face to the name on the report. How should you react? First of all, do not panic, but read the report carefully and ask two questions:

- *What is the thickness of the tumour?*
  The single most important factor in the prognosis of malignant melanoma is the tumour thickness at presentation (the Breslow thickness; see above). Thin tumours (less than 1 mm) have a very good prognosis, whereas thick tumours (over 3 mm) have a very poor prognosis. Figures for 5-year survival were given earlier in the chapter.
- *Has the tumour been completely removed and, if so, by what excision margin?*

With the answers to these two important questions, you can decide how to proceed. But remember that even if the excision is incomplete, you have *not* worsened the prognosis provided you act promptly.

Malignant melanoma, Breslow thickness less than 1 mm, completely excised with 2 mm excision margin

- This patient has an excellent outlook, with a 5-year survival figure of 98%.
- Further surgery is necessary to give a 1 cm margin of excision.
- Arrange an urgent dermatology outpatient appointment (1–2 weeks). Arrange to review the patient within the next few days, and give this appointment to the patient yourself at the consultation. Make sure the dermatologist receives a copy of the histology report before the patient is seen in outpatients. In England, use the '2-week wait' referral process.
- When you see the patient for review, explain the diagnosis in a very positive way. Many people still associate malignant melanoma with a very poor prognosis, and it is important to reassure the patient that early surgical excision leads to complete cure. Discuss the need and reasons for further surgery.

Malignant melanoma, Breslow thickness greater than 1 mm, completely or incompletely excised

In this group of patients, the outcome is likely to be not so good. The prognosis and management will depend on the Breslow thickness, the patient's age, the site of the lesion, the type of melanoma, and whether there is any evidence of metastatic disease. Previously, wide surgical excision, with or without lymph node dissection, was the treatment of choice in this group of patients. There is now good evidence that extensive surgery does little to influence the outcome. The recommended excision margin for most melanomas up to 2 mm in thickness is 1 cm. The necessary margin for thicker tumours is still debated. A reasonable management strategy is as follows:

- Arrange an urgent outpatient assessment (1–2 weeks) by a dermatologist or plastic surgeon. Make sure the referral contains a copy of the histology report. In England, this will be using the '2-week wait' process.
- Discuss the diagnosis with your patient in general terms. Try to be positive, but explain that your knowledge of the outlook is limited. Advise the patient of the referral you have arranged, and warn that further surgery may be necessary.
- Malignant melanoma is neither radiosensitive nor responsive to chemotherapy, so referral to a radiotherapist or oncologist at this stage is inappropriate.
- In England, all patients with malignant melanoma are discussed by the local skin cancer multidisciplinary team and a management plan agreed.

Solar (actinic) keratosis

Usually, you will elect not to excise these lesions. However, if you do remove them by curettage, the curettings should be sent for histopathological assessment. This will usually confirm your clinical diagnosis, and no further action will be required. It is reasonable to tell the patient that the lesion removed was due to sun damage and to take the opportunity of discussing the dangers of excessive sun exposure. The tendency for solar keratoses to be more active in the summer and less active in the winter is worth mentioning.

'Solar keratosis with mild/moderate dysplasia'

All solar keratoses show some degree of dysplasia, from mild through to severe. Provided the dysplastic change is confined to the epidermis, there is no cause for concern.

'Microinvasion'

If the word 'microinvasion' appears in the report, this may indicate an early SCC. Squamous cell carcinoma arising in a solar keratosis is usually very slowly growing.

- Refer the patient for a dermatological opinion within about 2–4 weeks. The histology will be reviewed and further surgery arranged as appropriate.
- The patient can be reassured but should be advised that the biopsy report has suggested the presence of very early skin cancer. Again, it is important to explain that this is non-melanoma skin cancer and that there is a possibility that a further very minor surgical procedure may be required. Stress that the outlook is excellent and that spread is very unlikely.
- If there is no evidence of a residual lesion and the patient is elderly and frail, arrange to review the patient at 3 months to check the scar. Advise the patient to seek advice if the lesion recurs at a later date. Refer if there is any evidence of recurrence.
- In England, all patients with SCC are considered by the local skin cancer multidisciplinary team and a management plan agreed.

Bowen's disease

This is sometimes reported as intraepithelial or intraepidermal dysplasia, i.e., dysplasia extending throughout the epidermis. If left, it can progress to SCC, although the period of latency may be many years and is unpredictable.

'Patch of Bowen's disease, completely excised'

- Review the patient and check that this was a solitary patch, that the scar has healed, and that there is no clinical evidence of residual tumour. You can either ask the patient to return for review at 3 months to look for recurrence or advise the patient to seek advice if the lesion recurs at a later date. Refer if the lesion recurs.
- Check the patient for other non-melanoma skin cancers.

- Reassure the patient that the lesion was harmless but that if it had been left, it might have progressed to a skin cancer many years later.
- Advise the patient to return early if the lesion recurs or if any other persistent or non-healing lesions develop.
- If on review you find other skin tumours, you should arrange dermatological assessment relatively urgently (about 4–6 weeks)—the next week if you discover a melanoma.
- If the patient's skin is generally sun-damaged, you may prefer to refer the patient to the dermatology outpatient department for a general skin examination.

'Patch of Bowen's disease, incompletely excised'

- This can be managed in a number of different ways depending on such factors as site, size of residual lesion, and age of patient.
- Refer for dermatological assessment within about 4–6 weeks.

Keratoacanthoma

A report of such a lesion will nearly always conclude:

'...although the clinical history and histological appearances support the diagnosis of keratoacanthoma, the diagnosis of squamous cell carcinoma cannot be completely excluded on this specimen.'

This report *must not* be filed and forgotten! Consider carefully how to proceed. Much will depend on your preoperative clinical diagnosis, the site of the lesion, the age of the patient, and whether or not excision has been complete. If the clinical diagnosis of keratoacanthoma is in any doubt, the lesion should be managed as an SCC.

'Keratoacanthoma, completely excised'

- No further surgery is necessary.
- Tell the patient that this was almost certainly a benign lesion but that occasionally it can recur. Advise the patient to attend for review once in about 3 months for you to check the scar, and to return earlier if the lesion recurs.
- If the lesion recurs, this suggests that the original lesion was an SCC. The patient should be urgently referred (for an appointment within 2 weeks). This type of SCC is more aggressive than that arising in a solar keratosis.

'Keratoacanthoma, incompletely excised'

- Because of the risk of missing and inappropriately treating an SCC, you may prefer to discuss the patient with the dermatologist. Alternatively, an urgent hospital referral may be appropriate, requesting the patient to be seen within 2 weeks.

- Further surgery or radiotherapy is usually indicated to remove any residual lesion. Occasionally, no further treatment is necessary and a wait and see approach can be adopted. This decision is best taken by a specialist.
- Reassure the patient that the lesion was almost certainly not cancerous, but that it was not completely removed and that it may rarely recur. Advise the patient that this lesion can sometimes turn out to be a type of skin cancer, again stressing the point that this is a good type of cancer to have and is nothing to do with 'mole skin cancer'. Even if it subsequently becomes clear that it was a skin cancer, the outlook is good.

Squamous cell carcinoma

The realisation that you have removed an SCC usually comes as an alarming surprise. You should consider the management in two stages. First is management of the lesion itself. Second, the rest of the skin should be checked for other non-melanoma skin cancers, which are known to develop and will need treating. All patients should be discussed by the multidisciplinary skin cancer team.

'Squamous cell carcinoma, completely excised'

- *Relax*. If the patient is elderly or frail, no further treatment is necessary. If the lesion is well differentiated and has been completely excised, no further treatment is usually needed, and recurrence is unlikely. Long-term follow-up for well-differentiated lesions is no longer advocated. Refer the patient if the lesion recurs. Ideally, check the rest of the patient's skin. In England and Wales, if a GP inadvertently excises an SCC, the patient will usually be discussed at the local skin cancer multidisciplinary meeting.
- If the tumour is moderately or poorly differentiated, even if it has been completely excised, it is preferable to seek the dermatologist's advice on further management as further surgery may be needed.
- In younger patients, with or without obvious sun damage, consider referral for a full skin check and education about non-melanoma skin cancer and sun avoidance. Referral is also an opportunity to review the histopathology and check the excision margins. Patients should be seen preferably within about 6–8 weeks of excision.
- Reassure the patient that the tumour has been completely removed. Explain that this is non-melanoma skin cancer that may invade locally but does not usually spread internally. Further surgery is seldom necessary. Warn the patient that other non-melanoma skin cancers may occur, and ask the patient to return if any other persistent or non-healing lesions develop.

'Squamous cell carcinoma, incompletely excised'

- This is not such good news, but there is still no need to panic. Refer the patient urgently as he or she will require further specialist assessment and treatment.
- In England, an individual treatment plan will usually be agreed when the patient is discussed by the multidisciplinary skin cancer team. You should therefore refer the patient and/or discuss the case with the dermatologist.
- A further small surgical procedure carried out by the dermatologist may occasionally suffice, but referral to a plastic surgeon or radiotherapist is sometimes necessary. This will be decided at the multidisciplinary skin cancer team meeting.
- Again, be positive in your consultation with the patient, discussing the issues raised in the previous example. You should also discuss the need for referral and further treatment.

Basal cell carcinoma

Basal cell carcinomas are very slowly growing, locally invasive tumours. Some GPs who are suitably trained and meet the criteria outlined in the national guidance may elect to excise them for those who are elderly and frail as this is more convenient for the patient. Basal cell carcinomas are sometimes discovered only after histopathological examination of an excised lesion. It is important to remember that if a patient presents with one BCC, there is a strong possibility of a second tumour developing within the next 5 years. Follow-up involves looking both for recurrence and for second tumours. The patient is also more likely to have other non-melanoma skin cancers and solar keratoses.

Where possible, surgical excision is the preferred option for BCCs, although other management options are sometimes indicated. If you remove a BCC, particularly multiple lesions, from a very young patient, it is worth referring the patient for a dermatological opinion to exclude the diagnosis of Gorlin syndrome (a familial cancer syndrome).

'Nodular basal cell carcinoma, completely excised'

- No further surgery is required.
- Reassure the patient that although this is skin cancer, it is the 'good' type of skin cancer that never spreads to any other part of the body and is not life-threatening. It is usually only a nuisance, but if left would continue to enlarge and invade locally.
- It is often useful to clarify that this is not 'mole' skin cancer. Many patients who have had a BCC removed will tell you at a later date that it was a melanoma.
- There is no real need for you to review the patient if the lesion has been completely removed.
- Either ask the patient to return if the scar changes or arrange an annual review if you feel the patient is unlikely to report with a recurrence or a new tumour.

'Nodular basal cell carcinoma, incompletely excised'

- Further surgery is indicated, but only to remove residual tumour.
- There is no urgency about referral, but 4–6 weeks is preferable.
- Depending upon the site, arrange referral to either a dermatologist or a plastic surgeon.
- Discuss the diagnosis and prognosis as outlined in the previous section.

'Morphoeic basal cell carcinoma' or 'Features of a morphoeic-type tumour are seen'

- This is a rarer type of BCC that is more difficult to manage, and recurrence is more likely.
- The margins of excision are often difficult to define both clinically and histologically.
- Refer to the dermatologist for further assessment (within 4–6 weeks). The patient will be discussed by the multidisciplinary skin cancer team and a management plan agreed.
- Give the patient positive advice about the diagnosis, as previously described, but warn about the need for further surgery or radiotherapy to prevent local recurrence.

'Multicentric/superficial basal cell carcinoma... the margin of excision is less than the distance between tumour nests'

- As the name implies, these are 'many-centred' and are often more extensive than is first apparent. They are more likely to occur on the trunk and are frequently multiple.
- Where the margin of excision is less than the distance between tumour nests, you cannot be sure that the tumour has been completely removed.
- In these tumours, there is a possibility of further residual tumour nests just outside the excision margin even if the histology report indicates complete excision.
- Refer the patient to a dermatologist, to be seen within 6–8 weeks.
- If the lesion has been clinically completely removed and the patient is elderly or frail, arrange reviews at 3 and 6 months. Annual review is only necessary if you think the patient would not report a recurrence.
- Once again, the patient can be reassured that there is no cause for concern and that this type of skin cancer grows slowly and is only locally invasive. Wherever possible, the patient should be instructed to check for recurrence and for other similar lesions, and to seek medical advice if worried about either.
- Hospital referral is indicated if a recurrence develops.
- Remember that superficial BCC has a range of treatment options (see page 131), including non-surgical treatments, and that extensive surgery is not appropriate.

Other unusual reports

If a fleshy lesion proves to be a neurofibroma or a Schwannoma, you should establish whether the lesion was solitary. Check the whole of the patient's skin, looking for café-au-lait patches and axillary freckling. If you discover features of neurofibromatosis, refer the patient for a full assessment. Remember, however, that a solitary neurofibroma may occur without the patient having neurofibromatosis.

Eccrine hydradenomas and syringomas are relatively rare benign sweat gland tumours that are sometimes removed without a preoperative diagnosis.

The bottom line

- If you remove lesions only when you are confident of the clinical diagnosis, the histological diagnosis will rarely cause any difficulty.
- If you do not understand the report, do not ignore it. Ask your dermatologist or histopathologist for help.
- If you receive an unusual or unexpected report, you should always evaluate it and decide a management plan before discussing it with the patient.
- In the case of a surprising report, for example Kaposi's sarcoma in a teenager with no predisposing factors for HIV infection, the histology should be reviewed before discussing the diagnosis with the patient. If the lesion proves to be benign, you will have saved the patient a period of unnecessary anxiety.
- Seek specialist advice if the histology report is particularly unusual or unexpected, for example a BCC in a 25 year old or a keratoacanthoma in a 30 year old. The skin lesion could be a marker of a familial cancer syndrome requiring screening for internal malignancy.

What is dermoscopy?

Chapter 10

Dermoscopy

Jonathan Bowling

INTRODUCTION

Chapter 9 described the range of skin lesions and provided information about how to manage them, making reference to the management of uncertainty when there is diagnostic doubt. This chapter provides an introduction to dermoscopy and how it can assist the clinician to help lessen diagnostic doubt.

WHAT IS DERMOSCOPY?

Dermoscopy is a technique recognised worldwide as proven, in the hands of suitably trained clinicians, to increase diagnostic accuracy for diagnosing skin lesions, both benign and malignant. The technique incorporates two of the fundamental principles for skin lesion diagnosis, namely illumination and magnification. By combining these principles in portable devices (dermatoscopes), greater information is available for diagnosis.

All clinicians managing patients with skin lesions should become familiar with dermoscopy, and there are a range of texts and educational tools available to develop skills in dermoscopy. Accessing these resources should be supported by good and ongoing clinical experience of using the technique.

DON'T FORGET ▶▶
Dermoscopy provides additional information to confirm a diagnosis. It should never be used in isolation, but forms part of the overall assessment of a patient and the skin lesion, which should include a history, examination, and dermoscopy.

Basic principles

The skin surface (stratum corneum) is not smooth, and therefore scatters light in all directions. If this scatter phenomenon can be overcome, light can penetrate deeper within the skin before reflecting back to the surface, thereby yielding greater information on the deeper structures lying within it. Dermoscopy uses light and magnification to achieve this by either the application of a surface interface medium, such as alcohol gel, and/or by the use of polarised light.

The usual principles for skin lesion diagnosis, namely the shape, size, and colour of a lesion, are revealed as relatively crude data upon which to base a diagnosis when dermoscopy is adopted and integrated into clinical practice. The technique reveals the diagnostic morphological detail within the lesion, thereby revealing its true biological potential.

Let's use an example to illustrate the point. An art dealer at an auction would not base his or her opinion on the size of the painting, the shape of the frame used, how long it has been hanging on a wall, or the number of colours used! Their opinion would be based upon the brushstrokes used (the artistic detail) to determine whether it is a genuine Monet, a Van Gogh, or a fake. Admittedly, however, these principles may not apply to all works of art!

Dermoscopy devices

There are three main types of device:
- Non-polarised contact devices.
- Polarised non-contact devices.
- Hybrid devices with both polarised non-contact and non-polarised contact modes.

There are subtle differences between polarised and non-polarised devices in terms of how some skin structures are seen. The choice of device is usually determined by a number of factors. For instance, if the technique is to be used for diagnosing individual lesions, for referral and/or biopsy, a device that allows the greatest information for diagnosis should be considered, namely one with the contact non-polarised mode. If the clinician wants to examine multiple lesions, however, a device with the polarised non-contact mode would be preferable, because of its ease and speed of examination.

A range of devices are available; these are in constant evolution and older devices are fast becoming obsolete. The choice of device will depend upon numerous factors, not least of which is personal preference.

WHAT ARE THE BENEFITS OF DERMOSCOPY?

Increasing the accuracy of diagnosis of benign lesions

Benign skin lesions are numerous and are frequently influenced by internal (inflammation) and external (trauma) factors. Greater confidence in identifying these common changes in benign lesions can result in fewer referrals to specialists and a reduction in the number of unnecessary skin surgery procedures. Not only is this good for patients because of the avoidance of unnecessary surgery, but it also leads to a better use of health-care resources.

The following section describes the four most common benign skin lesions that have typical dermoscopic features which can support and aid clinical diagnosis.

Seborrhoeic keratoses

These common lesions have a range of typical dermoscopic features that can help with diagnosis. These are shown diagrammatically in Figure 10.1.

Figure 10.2a shows the naked eye appearance of a typical seborrhoeic keratosis with the classical keratotic brown pigmented papules and plaques, while Figure 10.2b shows the dermoscopic features, which include comedo-like openings and milia-like cysts.

Haemangiomas and angiokeratomas

A diagrammatic representation of the typical dermoscopic features of haemangiomas and angiokeratomas is shown in Figure 10.3.

The typical naked eye appearance includes red/purple papules and plaques (Figure 10.4a), while the dermoscopic features include purple lacunes (Figure 10.4b).

Dermatofibromas

Dermoscopically, dermatofibromas are characterised by an obvious central scarred area. This is shown diagrammatically in Figure 10.5.

The typical clinical features of a firm dermal papule on an extremity are seen in Figure 10.6a, and the dermoscopic features, which include a peripheral pseudonetwork and a scar-like central area, are demonstrated in Figure 10.6b.

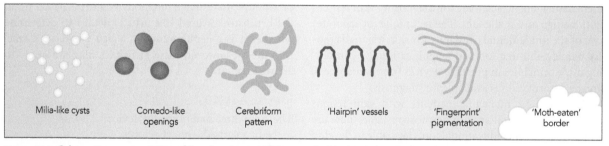

| Milia-like cysts | Comedo-like openings | Cerebriform pattern | 'Hairpin' vessels | 'Fingerprint' pigmentation | 'Moth-eaten' border |

Figure 10.1   Schematic representation of the dermoscopic features of seborrhoeic keratosis.

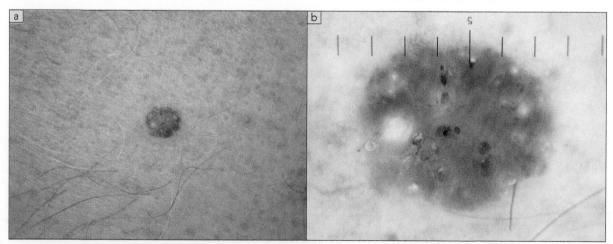

Figure 10.2   Clinical (a) and dermoscopic (b) features of a classical seborrhoeic keratosis.

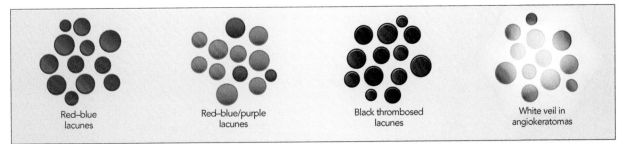

Figure 10.3 Schematic representation of the dermoscopic features of haemangiomas and angiokeratomas.

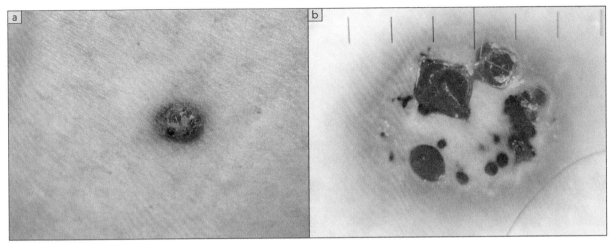

Figure 10.4 (a) Clinical and (b) dermoscopic features of an angiokeratoma.

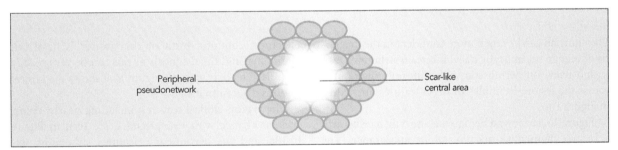

Figure 10.5 Schematic representation of the dermoscopic features of a dermatofibroma.

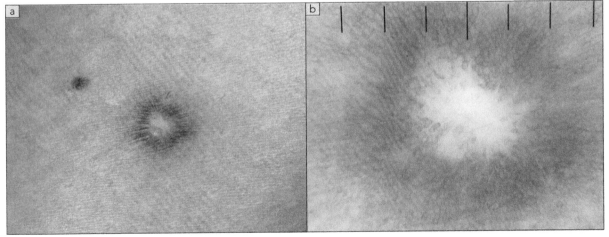

Figure 10.6 (a) Clinical and (b) dermoscopic features of a dermatofibroma.

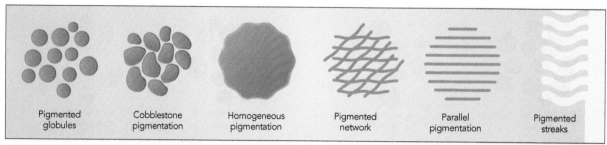

Figure 10.7 Schematic representation of the dermoscopic features seen in benign melanocytic lesions.

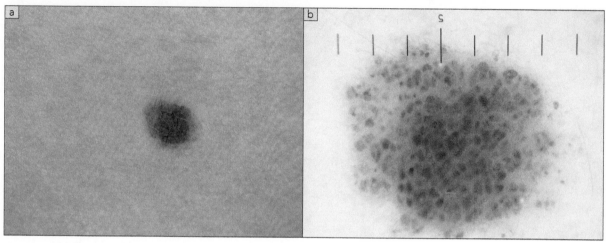

Figure 10.8 (a) Clinical and (b) dermoscopic features of a benign melanocytic naevus.

Benign melanocytic naevi

The clinician can be much more confident in the diagnosis of benign melanocytic naevi if certain structures seen within naevi on dermoscopy are uniformly distributed across the lesion. Examples of these features are shown in Figure 10.7.

Figure 10.8a shows a benign melanocytic naevus with a brown pigmented maculopapular appearance. The dermoscopic features (Figure 10.8b) include brown pigmented globular and central cobblestone pigmentation.

Increasing accuracy of skin cancer diagnosis

Skin cancers do not appear, they grow! Dermoscopic features seen in larger skin cancers are frequently seen in smaller tumours. As clinicians, we should endeavour to diagnose tumours at the earliest point in their evolution, thereby broadening the treatment options and subsequently reducing the morbidity from skin cancer and improving patient care. Dermoscopy is particularly helpful in supporting the diagnosis of basal cell carcinoma and malignant melanoma.

Basal cell carcinoma

The most common form of skin cancer is basal cell carcinoma, and the diagnosis of this can be very readily supported by dermoscopy. Figure 10.9 shows the typical features diagrammatically.

The typical clinical features, including pearly, cystic, nodular change with telangiectasia, are seen in Figure 10.10a, and the dermoscopic features, arborising telangiectasia and blue–grey ovoid nests, are shown in Figure 10.10b.

Malignant melanoma

Recognition of the dermoscopic features seen in malignant melanoma should result in an ability to diagnose melanoma at increasingly earlier stages of evolution. Figure 10.11 shows the typical features diagrammatically.

The typical clinical features, including an irregularly pigmented maculopapular lesion, are seen in Figure 10.12a, and the dermoscopic features, including an irregular pigmented network, globules, streaks, and pigmentation, are shown in Figure 10.12b.

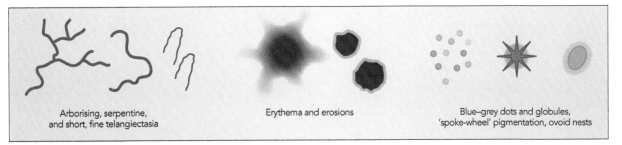

Figure 10.9 Schematic representation of the dermoscopic features of basal cell carcinoma.

Arborising, serpentine, and short, fine telangiectasia

Erythema and erosions

Blue–grey dots and globules, 'spoke-wheel' pigmentation, ovoid nests

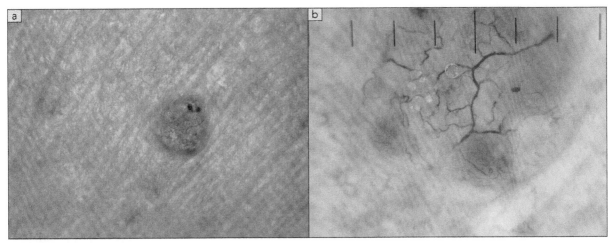

Figure 10.10 (a) Clinical and (b) dermoscopic features of a basal cell carcinoma.

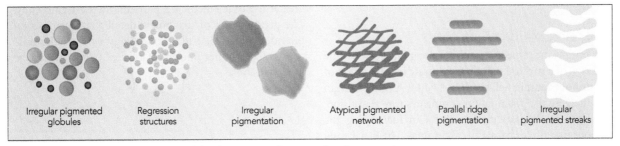

Figure 10.11 Schematic representation of the dermoscopic features of malignant melanoma.

Irregular pigmented globules

Regression structures

Irregular pigmentation

Atypical pigmented network

Parallel ridge pigmentation

Irregular pigmented streaks

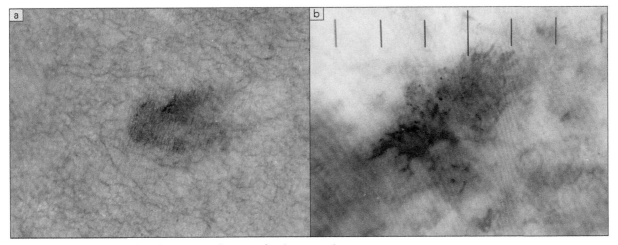

Figure 10.12 (a) Clinical and (b) dermoscopic features of malignant melanoma.

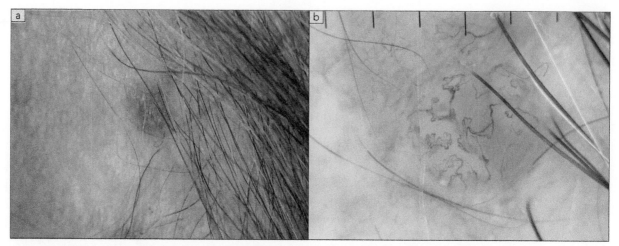

Figure 10.13 Basal cell carcinoma. (a) Naked eye view. (b) Findings on dermoscopy, demonstrating the extended margins of the tumour.

> **GOLDEN RULE** ✳
> Never base a clinical diagnosis on the presence or absence of one dermoscopic structure alone. The diagnosis should always be based upon the summation of information gained from the clinical history and the clinical and dermoscopic examination.

Improving skin cancer surgery

An important aspect of skin cancer surgery is the marking of a surgical margin as accurate identification of the tumour margin will result in a better surgical margin and increase the potential for complete surgical excision. Dermoscopy is particularly helpful in identifying the tumour margin for basal cell carcinomas. The facial basal cell carcinoma in Figure 10.13a shows a pearly papule on the left temple; dermoscopy (Figure 10.13b), however, clearly shows an extension of the vascular structures (arborising vessels) superiorly.

DERMOSCOPY: THE FUTURE

Dermoscopy allows the opportunity for suitably trained specialists and generalists to confidently diagnose a variety of skin conditions and not just skin tumours. In addition to extending the use of dermoscopy in general face-to-face skin examination, the future of skin lesion and skin cancer management is likely to incorporate a greater use of telemedicine, particularly teledermoscopy. The greater level of diagnostic detail that dermoscopy provides means that teledermatology with teledermoscopy is likely to become an established part of the triage of skin lesions.

DERMOSCOPY TIPS

- Use alcohol gel to avoid cross-contamination.
- Keep the devices fully charged.
- Examine as many lesions as possible!

FURTHER READING

Bowling J (2011) Introduction to dermoscopy. In *Diagnostic Dermoscopy: The Illustrated Guide.* Oxford: Wiley-Blackwell.

Chapter 11

Carpal tunnel syndrome, Dupuytren's contracture, trigger finger, and ganglia: knowledge

Tim T. Wang and Simon Eccles

INTRODUCTION

In this chapter, we consider the causes and consequences of these four wrist and hand conditions, followed by guidance for suitable management. There are numerous conditions that affect the wrist and hand that may be amenable to surgical intervention, but these have been chosen not only because they are commonly encountered, but also because correct management can have a significant influence on future hand function. Details of actual treatments can be found in Chapter 22.

CARPAL TUNNEL SYNDROME

Carpal tunnel syndrome (CTS) is caused by pressure on the median nerve as it traverses the wrist. This results in localised ischaemia, endoneural oedema, and finally axonal loss with Wallerian degeneration. This leads to numbness, tingling, weakness, or muscle wasting in the hand and fingers.

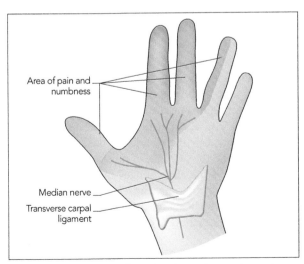

Figure 11.1 Distribution of pain/numbness in carpal tunnel syndrome.

The main symptom of CTS is intermittent numbness of the thumb, the index and middle fingers, and the radial half of the ring finger (Figure 11.1). In cases of proximal median nerve compression (also known as anterior interosseus nerve syndrome), patients commonly also present with weakness in flexor pollicis longus and in the flexor digitorum profundus to the index and middle fingers. This is clinically differentiated from true CTS by abnormal sensation over the thenar eminence as this is innervated by the palmar cutaneous branch of the median nerve, which arises 4–7 cm proximal to the carpal tunnel.

Causes

Traditionally considered most common in people performing repetitive hand and wrist movements, there is growing recognition that the condition is an inherited, slowly progressive, idiopathic peripheral mononeuropathy unrelated to work. Several medical conditions appear to trigger the onset of CTS:

- Obesity.
- Arthritis affecting the wrist.
- Acromegaly.
- Diabetes.
- Alcoholism.
- Hypothyroidism.
- Renal failure.
- Menopause, premenstrual syndrome, pregnancy, and the combined oral contraceptive pill.

There are common factors that appear to precipitate the onset of CTS in those prone to the disorder. These include occupations involving prolonged wrist flexion, most commonly heavy manual labour. Other triggers include:

- Sewing.
- Driving.
- Painting.
- Writing.
- Computer work with typing and using a mouse (although there are conflicting views on this).
- Using hand tools.
- Sports that involve gripping and frequent wrist movements.
- Playing certain musical instruments.

Epidemiology

CTS occurs most frequently in the 45–60 years age group. It is more common in women than men (3:1). The prevalence within the general population appears to be around 2.5–6.0% and increasing. It is also more common in white populations.

Clinical features

There is numbness of the palm, thumb, index finger, middle finger, and radial side of the ring finger, with weakness and wasting of the thumb. The pain almost always occurs at night or on waking. This is related to the fact that humans tend to sleep with flexed wrists as the strength of the flexor muscle groups outweighs that of the extensors.

With time, CTS may cause permanent nerve damage resulting in numbness, atrophy of the thenar eminence, and weakness of palmar abduction.

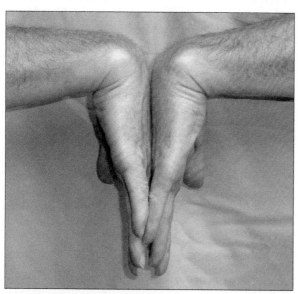

Figure 11.2 Phalen's test.

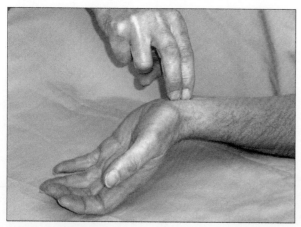

Figure 11.3 Tinel's test.

Diagnosis

Along with the history and examination, there are several simple tests that can help to confirm pressure on and irritation of the median nerve.

Phalen's sign

The patient is asked to flex the wrist gently as far as possible and then hold this position (Figure 11.2). A positive test is one that results in numbness (and/or pain) in the median nerve distribution within 60 seconds when the wrist is held in this acute flexion. The more quickly the numbness starts, the more acute the nerve compression.

Tinel's sign

Tinel's sign is a sign of neural regeneration. This is performed by lightly tapping the skin over the median nerve as it traverses the carpal tunnel to elicit a sensation of tingling or 'pins and needles' in the nerve distribution (Figure 11.3). It is less sensitive but slightly more specific than Phalen's sign. During early, acute nerve compression, ischaemia is localised, resulting in a negative Tinel's sign. Similarly, it will also be negative in late-stage disease predominated by axonal loss with no neural regeneration occurring.

However, the median nerve originates from the brachial plexus, running down the upper arm with the brachial artery through the cubital fossa and passing between the two heads of pronator teres before running down to the carpal tunnel beside the flexor muscles of the hand (Figure 11.4). It should be remembered that cervical nerve root entrapment at the C7 level will also give pain in the hand and numbness of the middle finger, so it is important to check the neck at the time of the initial examination.

Thus, any disturbance to the nerve along this route may mimic CTS. Patients may complain of pain radiating up the arm to the shoulder. If there is confusion about the origin of the nerve involvement, nerve conduction studies and electromyography may help to locate the problem (Figure 11.5).

Treatment

Measures to relieve pressure within the carpal tunnel vary from watchful waiting and trigger avoidance to elevating the wrist and/or wearing a wrist brace at night, through to injections of corticosteroids and finally surgical release. The decision of which treatment to use should be guided by the severity of the symptoms, the age of onset, and the presence of muscle wasting.

In young individuals (younger than 30 years) with mild unilateral symptoms, the condition may resolve within 6 months. Changing the computer keyboard or mouse action may relieve occupational triggers.

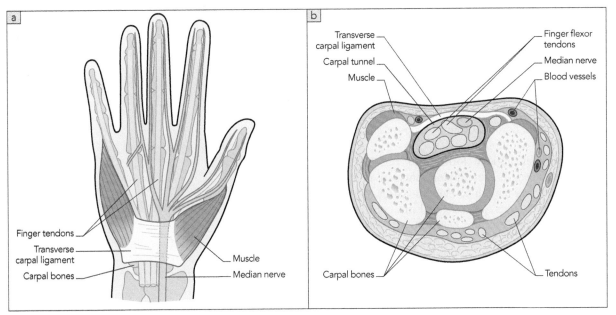

Figure 11.4 Carpal tunnel anatomy: (a) palmar aspect; (b) cross-section at wrist.

If a brace or splint is to be used (Figure 11.6), it should be for those with mild symptoms, particularly when the cause is temporary (e.g., pregnancy), and it should be designed to hold the wrist in a neutral position.

In the past, non-steroidal anti-inflammatory drugs and diuretics were advocated; however, the best evidence of effectiveness lies with injected corticosteroids and surgery.

In deciding the correct treatment for the individual it helps to classify the condition by severity (based on the British Society for Surgery of the Hand classification, undated):

- *Mild*—intermittent paraesthesia:
  – Nocturnal.
  – Position of hand.
  – Pregnancy.
  – Hypothyroidism.
- *Moderate*—constant paraesthesia:
  – Interference with activities of daily living.
  – Constant waking at night.
  – Reversible numbness and/or pain (perhaps by clenching and unclenching of the fist or shaking the hand).
- *Severe*:
  – Constant numbness or pain.
  – Wasting of the thumb muscles.
  – Weakness of the thumb muscles.

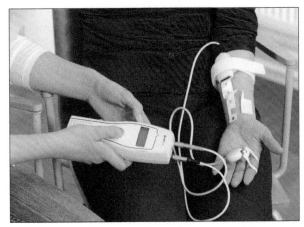

Figure 11.5 Electromyography equipment suitable for near-patient testing in primary care, seen with electrodes attached to the patient.

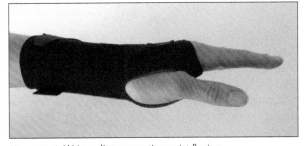

Figure 11.6 Wrist splint preventing wrist flexion.

Treatment choices

For those with mild symptoms, conservative measures such as wrist splints should be recommended; alternatively, treatment can be with corticosteroid injections.

For those with moderate symptoms, the initial options remain the same as for mild symptoms, but with the proviso that those with diabetes or symptoms lasting for over a year are more likely to need surgery.

For those with severe symptoms, those with diabetes, or when symptoms have lasted for more than a year, surgical treatment should be recommended (see Chapter 22).

DUPUYTREN'S CONTRACTURE

Causes

Dupuytren's contracture is a fibroproliferative disorder of unknown aetiology characterised by the formation of nodules, cords, and contractures of the connective tissue within the palm of the hand. It is named after the French surgeon, Baron Guillaume Dupuytren, who first described the condition in 1834.

The nodules initially form from fibroblasts that produce collagen. As these nodules increase in number and contract, they tend to develop into cords. With time, the connective tissue contracts, and this contracture in turn causes a fixed flexion deformity of one or more fingers.

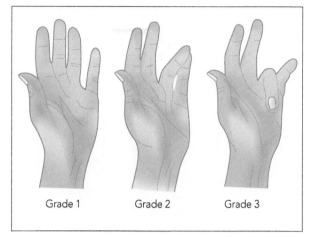

Figure 11.7 Appearance of Dupuytren's contracture.

Aetiology

The condition commonly affects patients of northern European ancestry, with 10–39% of patients having a family history through a proposed autosomal dominant mode of inheritance (McGrouther, 2005). It is more common in men than women, often occurring in later life. Up to 20% of men over 60 years old, and 20% of women over 80 years old, are affected.

Several conditions are associated with Dupuytren's disease, including diabetes mellitus, epilepsy, and alcoholic liver disease.

Clinical features

The most commonly affected digits are the ring and little fingers (Figure 11.7). Affected palmar fascia is known as a cord, where normal palmar fascia is referred to as a band (Figure 11.8). Flexion contracture of the meta-carpophalangeal joint (MCPJ) is caused by the pretendinous cord. The formation of central, spiral, and lateral cords is responsible for flexion contractures of the proximal interphalangeal joint (PIPJ).

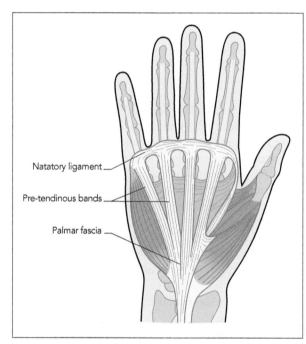

Figure 11.8 Diagram of digital and palmar fascia.

Diagnosis

Patients may initially present with a solitary nodule in their palm. This progressively extends to form palpable contractures overlying one or several rays and may extend into the fingers. Over time, patients develop fixed flexion contractures of their MCPJ and PIPJ, with resulting loss of function.

Clinically, this can be confirmed by Hueston's table-top test. The patient is asked to place the affected palm flat upon a table. If all fingers cannot be simultaneously laid flat upon the surface, the test is considered positive.

Treatment

Once there are 30° of contracture over a joint, interference with daily living becomes significant.

Traditionally, treatment has been limited to surgery (see Chapter 22). Surgery to correct Dupuytren's disease has a significant complication rate and is therefore not undertaken lightly. Patients opting for surgery must demonstrate progression of the disease and significant loss of function. This commonly presents as worsening joint contractures, one indication being MCPJ contracture reaching about 30°. In comparison, any degree of PIPJ flexion contracture is challenging to correct completely, and thus any degree of PIPJ involvement represents an additional indication.

Two types of surgery are available:

- *Fasciotomy*, in which the contracted tissue is cut to relieve the tension (used for mild contractures).
- *Fasciectomy*, in which the contracted tissue is excised (used for more extreme or recurrent contractures).

With fasciotomy, the procedure can be either closed or open. The closed procedure is called a needle fasciotomy and involves cutting the fibrous tissue via a percutaneous needle (Figure 11.9). Recurrence rates are, however, high, with 50% of patients showing recurrence of the contracture within 5 years. With an open fasciotomy, the fibrous material is divided via a skin incision.

Surgery more commonly involves removing fibrous tissue via an open approach—a fasciectomy. The amount of tissue removed can vary from partial excision to complete excision of the fibrous material or complete removal, including the overlying skin, followed by a full-thickness skin graft (dermofasciectomy). Recurrence rates are lower (around 8%) than with a fasciotomy, but recovery is more prolonged and there are more significant surgical complications.

Non-surgical treatments

A relatively new treatment involves injecting the enzyme collagenase from *Clostridium histolyticum* into the thickened cord (Figure 11.10). The collagenase breaks down the collagen within the cord, and initial results appear encouraging. The injection is deposited into the chosen cord. The digit is then kept still for 24 hours to allow localised enzymatic activity. At 24 hours, the clinician attempts to straighten the digit. This procedure disrupts the cord and should allow free movement. The treatment can be repeated twice at monthly intervals.

Alternatively, radiation therapy may delay progression of the disease and relieve symptoms. This treatment is currently available only in specialist centres, and long-term results have yet to be generally accepted. Physiotherapy, ultrasound, and oral drug therapies have all failed to show a beneficial effect.

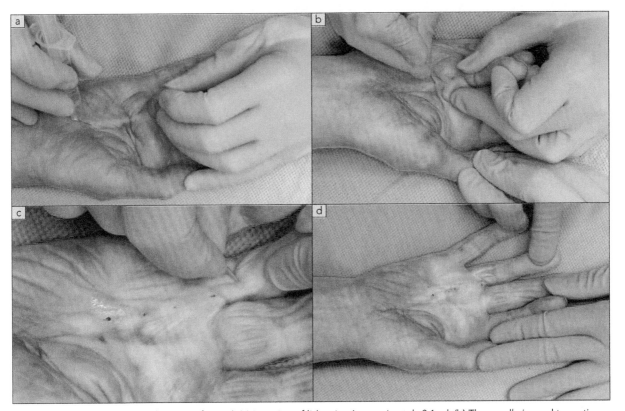

Figure 11.9 Needle fasciotomy being performed. (a) Injection of lidocaine (approximately 0.1 ml. (b) The needle is used to section the fibrous band. (c) The hand after the first sectioning. After the process, there will be two or three more similar puncture wounds. (d) After the procedure. A splint was applied to help with joint contracture but no physiotherapy was needed. The patient returned to normal activities the next day.

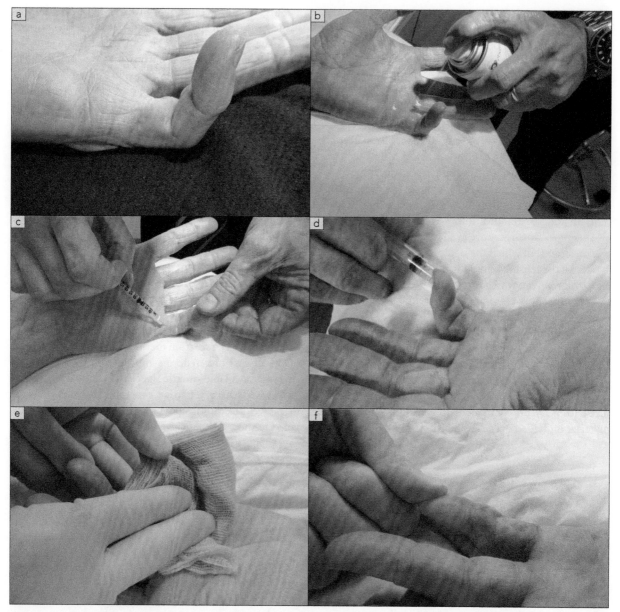

Figure 11.10 Collagenase injection for Dupuytren's contracture. (a) The little finger affected by a cord. (b) The skin is initially numbed with cryoanaesthesia prior to injection. (c) Injecting the collagenase (Xiapen). (d) After 2 days, local anaesthetic is infiltrated prior to (e) manipulation. (f) This results in full correction. (By permission of David Warwick, www.handsurgery.co.uk.)

TRIGGER FINGER

Causes

The flexor tendons of the fingers and thumbs cross specific fibro-osseous canals known as pulleys as they run from the MCPJs to the distal interphalangeal joints (DIPJs). These pulleys prevent bowstringing of the digital flexor tendons during finger flexion, which creates grip strength. There are a number of important annular pulleys (A1–A5) and less critical cruciate pulleys (C1–C3), the latter providing support and stability to the tendon (Figure 11.11).

Trigger finger or thumb occurs when there is either a swelling (nodule) of the flexor tendon or a narrowing of the A1 pulley causing the flexor tendon to become impinged as it passes through the A1 pulley at the metacarpal head (Figure 11.12).

Epidemiology

Trigger finger may be primary or secondary. *Primary* trigger finger affects females four to six times more commonly than males, with a lifetime incidence of 2.2% (Stahl *et al.*, 1997). In contrast, *secondary* trigger finger is frequently seen in patients with diabetes, gout, or rheumatic disease, and is associated with a worse prognosis (Wolfe, 2011). It most commonly occurs in patients aged in their 50s to early 60s. Congenital cases are caused by a nodule on the flexor tendon.

Clinical features

Because the tendon catches as it passes through the A1 pulley, the patient can experience difficulty with both extending and flexing the digit, but most commonly with extending it. When the tendon does manage to pass through the pulley, the digit flicks out into extension, often with significant pain (the releasing of the 'trigger'). Extension may require assistance from the contralateral hand. On flexion, some patients may have a similar problem in reverse.

Diagnosis

Trigger finger, or stenosing tenosynovitis of the fingers and thumb, is a common cause of pain and disability in the hand. Patients frequently complain of a dull pain around the affected MCPJ.

The term 'triggering' of an affected digit suggests that it adopts a flexed posture unable to be actively straightened. Commonly, however, as mentioned above, the finger or thumb can be straightened passively. On clinical examination, a nodule or 'click' is frequently palpable overlying the MCPJ as the affected digit is gently flexed and extended.

It is not uncommon for a locked trigger digit to be misdiagnosed as 'true locking' of the digit. In these circumstances, an injection of the local anaesthetic into the flexor sheath will frequently allow passive extension of the digit and confirm the diagnosis. In addition, pressure from the examiner's hand over the proximal aspect of the A1 pulley may allow the tendon to slip through, confirming that the digit is not locked.

There are no investigations that will confirm the diagnosis—instead it is confirmed by the history and examination.

Treatment

Although treatments including rest and splinting of the digit have been tried, the most universally agreed management plan is the trial of two or even three corticosteroid injections, followed by surgery if the condition is unresponsive. Corticosteroid injection can frequently alleviate symptoms and delay the need for surgery, and has a quoted success rate of between 50% and 92%. However, patients who have failed to improve with two corticosteroid injections, those with severe symptoms, or those who experience locking of their finger in a fixed flexion posture, will usually require operative release.

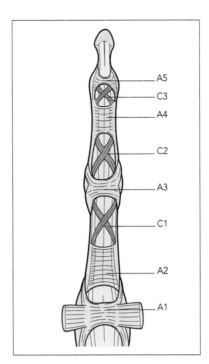

Figure 11.11 Digital flexor pulleys; annular (A1–A5) and cruciate (C1–C3).

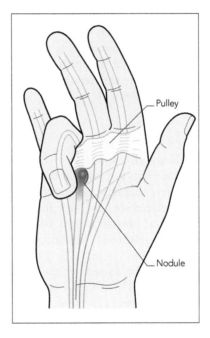

Figure 11.12 The tendon nodule in trigger finger.

GANGLIA

Causes

The cause of a ganglion is not fully understood, but it may be a degenerative process in the mesoblastic tissues surrounding the joint. Histologically, ganglia are composed of a thin connective tissue (collagen) capsule without a synovial or epithelial lining. The contents consist of glucosamine, globulin, and albumin in a hyaluronic acid-rich mucin.

Ganglia may arise from joints or tendon sheaths. Wrist joint ganglia are found most commonly on the dorsal aspect (scapholunate joint) or palmar (radiocarpal or scaphotrapezial joints) aspect of the wrist. They also exist as:

- Flexor sheath ganglia.
- Mucous cysts originating from the DIPJ.

Epidemiology

Ganglia are the most common soft-tissue tumours found in the hand and wrist, but their incidence is difficult to ascertain since many are asymptomatic and not brought to medical attention. Historical evidence, however, suggests an incidence of between 25 and 43 per 100,000 population. They occur more commonly in women and most commonly in the second to fourth decades. However, they are also common in children (but usually resolve within a year) and the elderly.

Clinical features

Ganglia are cystic swellings surrounded by a fibrous tissue wall, occurring in the vicinity of joint capsules and tendon sheaths. These are commonly associated with a constant aching pain, exacerbated by joint motion, although up to one-third of ganglia present without pain. Most have crystal-clear gelatinous contents, unless bleeding has occurred.

The most common site is the dorsum of the hand (60–80%; Figure 11.13), followed by the volar aspect of the wrist adjacent to the radial artery (15–20%). Smaller ganglia occur in the flexor sheaths of the fingers, dorsum of foot, ankle, and head of fibula.

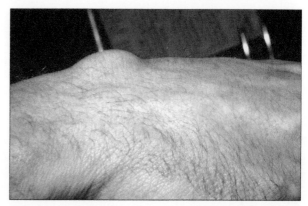

Figure 11.13 Typical ganglion on the dorsum of the wrist.

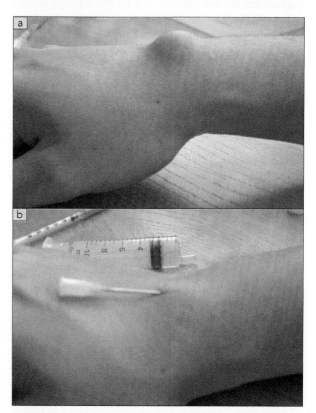

Figure 11.14 a) Dorsal wrist ganglion. (b) The same ganglion with a 19 G needle in it, and in the distance, the aspirating syringe containing the clear gel contents.

Diagnosis

The diagnosis is usually made clinically from the history and examination, although transillumination and needle aspiration may help to confirm it. Ultrasound and/or magnetic resonance imaging can be used to confirm the clinical diagnosis. The most important aspect to diagnosis is eliminating swellings due to alternative causes, such as extensor tenosynovitis or radial artery aneurysm.

Treatment

Untreated, many ganglia disappear spontaneously. In a 6-year prospective study, 33% of dorsal and 45% of volar ganglia resolved spontaneously. Many others appear not to trouble the patient and may be left alone.

Treatment is indicated if the patient is complaining of unacceptable symptoms—usually pain or limitation of function—or, on occasion, for aspiration of the clear gel-like material to confirm the benign nature of the swelling.

Many treatments have been advocated, but all carry a recurrence rate, and the patient should be advised of this accordingly:

- Simple rupture of the cyst by pressure occasionally succeeds (medical folklore often involved hitting the hand with a copy of the Bible).
- Aspiration with a large-bore (19 G) needle (Figure 11.14) can be employed, followed by splinting of the wrist.

There is evidence to show that the recurrence rate reduces with repeat aspiration (from greater than 50% after one to less than 20% after three aspirations). Aspiration and injection of sclerosant or hyaluronidase reduces recurrence, but not as effectively as surgery. There is no evidence that aspiration followed by injection of steroid confers any benefit over simple aspiration.

The British Society for Surgery of the Hand comment on two large studies that looked at treatment for volar and dorsal wrist ganglia over 5 and 6 years respectively (Dias and Buch, 2003; Dias *et al.*, 2007):

- No significant difference was identified between the groups that had received reassurance, aspiration, or surgery.
- Patient satisfaction was higher in the group that had received surgical intervention.

Treatment for symptomatic ganglia therefore remains controversial.

REFERENCES

Carpal tunnel syndrome

British Society for Surgery of the Hand (undated) Evidence for surgical treatment 1. Carpal tunnel syndrome (CTS). Available from: www.bssh.ac.uk/ education/guidelines/carpal_tunnel_syndrome.pdf (accessed July 2012).

Dupuytren's contracture

McGrouther DA (2005) Dupuytren's contracture. In Green DP, Hotchkiss R, Pederson W, Wolfe S, eds. *Green's Operative Hand Surgery*, 5th edn. Philadelphia: Elsevier.

Trigger finger

Stahl S, Kanter Y, Karnielli E (1997) Outcome of trigger finger treatment in diabetes. *Journal of Diabetes and its Complications* 11: 287–90.

Wolfe SW (2011) Tendinopathy. In: Wolfe SW, Hotchkiss RN, Pederson WC, Kozin SH, eds. *Green's Operative Hand Surgery*, 6th edn. Philadelphia: Elsevier, Chapter 62.

Ganglia

Dias J, Buch K (2003) Palmar wrist ganglion: Does intervention improve outcome? A prospective study of the natural history and patient-reported treatment outcomes. *Journal of Hand Surgery (Br)* 28: 172–6.

Dias JJ, Dhukaram V, Kumar P (2007) The natural history of untreated dorsal wrist ganglia and patient reported outcome 6 years after intervention. *Journal of Hand Surgery (Eur)* 32: 502–8.

FURTHER READING

Carpal tunnel syndrome

American Academy of Orthopaedic Surgeons (2008) Clinical practice guideline on the treatment of carpal tunnel syndrome. 2008. www.aaos.org/Research/ guidelines/CTSTreatmentGuideline.pdf (accessed July 2012).

Clinical Knowledge Summaries. Carpal tunnel syndrome—Management. Available from: www.cks.nhs. uk/carpal_tunnel_syndrome/management/scenario_ diagnosis#-344544 (accessed July 2012).

Ganglia

British Society for Surgery of the Hand. Evidence for surgical treatment 1. Wrist ganglion. Available from: www.bssh.ac.uk/education/guidelines/ganglion.pdf (accessed July 2012).

Chapter 12

Vasectomy: knowledge

Laurel Spooner and Tony Feltbower

INTRODUCTION

The ideal male contraceptive should be non-surgical, reversible, effective, not dependent on coitus, and should not alter androgen levels or libido. Several non-steroidal molecules and vaccines are being investigated in animal models, with the hope that male hormonal contraception may become a reality in the near future. In the meantime, vasectomy remains the gold standard for permanent male contraception, and this chapter will provide information on the technique. Details of the surgical procedure are in Chapter 23.

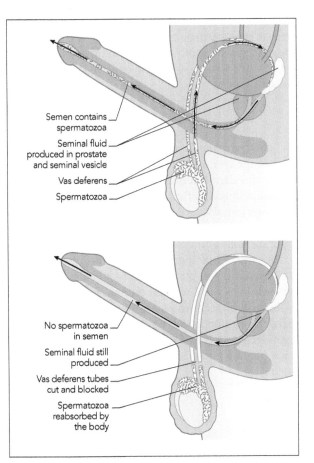

Semen contains spermatozoa

Seminal fluid produced in prostate and seminal vesicle

Vas deferens

Spermatozoa

No spermatozoa in semen

Seminal fluid still produced

Vas deferens tubes cut and blocked

Spermatozoa reabsorbed by the body

WHAT IS VASECTOMY?

Vasectomy is defined as a surgical procedure for male sterilisation for the purpose of permanent birth control. During the procedure, the vas deferens tubes (vasa deferentia) are divided and then occluded to prevent spermatozoa entering into the semen in the ejaculate (Figure 12.1). Therefore the semen does not contain spermatozoa, and the patient cannot father a child.

This procedure has been performed in one form or another for over 100 years. In the United Kingdom, it was only relatively recently (1968) that the first Family Planning Association vasectomy clinics opened. However, it was not until 4 years later, in 1972, that the UK National Health Service (NHS) Family Planning Amendment Act empowered local health authorities to provide vasectomies free at the point of delivery to the public. In other countries, male and female sterilisation was legalised as recently as 1983 (Turkey) and 1997 (Brazil). The main advance in male sterilisation has been in the development of non-scalpel vasectomy (NSV) in 1974 in China and more recently in other countries (1985 in the United States, and 1995 in the United Kingdom).

Before performing a vasectomy, the clinician needs a sound knowledge of the procedure. This chapter considers the following issues:

- Definition.
- Indications.
- Anatomy.
- Risks.
- Counselling.

In all other areas of minor surgery, the patient-care pathway includes clinical assessment, presumptive diagnosis, and surgery. Vasectomy is different because the patient undertakes his own assessment and diagnosis. In order for the patient to be fully informed, it is essential that the doctor offering a vasectomy service provides comprehensive counselling, so this is considered in some detail in this chapter. Surgical technique and post-vasectomy testing are considered in Chapter 23.

Figure 12.1 Anatomy (a) before and (b) after vasectomy.

INDICATIONS

The only ethical indication for vasectomy is for permanent, irreversible family planning.

ANATOMY

Spermatozoa are made in the testicles and mature in the epididymis. Each vas deferens originates at the tail of the epididymis and runs along the posterior border of the testis and the medial side of the epididymis, leaving the superior pole of the testis. It then runs in the posterior part of the spermatic cord upwards to the deep inguinal ring. Here, it loops back down and travels through the retroperitoneal space, between the base of the bladder and the rectum, to the base of the prostate gland, where it is joined by the duct of the seminal vesicle to form the ejaculatory duct.

At orgasm, semen is produced, made up of sperm and fluid from the prostate and seminal vesicles. The sperm contribute only about 10% of the volume of the seminal fluid, and there is no appreciable drop in the ejaculate volume after the vasectomy.

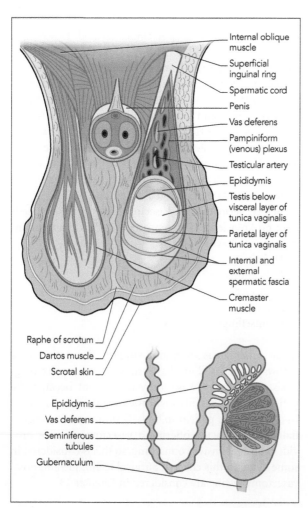

Internal oblique muscle
Superficial inguinal ring
Spermatic cord
Penis
Vas deferens
Pampiniform (venous) plexus
Testicular artery
Epididymis
Testis below visceral layer of tunica vaginalis
Parietal layer of tunica vaginalis
Internal and external spermatic fascia
Cremaster muscle

Raphe of scrotum
Dartos muscle
Scrotal skin

Epididymis
Vas deferens
Seminiferous tubules
Gubernaculum

Figure 12.2 Cross-section of scrotum, penis, and testicle.

Vas deferens

The thickness of the wall relative to the small size of its lumen gives the vas a hard, cord-like feel when palpated. It is essential to be able to identify the vas from the other linear structures that run in the spermatic cord to avoid inadvertent injury to these other structures when isolating it for exposure during surgery.

It is not unusual for the two vasa to be asymmetrical in diameter and/or position. Rarely, there is a unilateral absent of the vas due to congenital absence of the vas deferens (CAVD). This can be bilateral, but the patient will be infertile and therefore will not be presenting for contraception. Unilateral CAVD is associated with unilateral renal agenesis, and the genetic basis in this group is not well understood. The two approaches to this are either to request an ultrasound scan to look for the clinically absent vas, or to carry out a unilateral vasectomy and wait for the postoperative seminal analyses rather than explore the scrotum for the other vas.

The spermatic cord

The vas runs upwards from the superior pole of the testis in the posterior part of the spermatic cord. The cord is composed of arteries (testicular, cremasteric, and deferential), veins, lymph vessels, nerves, and the vas deferens. Therefore an anterior approach to the vas during vasectomy is associated with a risk of inadvertent injury to any of these structures unless care is taken to identify and apply surgical instruments on the vas and only the vas.

A vascular injury is associated with a primary haemorrhage and haematoma formation unless recognised and managed promptly. An injury to the testicular artery is associated with a risk of ischaemia and atrophy of the testis it supplies.

Scrotum

The scrotum is the sac that contains the testes and distal parts of the spermatic cords (Figure 12.2). It is made up of skin, the dartos muscle, and three layers of fascia that are continuous with the coverings of the spermatic cord. The inner fascial layer is very loosely attached to the outer covering of the testis, the tunica vaginalis. Therefore this tissue plane is easily dissected to access the vas.

However, an incision into the dartos muscle can be associated with significant bleeding, and meticulous haemostasis is required without thermal injury to the skin as this will impede wound healing. Some practitioners make the incision in the scrotal skin using cutting waveform electrosurgery with the advantage of better haemostasis but the potential disadvantage of slower wound healing.

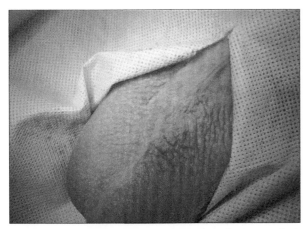

Figure 12.3 Typical postoperative appearance after non-scalpel vasectomy.

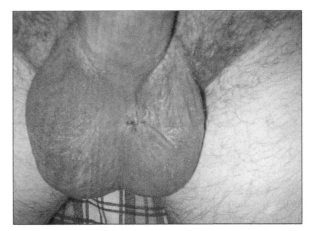

Figure 12.4 Marked bruising after vasectomy.

RISKS AND COMPLICATIONS

There are a range of risks and complications associated with vasectomy, and the most important will be considered here. It is important that the patient understands the common risks and the few rare serious complications associated with the procedure, as well as what can be done to minimise them. Figure 12.3 shows the typical appearance after an NSV.

Postoperative pain

Scrotal pain is common but is dependent on multiple factors, including the degree of disturbance of the tissues during surgery and the patient's pain threshold and tolerance. In general, there is a close correlation between pain and bruising and swelling.

Management

Simple oral analgesia should be sufficient, but aspirin-containing formulations should be avoided. With the principle that prevention is better than cure, it takes a weaker analgesic agent to prevent pain than to relieve pain when it is already present. Therefore, simple analgesia taken before the local anaesthetic has worn off is as effective as stronger analgesia taken later when the pain is severe. The prevention of bruising and swelling by early physical inactivity and the routine regular application of cold packs (see 'Management' below) after the operation results in a more pain-free immediate post-vasectomy period.

Bruising and swelling

This is normal, and there is individual variation despite surgical technique (Figure 12.4). In general, the more immediate postoperative physical exertion, the more bruising and swelling occurs. Superficial tracking can lead to the penis and scrotum appearing bruised. This is, however, usually painless and self-limiting.

Management

Cold compresses (gel packs, crushed ice, or bags of frozen peas) should be applied for 15–20 minutes every hour until bedtime on the day of surgery. Scrotal support with tight-fitting underpants or swimming trunks for the first few days is highly recommended.

Bleeding

Bleeding from the scrotal wound can occur, especially if the source is the dartos muscle or skin edges. If active bleeding at the end of the operation does not cease with pressure, haemostasis with electrocoagulation for the former or a horizontal mattress suture for the latter should be carried out.

Management

Rarely, the wound may need to be reopened to establish haemostasis.

Haematoma

The incidence of haematoma is related to the surgeon's experience and the surgical method used. An accomplished surgeon not using NSV methods should achieve results as good as one employing NSV. Most haematomas are caused by reactive haemorrhage from capillaries due to inadequate haemostasis. However, inadvertent venous or arterial injury will cause heavy primary haemorrhage and large haematomas, requiring prompt emergency management.

Management

Small haematomas will resolve spontaneously with time, but large ones may require surgical evacuation; this may demand referral to a local surgical unit.

Infection

The risk of infective epididymitis or epididymo-orchitis is reduced with NSV and seems to be independent of the surgeon's experience or the patient's activity levels.

Management

Oral antibiotics will usually suffice.

Blood in the ejaculate

This is rare but can occur, usually within 2 weeks of the procedure.

Management

Spontaneous resolution usually occurs. If it does not, further investigation is warranted.

Sperm granuloma

Sperm that leaks from the vasectomy site has highly antigenic properties and may stimulate an inflammatory reaction, forming pockets—firm balls of tissue about 1 cm in diameter—that trap sperm.

The formation of sperm granulomas is more likely in an 'open' vasectomy (see below). Granulomas typically occur in the second or third week in 60% of men who undergo vasectomy, but are troublesome in only 3–5% of cases.

Management

Most granulomas are asymptomatic and self-limiting. Fewer than 1% require active intervention, the options for this including steroid infiltration and surgical excision.

Congestive epididymitis

The onset of congestive epididymitis may be in the first year, and the condition usually clears up within a week when treated. The incidence is reduced by open-ended vasectomy in which the testicular end of the divided vas is not occluded. Heat and oral non-steroidal anti-inflammatory medication are helpful.

Post-vasectomy pain syndrome

The incidence of post-vasectomy pain syndrome is unknown due to the variable presentation of the condition and poor quality trials. It seems to be a collective title with many theories for its aetiology. As no one cause has been identified, treatment options are unclear, with conservative measures, including antibiotics and analgesia, being first line. Vasectomy reversal has a success rate of up to 84%. Epididymectomy has a success rate of up to 90%, but requires more specific diagnosis. Microsurgical denervation has a success rate of up to 96% in meticulously selected cases.

Recanalisation

This can be divided into early or late recanalisation.

Early recanalisation

This occurs within weeks of the surgery and is detected by the post-vasectomy seminal analyses, provided they are carried out at a long enough interval after the operation. The minimum interval recommended by the national guidelines is 8 weeks, although this may be too soon for many men to achieve azoospermia and it is more common to test at 16 and 18 weeks; only 87% of men achieve azoospermia at 12 weeks.

Late recanalisation

This occurs after clearance has been given on the basis of azoospermia on analysis. The incidence quoted by the Royal College of Obstetricians and Gynaecologists is 1 in 2000. Technical methods of occlusion used may affect failure rates.

Management

Repeat vasectomy should be discussed with the patient.

COUNSELLING

Before the procedure is performed, the patient should receive enough written and verbal information to be able to provide signed, informed consent for the procedure. Where there is a stable relationship, it is preferable to see both the patient and his partner together, although in the United Kingdom her consent is not a legal necessity. The information discussed, ideally with the couple, should include the full range of other reversible methods of contraception.

The information should be accurate, impartially printed or recorded, in translation, where appropriate and possible. It is essential that the patient has enough time to study the information before signing the consent form and undergoing the procedure. Chapter 2 discusses the importance of informed consent and the requirements necessary to ensure that the consent process has been correctly followed. Particular care should be taken if the referral pathway requires written consent to be sought by the doctor referring the patient for the procedure, rather than the clinician performing the operation. If the referring clinician obtaining the consent has inadequate knowledge of the procedure and was not aware of the limits of his or her competence in giving the patient sufficient information about the risks of vasectomy, the consent may be invalid.

It is important to emphasise that vasectomy has to be regarded as permanent and irreversible. This is particularly important when counselling people under 30 years of age or childless people who request sterilisation. The failure (pregnancy) rate is about 1 in 2000. Some men do undergo vasectomy reversal, perhaps because they have a different partner or have lost a child, but it is not always successful. In the United Kingdom, this is potentially a very expensive procedure and it is unlikely to be funded through the NHS.

The risks of vasectomy discussed should include failure, irreversibility, pain, bleeding, scar formation, infection, and sperm granuloma. The information should also include advice on how the patient can minimise these risks and reduce postoperative pain, how to recognise when and where to seek medical help, and the necessity of post-vasectomy seminal analysis to confirm sterility. An example of a patient information leaflet can be found in the Appendix to this chapter. Every surgeon must ensure that appropriate and timely information is provided to their patients and adapted to the particular circumstances of their own vasectomy service.

PRACTICAL CONSIDERATIONS

- Many vasectomy services offer a 'one-stop shop' in which the patient is seen and counselled on the same day as the operation. Where this occurs, it is important to provide an informative leaflet to the patient at the same time as the vasectomy appointment is arranged.
- It is also good practice to provide a copy of the consent form in advance so that the patient and his partner have an opportunity to consider both the information and the consent process before the operation. It is essential that the patient and partner have opportunities to ask further questions and express any concerns or anxieties they might have.
- The main disadvantage of a 'one-stop shop' approach is that patients may not feel they have had sufficient time to reconsider. This concern is minimised by providing the relevant leaflets beforehand.
- If asked, further information regarding specific risks can be provided for any of the potential complications, perhaps emphasising that it is very unlikely any of them will be severe. The most difficult complication to quantify is post-vasectomy pain syndrome, with literature quoting rates anywhere from 0.5% up to 30%. However, most surgeons will say that they are aware of very few cases of post-vasectomy pain syndrome being severe enough to significantly interfere with and affect everyday living or to require additional treatment.

FURTHER READING

Family Planning Association (2011) A history of family planning services factsheet. Available from: > www.fpa.org.uk/Professionals/Factsheets/historyoffamily-planning (accessed July 2012).

APPENDIX 1: SAMPLE PATIENT INFORMATION GUIDE

Patient's Guide To Non-Scalpel Vasectomy and Pre/Postoperative Care

Name of clinic: ....

Address of clinic: ....

....

Tel: .... E-mail: ....

HAVING A VASECTOMY

This leaflet has been prepared to guide you through your visit to us for your vasectomy and through the immediate postoperative period. If you have any questions that are not answered or if you would like to discuss a special problem, please do not hesitate to telephone.

If you change your mind, or wish to postpone your operation, please let us know as soon as possible so that the appointment can be offered to someone else.

We want to ensure you receive the best possible treatment and care while you are with us. We are aiming to improve our services wherever we can, and we welcome any comments or suggestions you may have.

Your appointment to have your vasectomy is:

Time: ....

Date: ....

- You will be having a local anaesthetic; it is a good idea to have a light meal before attending.

- You should aim to be collected from the surgery by car, or you can order a taxi (at your own expense) when it is time to leave. You should *not* drive home, so please arrange for someone to collect you and be with you for the rest of the day.

- The surgeon will spend a few minutes talking with you before the operation to explain details again and to answer any final questions you may have. Your partner is welcome to attend at this time and can stay with you during the operation if you wish.

More information can be obtained on the web at: www.aspc-uk.net/www.eguidelines.co.uk

Why choose vasectomy?

People ask for vasectomy when they are sure that their family is complete or they do not want children. It is one of the most effective forms of permanent contraception. However, it should always require very careful thought beforehand as it must be recognised that personal circumstances can change (e.g., a tragedy to existing children, or a new partner in the future), and that reversal operations are not always successful, are not usually available on the NHS, and are very expensive.

Who can have a vasectomy?

Any man can have a vasectomy regardless of age, or whether he is married, single, divorced, widowed, childless, or with a family. If you have a permanent partner, her consent is not legally required, but it is recommended that your decision is discussed with her and that she agrees with it.

How effective is vasectomy?

Vasectomy is over 99.9% effective, but the operation occasionally fails if one or both tubes rejoin, even after the 'all clear' has been given, and pregnancy can occasionally happen, even years later.

Am I suitable for vasectomy?

Anyone can have a vasectomy, but some medical conditions may make the procedure more difficult. In particular, you must let your GP and the surgeon know if you have had any operations or infections in the genital area (including hernias) and if you have any known abnormality of the urogenital system (e.g., kidneys, bladder).

Are there risks?

- There can be sperm in the ejaculated fluid for many months after the operation. You must continue to use contraception until postoperative sperm tests (starting at about 4 months) have been carried out, you have had at least one satisfactory sperm test, and the surgeon or your GP have given you the 'all clear'. You will be given further information about this after the operation and before you go home.

- After the procedure, care should be taken with bathing for about 7 days. Although the operation area may be slightly bloodstained, it is better not to wash for 24 hours. It is then best not to soak in a bath, but to have showers, letting the water run over the area. If you do not have a shower, kneel in a bath and sponge water over the area. Do not use excessive soap or shampoos, or any talc.

- Sexual intercourse can be resumed when comfortable. However, it is essential to continue using contraception until there are no more live sperm in the ejaculate. This will be shown by tests carried out starting 4 months after the operation.

- Vasectomy has no effect on masculinity, or on sexual arousal performance or orgasm. Sperm continue to be produced by the testicles, but the passage to the penis is blocked, so they are reabsorbed into the body.

- It is important that you must continue to take precautions against pregnancy until you have been given the 'all clear' following the semen specimen results.

- It can be reassuring to know that many people who have had a vasectomy say their sex life has improved because the fear of pregnancy has been removed.

- Important complications that you should be aware of include infection and excessive bruising (both common to any operation, but rare for a non-scalpel vasectomy [NSV]), which can delay the healing process. Some men develop a chronic testicular pain syndrome, sometimes years later. The incidence of this varies from 0.5% to 30%, it is very rarely severe, but it may require further medical or surgical treatment.

- *Post-vasectomy semen analysis.* You will be required to give at least one specimen after about 4 months. The greatest risk of rejoining of the tubes is in the first 4 months after the operation.

Non-scalpel vasectomy

How is the procedure done?

- Sperm make up approximately 5% of the fluid ejaculated at orgasm. The purpose of the operation is to stop the sperm being ejaculated by sealing and cutting the tubes (the vas deferens) that carry the sperm from the testicle to the fluid. The fluid originates in glands at the base of the penis, and the quantity produced is unaffected by the operation. After the operation, the sperm cannot 'get through' and are merely absorbed back into the body.

- You will be given a small injection of local anaesthetic into the skin of the scrotum. A tiny opening (rarely, two may be needed) is made, and a piece of the tube leading from each testicle is isolated, sealed, and cut so that sperm can no longer get through.

- The operation takes about 15 minutes, with perhaps 10 minutes before and after for preparation and finishing, but you will be at the surgery for at least 30 minutes after your operation before being allowed to leave.

Before your operation

- It is important that you have discussed thoroughly with your partner whether vasectomy is the right method of permanent contraception for both of you. Your own GP should have discussed with you alternative forms of contraception that might be suitable, in particular those known as LARCs (long-acting reversible contraceptives) as some of these are also quite reliable and can, of course, be reversed, thereby restoring fertility and the ability to have more children.

- It is not necessary to shave your scrotum beforehand. However, immediately before coming in for the operation, please wash the genital area thoroughly with soap and hot water, and keep warm. Bring a dressing gown with you to wear when walking from the consulting room to the operating room and afterwards to a recovery room.

- Eat a light meal before arriving at the surgery.

- Your partner is welcome to attend with you for any part or all of the consultation and/or operation.

- Remember to make arrangements for someone to accompany you home afterwards, as you should not drive yourself.

Patient information guide *continued*

After your operation

- Following a local anaesthetic, you can leave the surgery after a short rest. You should not drive home but ideally arrange for someone to collect you and be with you for the rest of the day.

- You are likely to experience some pain or discomfort during the first few days, and occasionally some swelling develops. It is sensible to plan to relax at home for a few days before returning to work. We advise that you avoid strenuous exercise, heavy lifting, or driving long distances for 1–2 weeks.

- To minimise swelling and discomfort, it is advisable to wear tight-fitting underpants, swimming trunks, or a jock strap (brought with you on the day of your operation). You should continue to wear these day and night for about 1 week. If you have a heavy manual job, you may need to take more time off work if 'light duties' are not available.

- About 1–2 hours after the operation, when the local anaesthetic wears off, you will normally have some discomfort or pain. It is OK for you to take your usual painkillers, e.g., paracetamol, ibuprofen, or co-codamol, in the normal dosages (these are all available from the chemist without needing a prescription) but avoid aspirin unless essential. Use of an ice pack on the scrotum for 10–20 minutes every 1–2 hours for the first day can help to reduce swelling and discomfort. Remember to place a tea towel (or something similar) between the ice pack and the skin.

- Some swelling (up to the size of a testicle) and bruising of the scrotum and testicles is normal, but if it is severe during the first few hours after the operation you should contact the surgeon. If you are unable to contact him or her, please contact a doctor through your own surgery.

- Where the tubes have been cauterised and cut, some scar tissue will form. This may be felt as a slightly lumpy, sometimes tender, area just above the testicle. This is quite normal, but if you do become concerned about any unusual lumps, see your GP.

- There are no stitches to remove, and there is only a small cut that will heal itself, although it may gape open a little and cause a slight bloodstained discharge. You only need to seek medical advice if this is persistent, excessively smelly, or inflamed. You may also notice slight bloodstaining the first few times you ejaculate.

- Sperm can live for up to 70 days or longer and will still be released for a variable length of time after the operation when you ejaculate. In order to empty the 'reservoir' of live sperm within this period of time, it is recommended that you have intercourse/ejaculate on average three times a week.

- Sometimes it is found that, even with this frequency of intercourse, some men take longer to clear their 'reservoir' of live sperm, and you should not worry if you are asked for further specimens. Evidence shows that one fresh sample at 4 months that is completely clear of all sperm is sufficient. If small numbers of dead sperm persist, you may be given the 'all clear' after about 7 months. However, you must wait until this is confirmed by your own GP or by the surgeon.

- *Until you have received confirmation from your own GP or the surgeon, you should continue to take contraceptive precautions.*

- No assurance that you have become infertile can be given without these tests, and no responsibility will be accepted for failure of the operation if the required semen specimens are not submitted for analysis at the appropriate times.

The approximate date (not before) for your first semen specimen collection will be:

....

A letter will be sent to you in about 4 months' time to remind you. Full instructions regarding request forms and sample pots and where to take the samples will be included in the letter.

Your own GP and the surgeon will have access to the results.

Chapter 13

Toenail problems that may require surgery

Ian Reilly

INTRODUCTION

This chapter describes the normal anatomy of the nail and some of the common problems affecting the toenails that might require surgery. No attempt is made to consider the range of inflammatory problems that might affect the nails, and readers are referred to specialist nail texts for this information. Toenail surgery techniques are then discussed in Chapter 24.

ANATOMY AND PHYSIOLOGY OF THE NAIL

Function of nails

The human nail serves a number of functions, some of these being less important for toenails than for fingernails. The more important functions of human nails are as follows:

- To aid with dexterity.
- For peripheral sensation through aiding plantar/palmar pressure responses.
- Scratching.
- Protection of the distal surface of the digit.
- Cosmetic appearance.
- As an important indicator of disease (local and systemic).

Anatomy of the nail
The nail plate

Figure 13.1 illustrates the anatomy of the human nail. The hard nail plate forms the basis of the majority of the nail apparatus. The nail plate extends from the nail matrix (also called the root), emerges at the proximal nail fold, and reaches to the distal free edge or hyponychium.

It is very important to recognise that both the nail matrix and the nail bed are important in terms of growth of the nail. Damage to either is not always predictable but can lead to permanent disfiguration of the shape and contour of the nail plate. When treating a nail problem by destroying the nail using a nail-ablation procedure (see Chapter 24), some authors believe it is necessary to destroy both the matrix and the nail bed, whereas others state that the nail bed does not require ablation when removing nails.

The majority of the nail plate is produced by the germinal matrix, which extends for several millimetres proximal to the nail fold. As the nail plate emerges and grows across the nail bed, additional material derived from the nail bed is added to the nail plate, which makes the plate thicker. The undersurface of the nail plate is grooved to help with anchoring it to the nail bed. Damage to the nail bed, or loss of its normal smooth surface, can result in a nail plate with an irregular or interrupted contour. Melanocytes in the matrix create pigment in some nail plates.

Cuticle (eponychium), hyponychium, and lunula

The structure of the nail is seen in Figure 13.1. The cuticle or eponychium is a thin layer of cells at the proximal nail fold that extend onto the dorsal surface of the nail plate. The function of this is to form a waterproof barrier between the nail plate and the skin of the digit. The hyponychium links the distal underside of the nail plate to the skin at the distal end of the digit and has a function similar to the eponychium.

The small-celled and relatively bloodless area at the base of the nail that forms a crescent shape is called the lunula. The lunula is the clinical representation of the nail matrix.

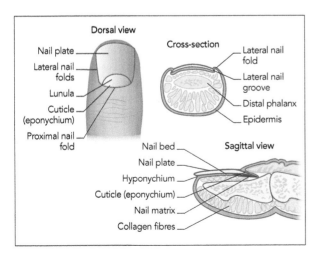

Figure 13.1 Anatomy of the nail.

Nail colour

No skin pigment usually appears in the nails because of their normally translucent nature: their appearance is usually pink due to the colour of the nail bed beneath, which is richly supplied with blood vessels.

Nail growth

Nails grow at widely varying rates in different individuals. The rate of growth depends upon blood supply and oxygen tension, trauma, inflammation, the temperature of the skin, the presence of local or systemic disease, and the state of general health. Typically, fingernails grow faster than toenails, at a rate of around 3 mm per month. Toenails typically grow at a rate of 1 mm per month. It therefore takes around 6 months for a fingernail to grow from the matrix to the free edge, whereas a toenail can take around 12 months to be completely replaced.

COMMON TOENAIL PROBLEMS THAT MAY REQUIRE SURGERY

Ingrown/ingrowing toenail

An ingrown toenail occurs when the side of a toenail begins to cut through the surrounding skin, which is known as the ungual labia or nail fold (Figure 13.2). The ingrown/ingrowing toenail (IGTN), or onychocryptosis, is one of the most commonly seen foot problems in primary care (Dockery, 2001) in the United Kingdom. The condition occurs when the nail plate punctures or traumatises the skin at the side of the nail, giving rise to pain and inflammation. This break in the continuity of the skin provides a portal of entry for microorganisms and therefore paronychia often accompanies an IGTN.

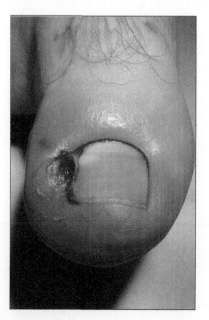

Figure 13.2
Ingrowing toenail.

Incidence

Ingrowing toenails can occur at any age, but it is typically the younger patient who is affected, most IGTNs being seen in the 10–40-year age group. Those seen in elderly patients often arise as a complication of other nail disorders, as described later. They occur twice as often in males as in females, and it is usually the lateral side of the hallux that presents as the sulcus is compressed by the second toe.

Aetiology

A range of factors may predispose to the development of an IGTN. These include:

- *Suboptimal nail care in adolescents.* Typically, a tear to the nail plate leaves an irregular or sharp shoulder of nail. This is evidenced by the prominent section of nail so often found at the time of surgery. Nail-pickers (onychotillomania) are even more at risk. Overgrowth or hypertrophy of the ungual labia or softening of the nail plate, as seen in the hyperhidrotic foot of younger patients, will predispose to the development of IGTN.
- *Trauma.* Trauma can also cause the nail to ingrow, as can overly tight hosiery and footwear. Underlying nail disease can cause IGTNs, and soft tissue or bony hypertrophy can also play a part.
- *Biomechanical alterations,* pathological curvature of the nail plate, surgical iatrogenic conditions, excessive weight, and the first toe being longer than the others have also been implicated.
- *Peripheral neuropathy* leading to loss of sensation and ischaemia; this in turn leads to frailty of the tissues, both of which put elderly and/or diabetic individuals at increased risk of developing nail penetration and infection. Other nail dystrophies that are separate from IGTN, but predispose to true penetration, are disorders of thickness and onychomycosis (see below).

Pathology

Penetration of the skin is only the start of the process. The body responds to the injury (in part) by producing granulation tissue. As the nail continues to grow forward, the granulation tissue hypertrophies. This hypergranulation tissue now complicates painful IGTN, typically accompanied at this point by a chronic paronychia. In neglected cases, the sharp edge of nail can exit the apex of the toe, further increasing the ingress of microorganisms. Rarely, systemic infection and osteomyelitis can occur secondary to IGTN.

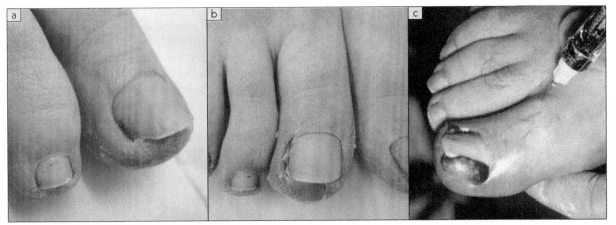

Figure 13.3 Ingrowing toenail stages: (a) Stage 1—erythema and swelling; (b) Stage 2—infection; (c) Stage 3—granulation tissue.

Stages of ingrowing toenail

Various authors have attempted to stage the process. Siegle and Stewart (1992) classified IGTN as follows (Figure 13.3):

- Stage 1: Erythema and swelling of the lateral nail fold.
- Stage 2: Infection with accompanying oedema and drainage.
- Stage 3: Chronic infection characterised by hypertrophy of granulation tissue along the lateral fold.

Management

The podiatrist and/or GP is often the first clinician to see a symptomatic presentation of this problem, and the expert treatment of early IGTNs is a core podiatric skill. In the early stages, conservative nail-cutting may be all that is required. However, the effectiveness of this management will depend on the shape of the nail plate, the size of the spicule, the level of infection, and the amount of granulation tissue. In more advanced or recurrent cases, permanent eradication of part or of the whole of the nail plate may be required, and Siegle and Stewart have suggested the following schema.

- Stage 1: *Inflammatory redness and swelling.*
  This will usually respond to non-operative treatments as follows:
  - Packing the nail edge with cotton wool.
  - Reducing the central thickness of the nail plate to reshape the nail profile.
  - Taping back the surrounding tissue.
  - Use of an interdigital spacer to reduce pressure from tight digits.
- Stage 2: *Inflammatory secretion.* Here the toe is infected. Stage 1 treatments combined with antibiotic therapy may resolve the problem. If not, surgery is often required.
- Stage 3: *Granulation tissue formation.* This mass of tissue overlies the nail and bleeds easily if traumatised. Surgery is the treatment of choice at this stage. Nail surgery options are detailed in Chapter 24.

Involuted nails

These are nails with increased transverse curvature of the nail plate (Figure 13.4). They not only predispose to penetration and the development of IGTN, but also make conservative and surgical treatment more difficult. Involuted nails may be painful and require removal in their own right as they often cause the build-up of excess dead skin and/or corn (onychophosis/onychoheloma) in the nail sulci, which can be acutely painful and hence require treatment beyond simple nail-cutting (Haneke, 2002).

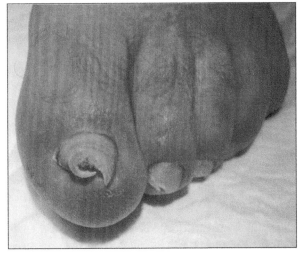

Figure 13.4 Involuted nails.

Hypertrophic nail conditions

Onychauxis and onychogryphosis are disorders of the nail that involve distortion and thickening (hypertrophy) of the nail plate. Both conditions can lead to complications and may be a source of discomfort and distress to those affected by them.

Onychauxis

Onychauxis (Figure 13.5) is a condition in which the nail plate is vertically thicker than normal without deformity (James *et al.*, 2006).

Aetiology

Onychauxis often arises secondary to some other disorder that has affected the germinal matrix of the nail or the nail bed. Examples are as follows:

- Trauma from tight-fitting footwear or from single acute trauma (e.g., stubbing the toe or dropping a weight on it).
- Circulatory changes such as peripheral vascular disease and microangiopathy.
- Infection, including onychomycosis, chronic paronychia, and cellulitis.
- Inflammation, such as chronic onychocryptosis, chemical injury, or psoriasis.

As the nail plate becomes thicker, a colour change in the nail is often seen. This is thought to be related to an increased density of the nail plate, which often results in the nail plate appearing more yellow or even brown in colour. Onychauxic nails are characteristically uniformly thickened, and there is usually minimal distortion to the longitudinal growth axis of the nail. Typically, the onychauxic nail appears like a normal nail but is thicker than normal. Very often the longitudinal growth of the nail is slow, and this may be the result of circulatory deficit, matrix damage, or both.

Onychauxis is problematic in that the thickened nails are difficult for patients to trim. Domestic nail scissors or clippers are generally inadequate for this task. This often results in patients presenting to their GP, nurse, or podiatrist for professional advice. In many instances, severe cases of onychauxis will warrant treatment from a foot health professional (foot-care assistant or podiatrist) as necessary.

The thickened nail plate can provide an ideal environment for the growth of microorganisms, particularly dermatophytes and yeasts. This can lead to further damage to the nail plate, germinal matrix, and surrounding skin. Further discoloration, affecting the cosmetic appearance of the nail, is also a consequence of dermatophyte and yeast infection. Fungal infection of this type can lead to a build-up of debris underneath the nail plate and in the nail sulci.

In patients with peripheral vascular disease and devitalised tissues, a thickened nail plate coupled with footwear pressure can result in other problems. These include onychophosis (a localised or diffuse hyperkeratotic tissue that develops on the lateral or proximal nail folds, within the space between the nail folds and the nail plate), subungual corns, and subungual ulceration. These conditions can be the cause of significant pain and discomfort for patients. In addition, subungual ulceration can result in secondary infection. Vascular disease may be both a causal factor in the distortion or hypertrophy of the nail plate and may also increase the risk of more serious complications.

Footwear evaluation is an important part of the management strategy for onychauxis. Poorly fitting footwear is often a causal factor in people with onychauxis, with the secondary problems of hyperkeratosis and ulceration more likely to occur unless the footwear is appropriately modified.

Onychogryphosis

Onychogryphosis is similar to onychauxis in that it is characterised by a thickening of the nail plate (Figure 13.6). However, unlike onychauxis, there is longitudinal distortion of the nail plate (James *et al.*, 2006). The nail plate often curves and may in severe cases resemble a ram's horn. Onychogryphosis represents a grossly distorted, deformed, and thickened nail plate.

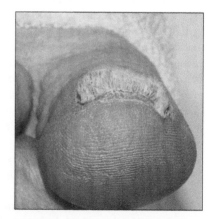

Figure 13.5
Onychauxis.

Figure 13.6
Onychogryphosis.

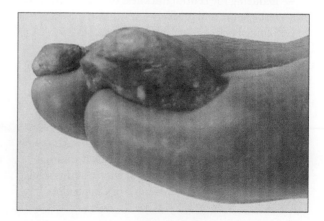

The deformity and asymmetry of the nail-plate thickening is thought to be due to asymmetrical damage to the nail matrix and/or nail bed, together with the effect of extrinsic factors (e.g., footwear) on the pattern of nail-plate growth. In severe cases of onychogryphosis, the nail is long and thickened, and curves to the limits of the shoes. In some cases when the patient removes his or her shoes, the shape of the nails describes the outline of the toe-box of the shoe. These severe deformities are common in the elderly or infirm who cannot manage their own foot-care.

Complications associated with onychogryphosis are similar to those of onychauxis, with the additional risk of trauma to adjacent tissues from the deformed nail plate. As the deformed nail plate continues to grow, it is likely to impact on other tissue, such as the surrounding skin, adjacent toes, and so on. This may then lead to trauma to these tissues, resulting in hyperkeratosis, ulceration, and infection.

Accommodating feet with severely thickened and/or deformed toenails in shoes can be a significant problem for many patients. The patient may modify footwear to accommodate the nail deformity.

The risk from ill-fitting shoes of periungual and subungual complications is greater for onychogryphosis than onychauxis because of the problems arising from the deformity. The risk of complications arising from damage to adjacent tissues is also significant.

Management of onychauxis and onychogryphosis

In most cases, these conditions cannot be cured, as it is not possible to permanently restore the nail plate to a normal structure and function. This would require repair of the damaged germinal matrix and nail bed, which is beyond the scope of current therapy. However, it is possible to manage these disorders and to temporarily restore normal structure and function to the nail plates. It should, however, be recognised that long-term care of these disorders is reliant on frequent maintenance of the nail plate. After initial professional input, it may be possible for patients or carers to undertake this maintenance themselves.

In cases of onychauxis or onychogryphosis where the viability of tissues is good and the patient is in good general health, surgery to remove the affected nail plate(s) may be indicated. Ideally, the nail plate should be completely removed and the germinal matrix and nail bed treated with phenol to prevent recurrence.

Tumours of the nail and distal digit

Tumours of the nail apparatus and adjacent structures are not uncommon. Most of the lesions seen are benign, but a good understanding of the range of pathology that presents will aid in the overall diagnosis and management of such problems. The clinician will need to consider whether the lesion can be operated on in an outpatient setting or whether referral to the local hospital is more appropriate. This section considers the more common benign and malignant lesions and includes a description of common melanocytic lesions of the nail.

Periungual and subungual warts

The most common tumour involving the nail is the viral wart, which can involve either the nail fold or the digit pulp (Figure 13.7). These are benign, fibroepithelial tumours caused by the human papilloma virus, and most will resolve spontaneously. Periungual warts are more common in nail biters and those involved in wet work. A range of treatments are available but their efficacy is poor (see Chapter 9 for more information about viral warts).

The main differential diagnosis in older patients is squamous cell carcinoma, but the latter is much more destructive and often painful. Warts are more common and much more difficult to manage in people who are immunosuppressed. Despite the bulky warts, the adjacent nail structure tends not to be distorted (unlike myxoid cysts; see Chapter 9).

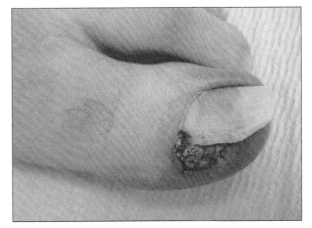

Figure 13.7 Periungual wart.

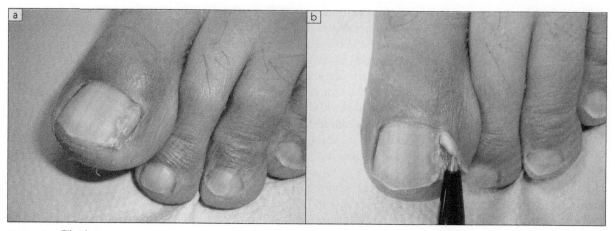

Figure 13.8 Fibrokeratoma.

Fibrous and fibroepithelial tumours

A large variety of clinical presentations of fibrous tumours may be seen in the subungual and periungual areas of the digits. The most common of these are fibromas, which usually develop as painless, slow-growing nodular tumours. They are either firm or elastic in consistency, and may be spherical or oval in shape. They can develop in any subepidermal structure and if seen in association with the nail matrix, will often cause nail dystrophy.

Histological variations include the true fibromas (fibrous dermatofibromas) and histiocytomas, although the latter are uncommon in the nail area. Acquired periungual fibrokeratomas are benign, spontaneously developing symptomatic nodules with a hyperkeratotic tip (Figure 13.8). Double and triple lesions are seen. Multiple periungual fibromas occur in tuberous sclerosis.

Vascular tumours

Glomus tumours

Glomus tumours most commonly occur in the subungual region of the fingers, with females more commonly affected than males (Figure 13.9). The main symptom is an acutely tender point in the nail plate triggered by pressure, trauma, or temperature change. The pain is intense and pulsatile, frequently radiating up into the arm and shoulder.

This history should alert the clinician to the possibility of a glomus tumour, although the clinician should remember that the lesion can be hidden under the proximal nail fold and can therefore be difficult to see. A visible bluish-red discoloration, usually of the matrix, should be looked for.

Treatment is by excision. It is often necessary to remove the nail first to identify the location of the lesion.

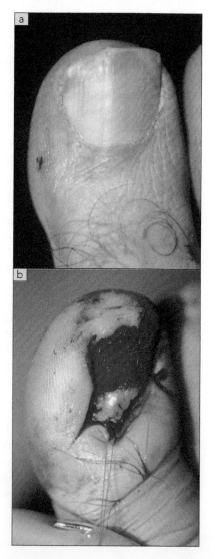

Figure 13.9
Glomus tumour beneath big toenail. (a) Preoperatively, the clue is the slight bulge in the nail plate and a history from the patient of a very localised pain. (b) At surgery, the tumour can be seen to bulge beneath the matrix.

Pyogenic granuloma

These are benign eruptive haemangiomas that typically present after minor penetrating skin trauma (Figure 13.10). They are commonly located at the proximal nail fold but may develop distally if the trauma causes onycholysis.

These lesions typically bleed easily and can be painful. The differential diagnosis includes amelanotic melanoma and squamous cell carcinoma. They are considered in more detail in Chapter 9.

Other vascular tumours

A range of haemangiomas, venous malformations, arteriovenous malformations, and arteriovenous fistulae can occur in the nail bed and distal digits. These are rare, and readers are referred to more specialist texts for consideration of these lesions.

Subungual exostoses

These are benign bony outgrowths of the terminal phalanx and most commonly occur on the great toe (Figure 13.11). The subungual exostosis first described by Dupuytren is a relatively common lesion of the nail plate area. It is commonly seen in the younger patient, occurring more commonly in females than males. It is thought that trauma, often repeated microtrauma, may be an aetiological factor. Most subungual exostoses arise from the dorsal lateral aspect of the tip of the distal phalanx, elevating the nail plate as the exostosis grows. The diagnosis is confirmed on radiography. Treatment is by excision with or without removal of the nail plate depending on the difficulty of gaining access to the bone.

Keratin cysts

Implantation cysts, also known as epidermoid or traumatic cysts, can occur in the terminal phalanx secondary to trauma with implantation of epidermal cells into the subcutaneous tissue or bone. The trauma may have occurred many years previously and may not be remembered by the patient. Such lesions can be seen postoperatively in close proximity to surgical wounds. As the epidermal island grows, the lesion enlarges and the digit can become clubbed in nature. Pain is of late onset, caused by compression of the bone.

Treatment is by enucleation of the lesion and its entire membrane, which will reveal a cyst filled with keratin and an epidermal lining. Subungual epidermoid inclusions (epidermal buds) develop from the ridges of the nail bed epithelium; they rarely become large enough to cause symptoms.

Keratoacanthoma

This typically is a painful, rapidly enlarging lesion occurring in the distal nail bed, where its growth causes separation of the nail plate from the nail bed. This onycholysis precedes the appearance of a crusted nodule, and the distal digit can be red and swollen. The hallmarks of the keratoacanthoma are its rapid growth over a period of just weeks and its glassy keratinocytes on histology, differentiating it from a squamous cell carcinoma.

The radiographic appearance of a subungual keratoacanthoma consists of a punched-out area of bone destruction in the terminal phalanx with well-circumscribed margins. Although there are some similarities to

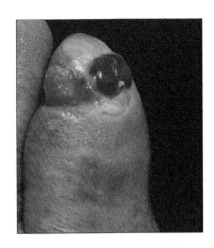

Figure 13.10 Pyogenic granuloma on the little toe. This is clinically indistinguishable from a squamous cell carcinoma and an amelanotic melanoma.

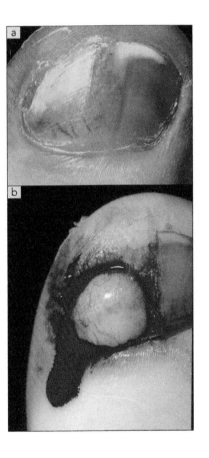

Figure 13.11 Subungual exostosis. (a) The tumour lies beneath the nail and has a hard texture if tapped with an instrument. The vascular pattern can be see through the nail. (b) At surgery, the rounded mass of the cartilaginous cap can be seen. The tumour will extend beneath the matrix and require careful surgery to avoid damage during removal.

the keratoacanthomas seen elsewhere on the body, there is no indication that nail keratoacanthomas involute, and they seem to be unrelated to cumulative sun exposure. Treatment is by surgery, either curettage or Mohs' micrographic surgery depending on the size and symptoms of the lesion.

Squamous cell carcinoma

Although non-melanoma skin cancer is the most common form of skin cancer (see Chapter 9), this rarely affects the nail unit, but Bowen's disease (in-situ squamous cell carcinoma) and invasive squamous cell carcinoma do occur. Clinical features include hyperkeratotic warty changes, erosions, swelling of the distal portion of the digit, and sometimes secondary infection (Figure 13.12). Diagnosis is often delayed because the typical features of squamous cell carcinoma seen elsewhere on the body are lacking. Treatment is surgical excision, and Mohs' micrographic surgery is often the treatment of choice.

Melanocytic lesions of the nail

It is important to have an understanding of the causes of nail pigmentation in order to be able to assess when nail biopsy might be necessary to confirm or exclude malignancy.

Longitudinal melanonychia

A subungual benign melanocytic naevus will cause longitudinal melanonychia. This is a linear longitudinal pigmented streak in the nail (Figure 13.13). The other very common cause of longitudinal melanonychia is racial variation, with 77% of Afro-Caribbean individuals over the age of 20 having this condition.

Malignant melanoma

Subungual malignant melanoma is rare and accounts for just around 3% of all malignant melanoma in white patients (see Chapter 9). In contrast, the tumour accounts for 20% of melanomas in Afro-Caribbean individuals. It is generally considered to be a disease of the elderly, the mean age of incidence being in the sixth decade. Subungual melanoma presents with a black or dark brown periungual pigmentation and longitudinal melanonychia.

The differential diagnoses include subungual haematoma and benign longitudinal melanonychia. Diagnosis is difficult and is often delayed, and many patients present with thick tumours and advanced disease because of this delay. About 20–25% of subungual melanomas are amelanotic (Figure 13.14), making diagnosis challenging.

The 5-year survival rate for subungual melanoma is poor compared with that for melanoma seen in other sites. Treatment is by surgical excision, although there is some controversy in the literature over the amount of surgery required, depending on the thickness of the melanoma itself. Amputation of the digit is usually required. An early diagnosis permits more conservative excision.

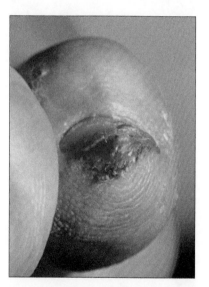

Figure 13.12 Squamous cell carcinoma. The subtle fleshy masses cause bleeding when patients cut their toenails. In other respects, they cause very few problems, although they can ooze. Squamous cell carcinoma of the nail unit will present with different features depending on where in the nail unit it is located.

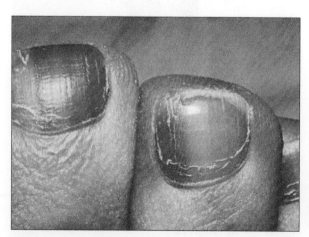

Figure 13.13 Longitudinal melanonychia. A pigmented longitudinal streak is a risk factor for melanoma. The likelihood of this diagnosis is less if there are multiple pigmented streaks or if the patient has dark skin.

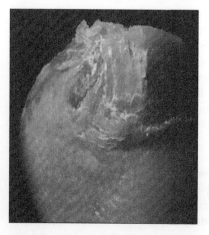

Figure 13.14 Subungual malignant melanoma. This melanoma is partly within the digit pulp and partly within the nail bed. It is amelanotic, which is common for melanoma of the nail unit and can lead to delay in diagnosis.

REFERENCES

Dockery GL (2001) Nails. In: Banks AS, Downey MS, Martin DE, Miller SJ, eds., *McGlamry's Comprehensive Textbook of Foot and Ankle Surgery*, 3rd edn. Philadelphia: Lippincott Williams & Wilkins, pp. 203–29.

Haneke E (2002) Ingrown and pincer nails: Evaluation and treatment. *Dermatologic Therapy* 15: 148–58.

James WD, Berger TG, Elston DM (2006) *Andrews' Diseases of the Skin: Clinical Dermatology*, 10th edn.) New York: Saunders Elsevier.

Siegle RJ, Stewart R (1992) Recalcitrant ingrowing toenails. *Journal of Dermatologic Surgery and Oncology* 18: 744–52.

Heifetz CJ (1937) Ingrown toenails: A clinical study. *American Journal of Surgery* 38: 298.

Krull EA, Zook EG, Baran R, Haneke E (2001) *Nail Surgery, A Text and Atlas*. New York: Lippincott Williams & Wilkins.

Lewis BL (1954) Microscopic studies of fetal and mature nail and the surrounding soft tissue. *Archives of Dermatology and Syphilis* 70: 732–44.

Martínez-Nova A, Sánchez-Rodríguez R, Alonso-Peña D (2002) A new onychocryptosis classification and treatment plan. *Journal of the American Podiatric Medical Association* 97: 389–93.

Mozena JD (2002) The Mozena classification system and treatment algorithm for ingrown hallux nails. *Journal of the American Podiatric Medical Association* 92: 131–5.

Rounding C, Bloomfield S (2003) Surgical treatments for ingrowing toenails. *Cochrane Database of Systematic Reviews* (1): CD001541.

Scher RK, Daniel CR (2002) *Nails: Therapy, Diagnosis, Surgery*. Philadelphia: WB Saunders.

Zaias MN, Daniel CR III (2002) Nails in systemic disease. *Dermatologic Therapy* 15: 99–106.

FURTHER READING

Baran R, Dawber RPR, de Berker DAR, Haneke E, Tosti A (2008) *Baran and Dawber's Diseases of the Nails and Their Management*. New York: Wiley-Blackwell.

Crawford F, Hart R, Bell-Syer SEM, Torgerson TJ, Young P, Russell I (2001) Athlete's foot and fungally infected toenails. *British Medical Journal* 322: 288–9.

PART 3

Essential generic skills

Chapter 14

Communication

INTRODUCTION

As in any other branch of clinical practice, anyone performing local anaesthetic surgery should have expert communication skills. This chapter reminds clinicians of the importance of effective communication and provides useful information on how to optimise communication in this particular setting. Considering the experience of minor surgery from the patient's perspective is particularly helpful in making the process more enjoyable for both patient and staff.

OVERVIEW

The best clinical communicators follow both verbal and non-verbal cues in order to gauge their patients' needs and to relax and reassure them. Relaxed patients tend to feel less pain (Syrjala *et al.*, 1995), bleed less, and have fewer complications. The whole surgical team should be integrated into the communication process and not be afraid to voice their opinions and provide appropriate information and support as part of a coordinated unit.

Although it may be attractive to view the role of surgeon as solely that of a technician, this is not appropriate in the context of minor surgery when patients are aware of everything that is taking place and may be very anxious. It is essential to keep patients fully informed of what is happening and what is likely to happen next. Most importantly, it is essential to make patients feel confident in your ability to perform the procedure and deal with any unexpected situation that may arise.

BEFORE THE PROCEDURE

Recognising Ideas, Concerns, and Expectations (ICE)

There are a variety of reasons why a patient may present at an operating session:

- A lesion has been noticed by the patient or an acquaintance.
- A lesion has been noticed in a medical consultation.
- The lesion may be causing the patient concern or distress.
- The procedure has been requested by you or by a colleague.

These different scenarios may lead to a variety of ideas, concerns, and expectations on the part of patients about what they have, what you are going to do, and what is going to happen afterward. It is important that you understand these ideas, concerns, and expectations in order that any consent to proceed is informed consent, and to ensure there are no misunderstandings before knife reaches skin. In some, but not all, situations, the patient will be well known to the surgical team, but where this is not the case, it is particularly important to establish a rapport quickly and listen carefully to any of the patient's anxieties because the surgeon needs to be able to confirm the patient's informed consent to the procedure (see Chapter 2).

Introductions

It is very important for the surgical team to introduce themselves properly to the patient by name and role. The introduction also allows for correct identification of the patient and of the part of the body to be operated on, as well as the indications for surgery. The patient should be given an opportunity to express any worries. Key questions that will help with understanding their ideas, concerns, and expectations (using the aide-memoire ICE) might include:

- What procedure is the patient expecting to be undertaken?
- Does he or she have any concerns about the procedure, the lesion, and/or the diagnosis?
- What does the patient expect the outcome to be in terms of restriction of activities after the procedure and the likely scar/cosmetic outcome?

Exposing the operation site

It is important to allow patients to remove their outer garments (ideally in a changing room, but at the very least in an area where they are not overlooked) and to reach the operating table in a state of dignity with modesty preserved. Within hospital settings, surgical gowns are usually provided, and GPs should consider how to allow patients to maintain their modesty if a supply of gowns is not available. This is where a suitably trained assistant is invaluable.

Once the patient is positioned on the table, it should be possible to expose the area required with as little undressing as possible, especially if surgical drapes or towels are made available. Some patients do not mind being exposed, whereas others find it very challenging and feel vulnerable in the foreign environment of an operating room. A good surgeon is able to judge patients' reactions and adjust his or her approach accordingly.

An adequately exposed surgical field is important for the surgeon but potentially increases embarrassment for the patient. Obscuring the patient's face with an operating drape denies the surgeon the opportunity to see the patient's reactions and to pre-empt any problems. These issues will need to be weighed up for different patients and managed sensitively, but without compromising on safety.

DURING THE PROCEDURE

During the operation, communication needs to be able to take place at different levels.

Between surgeon/assistant and patient

This communication should be reassuring and instil confidence. A relaxed patient will tend to bleed less, feel pain less, and take in advice better. The surgeon and assistant should agree in advance their role within this process as it is equally important that neither is distracted from their role. Some patients like to talk during the procedure; others prefer to be silent and listen to a conversation between surgeon and assistant. Try to work out which the patient would prefer.

It is a good idea to give the patient an indication of what you are doing, without so much detail that they feel faint! Again, engage the patient in the process, but judge individual needs. Encourage patients to let you know if they feel pain, feel faint, and so on, without constantly enquiring, as this can be unsettling in itself.

Between the surgeon and assistant

A good team will be able to organise most procedures without causing any alarm to the patient or to each other. To achieve this, there should be some useful code phrases such as:

- 'More swabs please' or 'Please put on some gloves' is a useful coded message to the assistant to prepare for haemorrhage by ensuring there is plenty of gauze to hand, and by putting on gloves to apply pressure.
- 'May we have the fan on?' or 'Are you feeling all right?' when uttered by the surgeon, alerts the assistant to prepare for a vasovagal attack, by lowering the operating table head, raising the patient's legs, or using a fan or air-conditioning to cool the patient.

Avoid certain words

There are some words that both surgeon and assistant should avoid, such as 'Oops' or 'Sorry'. It is easy to say these words if a swab or instrument is dropped. To the patient, however, this can easily suggest something has gone wrong with their surgery, and they may lose confidence in the surgeon and become anxious.

POSTOPERATIVELY

Chapter 8 discusses postoperative care in detail. It is very important that the patient receives written and verbal information about the following:

- Postoperative pain and bleeding.
- Looking after the wound, dressings, and washing.
- Follow-up arrangements in respect of suture removal and histopathology results.
- Contact details should there be any problems.
- It is essential to confirm that the patient has understood this information.

> **GOLDEN RULES** ❋
> - Introduce yourself and establish a rapport.
> - Understand the patient's ideas, concerns, and expectations.
> - Make sure that the patient fully understands the procedure and what it will involve.
> - Have a confident and reassuring manner at all times, even if things go wrong.

REFERENCE

Syrjala KL, Donaldson GW, Davis MW, *et al.* (1995) Relaxation and imagery and cognitive-behavioral training reduce pain during cancer treatment: a controlled clinical trial. *Pain* 63(2): 189–198.

Chapter 15

Local anaesthesia and minor surgical procedures

INTRODUCTION

Chapter 1 describes the equipment and the different types of anaesthetic agents that the surgeon may need to perform the range of procedures considered in this book. This chapter describes the different techniques that may be used, with an emphasis on infiltration, digital blocks (also known as ring blocks), and regional nerve blocks. Topical/surface anaesthesia is considered in Chapter 7. Sometimes more than one technique is used, for example surface and infiltration anaesthesia.

GOLDEN RULES ❋
The key points in ensuring effective anaesthesia are as follows:
- Use the correct type and quantity of anaesthesia.
- Anaesthetise the whole surgical field.
- Allow sufficient time for the anaesthetic agent to take effect.
- Never exceed the maximum safe dose for anaesthetic agents.

INFILTRATION ANAESTHESIA

This section describes the technique of infiltrating the skin with a local anaesthetic agent, the most commonly used technique for minor surgery. Tips for reducing the pain of injecting into the tissues are included at the end of the section. Local anaesthetic can be infiltrated either intradermally or subdermally. Commonly, a mixture of both techniques of administration is used, particularly when removing large epidermoid cysts or lipomas.

Intradermal injection
This involves injecting very superficially into the dermis. Insulin syringes and dental syringes are particularly useful for this type of anaesthesia as the fine needle reduces the pain (see Chapter 1 for a discussion of advantages and drawbacks of different needles and syringes). The technique has the following advantages and disadvantages:
- The local anaesthetic effect is rapid.
- If combined with adrenaline (epinephrine), the vasoconstriction causes skin blanching, the centre of which gives an indication of which areas are anaesthetised prior to surgery.
- The main disadvantage is that this technique is painful because the liquid is being injected into tissues that do not readily stretch. If, however, the infiltration is undertaken slowly, and with the small volumes of anaesthetic required, it is possible for this to be an almost painless procedure.

Subdermal anaesthesia
This technique requires injecting deep to the dermis, including into the subcutaneous fat. It has the following advantages and disadvantages:
- The technique is less painful as the tissues are less tight and larger volumes can be infiltrated with minimal pain.
- The onset of anaesthesia is delayed, it may be patchy, and the anaesthetised area may need to be mapped out.
- Larger-gauge needles may be necessary in order to pierce the dermis and reach the subdermis without bending the needle. This may cause more pain as the needle passes through the dermis.

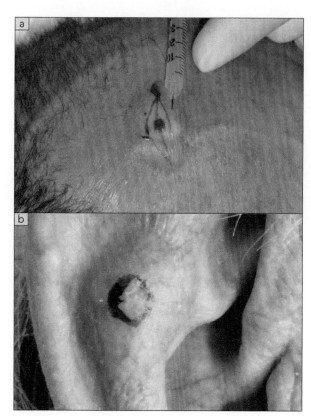

Figure 15.1 Hydrodissection over (a) the temporal artery and (b) the cartilage of the ear.

Hydrodissection

A further infiltrative local anaesthetic technique sometimes used in specific situations is so-called hydrodissection. This is where a larger volume of anaesthetic is injected under the lesion than is strictly needed for anaesthesia (Figure 15.1). The volume of liquid lifts the lesion away from underlying structures and facilitates surgical removal. Common areas where this can be helpful include the temporal area (to avoid the temporal artery) and the dorsum of the hand to avoid tendon sheaths. Care should be taken not to inadvertently inject the local anaesthetic agent into the structure being avoided.

Infiltrating the skin
Before you start

Confirm with your patient which lesion or lesions you are going to treat. It is recommended that you mark the lesion with a marker pen. This is particularly important if it lies deep to the skin. Once you have infiltrated a lesion, it is sometimes difficult to identify it, which is why preoperative marking is important.

Even with complete pain control, patients may still be aware of pressure at the operation site. An anxious patient may perceive this sensation as pain. It is therefore vital to help the patient feel at ease. The following are important:

- Establish a rapport.
- Make sure the patient fully understands the procedure and what it will involve.
- Develop a confident and reassuring manner.
- Warn the patient that, as you start, they will feel a sharp scratch or prick when you inject through the skin and that, if you are injecting intradermally, there may be some further discomfort, which will soon subside.

Techniques for infiltrating the skin: fan and encirclement

For small lesions, a fan-like approach, using two skin punctures at opposite sides of the lesion, is often sufficient (Figure 15.2a). For larger lesions, encircling is more appropriate. Anaesthetic is injected around the lesion, each time through skin that has already been numbed (Figure 15.2b). It is important to infiltrate all round the lesion and *deep* to it (Figure 15.3).

In vascular areas such as the scalp, keep the number of puncture points to a minimum in order to reduce bleeding. If you are using a dental syringe with a long fine needle, you will usually be able to manage with two punctures.

Figure 15.2 Techniques for infiltrating the skin: (a) fan approach and (b) encirclement.

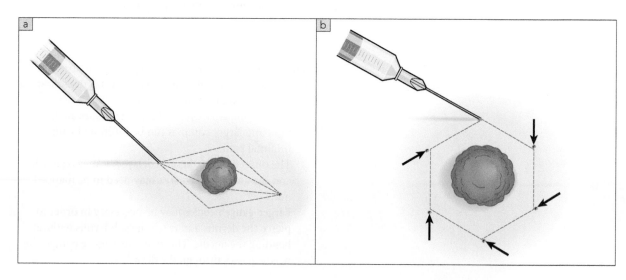

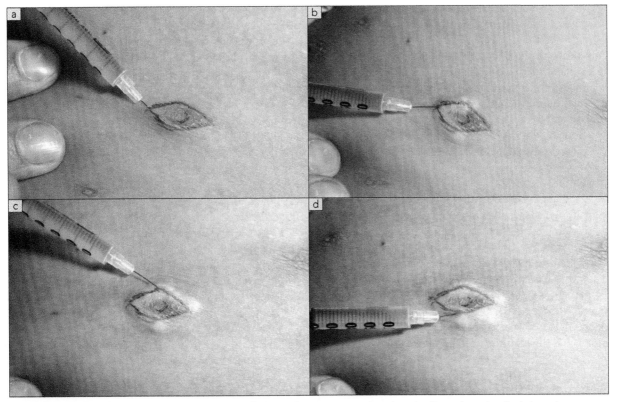

Figure 15.3 Infiltrating with local anaesthesia using a fan/encirclement approach and a mix of intradermal and subdermal infiltration.

Checking the efficacy of your anaesthesia

Although lidocaine works very quickly, its action is not instantaneous. If you do not allow enough time for it to take effect, you will soon lose the patient's confidence. Explain that you are going to demonstrate that the injection is working. When you touch the skin with an instrument, the patient should notice a difference between normal and anaesthetised skin. If they do not, give more anaesthetic until the patient is reassured that anaesthesia is complete.

Tips for reducing pain when performing infiltration analgesia

The pain of injecting is affected by the following factors, which can be influenced by the operator:

- The size (gauge) of the needle.
- The sharpness of the needle tip.
- The speed of injection (tissue distension is painful).
- The chemical being injected.
- The tonicity, pH, and temperature of the solution.

The operator can therefore reduce the pain of local anaesthesia by:

- Making sure the local anaesthetic solution is at body temperature.
- Injecting through a fine-bore needle with a sharp bevelled end.
- Using a solution as near isotonicity and neutral pH as possible.
- Injecting slowly to avoid tissue swelling and thereby reduce pain.
- Using a buffered preparation (see Chapter 7 for details) to produce an anaesthetic solution with a near-neutral pH.

DIGITAL AND REGIONAL NERVE BLOCKS

Any nerve in the body can be 'blocked' by infiltrating local anaesthetic around it. Ring and regional blocks are examples of this technique. Digital (or ring) blocks and regional blocks allow a smaller amount of local anaesthetic agent to be used, thereby:

- Reducing the risk of systemic toxicity.
- Allowing successful local anaesthesia of larger areas.
- Avoiding distortion of a surgical site due to the volume of anaesthetic.
- Reducing the need to inject into a particularly painful or dense area.
- Avoiding the likelihood of rupturing a cyst.

The only caution is to ensure that the local anaesthetic is not injected into the nerve itself, which could result in permanent damage to the nerve. It is therefore important, if the patient complains of pain in the distribution of the nerve during injection, that the needle be withdrawn and the injection tried again at a different site.

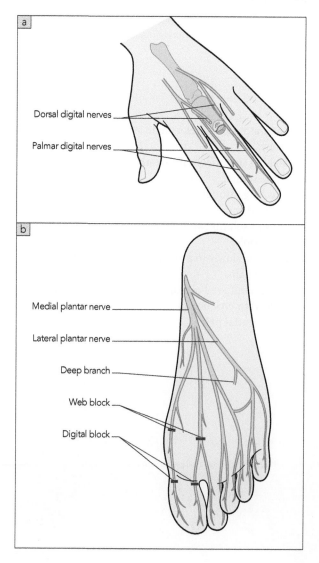

Digital block

Here, the anaesthetic agent is injected circumferentially around the surgical site without directly injecting the area to be operated. Although 1% or 2% lidocaine (*without adrenaline*) is most often used for this type of block, mixing it with bupivacaine may allow prolonged anaesthesia and thereby pain relief for procedures such as a nail resection.

Digital nerve block

This is a very useful technique for any procedure on a finger or toe. The digital nerves run along each side of the digit close to the bone, but there are often additional fibres that run much more superficially.

Finger digits are innervated by four digital nerves (Figure 15.4a):

- Two superior or dorsal nerve branches (branches of the radial and ulnar nerves).
- Two inferior or ventral/palmar nerve branches. (branches of the median and ulnar nerves).

Toe digits are similarly innervated (Figure 15.4b):

- Two dorsal nerve branches (branches of the peroneal nerve).
- Two ventral or plantar branches (branches of the tibial nerve).

Technique of digital nerve block

Insert the needle into the dorsolateral aspect of the digit just under the dermis and just distal to the metacarpophalangeal or metatarsophalangeal joint (Figure 15.5). Angle the needle towards the palm or sole and inject 1–2 ml of local anaesthetic along one side of the digit. Withdraw the needle and then repeat the procedure on the opposite side of the digit. The fluid will diffuse around the nerves. Further local anaesthetic can also be injected horizontally along the dorsal aspect of the digit (about 1 ml) to pick off any dorsal fibres.

Avoid injecting too much fluid—this may cause pressure ischaemia as digits have limited distensibility. A volume of 1–2 ml is usually all that is required, provided that you wait long enough for it to take effect. The use of adrenaline is contraindicated when performing a digital block.

It takes time for the local anaesthetic to infiltrate both the dorsal and the ventral digital nerves (10–30 minutes, depending upon the anaesthetic). Always test the surgical site for complete numbness before beginning the procedure. The patient will often be able to feel movement and pressure, but there should be no pain.

Figure 15.4 (a) Finger and (b) plantar digital nerves. The digital nerves travel down each side of the phalanges.

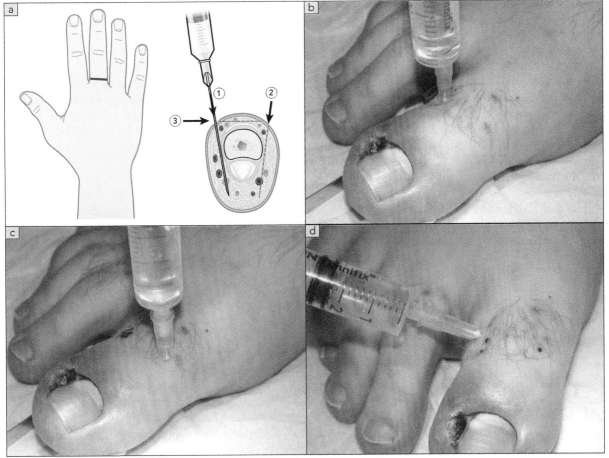

Figure 15.5 (a) Diagrammatic representation of a digital block. (b–d) Digital block technique: (b) and (c) correspond to 1 and 2 in (a); (d) corresponds to 3 in (a) .

Use of a tourniquet

A tourniquet is not a requirement when performing a digital ring block, but it may help to increase the duration of the digital block and aid haemostasis. The tourniquet should be left in place for as short a time as possible, ideally less than 10 minutes. The tourniquet should be placed tightly enough to prevent arterial flow. If it is not tight enough, only the veins are compressed and, with continued arterial flow, the digit will become engorged and bleeding will increase rather than decrease.

> ### GOLDEN RULES ⁕
> For digital nerve blocks:
> - Never use a local anaesthetic containing adrenaline; this can result in the loss of a finger or toe and is indefensible.
> - Always wait long enough before starting the procedure.
> - Never inject directly into the nerve.
> - Never give digital ring blocks to patients with diabetes or peripheral vascular disease.

Regional nerve block

The most commonly used regional nerve blocks (posterior tibial, radial, ulnar, and median nerves) are described below. Amide local anaesthetic agents are most often used for regional blocks. Higher concentrations, usually 2% lidocaine, are advantageous in producing a larger concentration gradient, which promotes diffusion into the nerve. *Adrenaline is not recommended* because any vasoconstrictive effect will be limited to the nerve (which may result in ischaemic damage) and there will be no beneficial vasoconstrictive effect at the operation site.

Several factors must be considered when a regional nerve block is performed:
- Most important is the anatomy. The surgeon must always know the anatomical landmarks and the location of the nerve to be blocked, keeping in mind individual variation.
- The local anaesthetic should be injected subcutaneously as most nerves lie subdermally.
- Aspiration should always be performed before injecting the local anaesthetic.
- A 25 G needle is recommended for regional blocks as it is difficult to aspirate through a smaller needle to ensure that a vessel has not been entered.

- The length of the needle required is determined by the estimated distance from the injection site to the nerve root targeted for the block.
- Never inject directly into the nerve; if nerve pain is experienced by the patient, the needle should be withdrawn and the site of injection changed.

Posterior tibial nerve block

One of the most useful nerve blocks is the posterior tibial nerve block. As a method of producing anaesthesia of the sole of the foot, it is ideal. In this area, the skin is particularly thick, and injections through the horny layer cause intense pain.

The posterior tibial nerve is a branch of the sciatic nerve. It passes distally along the posterior calf in company with the posterior tibial vessels to the interval between the heel and the medial malleolus, where it ends under the cover of the flexor retinaculum by dividing into the medial and lateral plantar nerves, which between them supply the sole of the foot. The posterior tibial nerve may be blocked as it passes behind the medial malleolus, before it divides.

Technique

A point is chosen exactly midway between the medial malleolus and the Achilles tendon at the level of the ankle, and the overlying skin is cleaned with antiseptic. A sterile syringe with 25 G needle is used with 5 ml 2% lidocaine. A small weal of local anaesthetic is raised at the point between the medial malleolus and the Achilles tendon, and the syringe is then directed at 45° in a horizontal plane, aiming the needle at the underlying bone (Figure 15.6). When the bone is reached, the needle is withdrawn 2 mm, and the plunger is gently withdrawn to check that the needle is not inside a vein. Then 2–5 ml of local anaesthetic solution is injected around the posterior tibial nerve, and the needle is withdrawn.

Anaesthesia of the sole of the foot gradually develops over the ensuing 10 minutes and will last for up to 2 hours. Because the overlying skin at the ankle is so much softer than the horny layers on the sole of the foot, an injection may be given painlessly at this site. The method is particularly useful for suturing lacerations on the sole of the foot or for the treatment of intradermal lesions.

Remember that proprioception depends on sensory impulses received from the soles of the feet. Therefore it is inadvisable to perform a posterior tibial nerve block on both feet simultaneously or the patient may be unable to maintain his or her balance.

Ulnar nerve block

The ulnar nerve at the wrist lies lateral to the tendon of the flexor carpi ulnaris, which runs distally along the ulnar border of the arm and is inserted into the pisiform bone. The nerve can usually be palpated as it passes lateral to this tendon proximal to the pisiform bone. Remember that the sensory distribution of the ulnar nerve is such that only the little finger can be totally anaesthetised with an ulnar nerve block.

Technique

Using 2% lidocaine, a small weal is raised in the skin overlying the nerve at the wrist, and the needle is inserted perpendicularly, lateral to the tendon over the nerve (Figure 15.7a). As the needle penetrates the deep fascia, it may touch the nerve, causing paraesthesia. A volume of 5 ml 2% lidocaine should then be injected. The dorsal sensory branch of the ulnar nerve frequently arises proximal to this point, so in order to block this as well, a further 5 ml 2% lidocaine should be injected subcutaneously from the medial side at the level of the ulnar styloid, extending under the skin to the middle of the back of the wrist (Figure 15.7b).

As with other nerve blocks, sufficient time should be allowed for the local anaesthetic to be absorbed by the nerve. It is also important not to inject the anaesthetic directly into the nerve; should the patient complain of pain, the needle should be either withdrawn or repositioned and the injection reattempted.

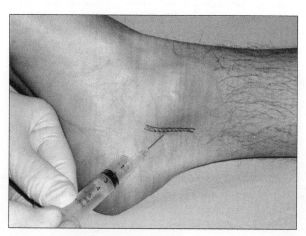

Figure 15.6 Posterior tibial nerve block.

GOLDEN RULES ✳

For regional nerve blocks:
- Never use a local anaesthetic containing adrenaline.
- Always wait long enough before starting the procedure.

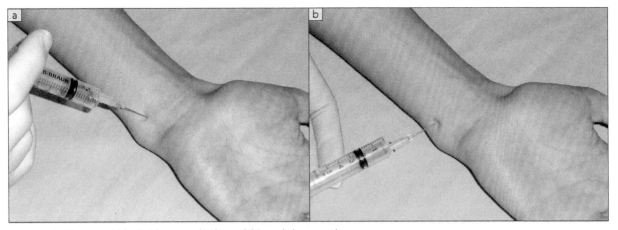

Figure 15.7 Ulnar nerve block: (a) perpendicular and (b) medial approach.

Radial nerve block

The radial nerve supplies the sensation over the dorsum of the lateral part of the hand. It accompanies the radial artery in the forearm, and then separates about 7 cm above the wrist, passing deep to the tendon of brachio-radialis muscle and subsequently dividing into digital branches.

Technique

To block the radial nerve, it is important to first identify the 'anatomical snuff box' by fully abducting the thumb, revealing a depression over the base of the first meta-carpal. This space is bounded anteriorly by the tendons of abductor pollicis longus and extensor pollicis brevis together, and posteriorly by the tendon of extensor pollicis longus.

Using 5 ml 2% lidocaine, a small weal should be created in the skin overlying the anatomical snuff box, followed by injecting about 3 ml subcutaneously into the anatomical snuff box (Figure 15.8). After this a further 2 ml of 2% lidocaine should be injected subcutaneously over the lower end of the radius. Allow sufficient time (10 minutes or more) for the anaesthetic to work.

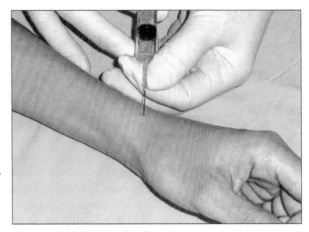

Figure 15.8 Radial nerve block.

Median nerve block

The sensory distribution of the median nerve supplies the palmar surface of the hand including half of the thumb, the palmar surface of the first and second fingers, and half of the palmar surface of the third finger (ring finger). At the wrist, the median nerve lies between the tendon of flexor carpi radialis laterally and the flexor digitorum sublimis and palmaris longus tendon medially.

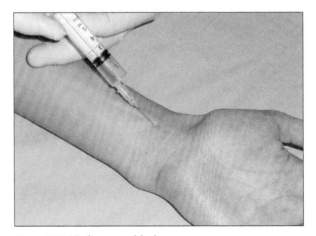

Figure 15.9 Median nerve block.

Technique

The needle should be inserted just lateral to the palmaris longus tendon, a weal raised in the overlying skin, and then 5 ml 1% lidocaine injected around the nerve (Figure 15.9). Again, allow sufficient time for the local anaesthetic to be absorbed (10–15 minutes).

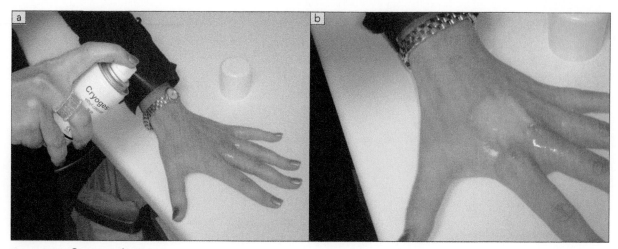

Figure 15.10 Cryoanaesthesia.

Cryoanaesthesia

Cryoanaesthesia refers to the external application of cold to the skin to produce numbness. This type of anaesthesia has a limited role following the development of local anaesthetic creams. Historically, ice was applied directly to the skin for 30–60 seconds to provide superficial short-duration anaesthesia for the 'painless' injection of a local anaesthetic.

Refrigerant sprays, such as ethyl chloride and dichloro-tetrafluoroethane (e.g., Histofreezer®), are still useful for anaesthetising superficial abscesses prior to incision and drainage. In the presence of infection, for example an abscess, the acidic tissue pH renders common local anaesthetic agents such as lidocaine relatively ineffective. After a frost is produced on the skin, a 10–12-second period of anaesthesia occurs before the skin temperature and sensation return to normal (Figure 15.10). The procedure therefore needs to be carefully coordinated so that the incision is completed before the effect of the cryoanaesthetic wears off.

These methods used to be recommended for children, but with the advent of topical anaesthetic creams, very fine-bore (30 G) needles and isotonic (0.5% lidocaine) or buffered anaesthetic, they have been largely superseded. Indeed for *children*, it is possible to mix 1% lidocaine 50:50 with normal saline. This is isotonic, produces minimal sting, and, if suturing a laceration, can be injected painlessly through the cut sides of the wound. Such weak solutions have a short duration of action, so need to be followed by infiltration with the usual type, concentration, and quantity of anaesthetics.

Resuscitation

INTRODUCTION

Chapter 1 discussed the recommended resuscitation equipment that should be available to manage emergencies. This chapter describes the potential causes of collapse during or after minor surgery and provides simple straightforward advice for their management.

OVERVIEW

Causes of collapse during or after minor surgery include the following:

- Reflex syncope/vasovagal episode (faint), which is by far the most common.
- Anaphylaxis.
- Cardiopulmonary arrest.

Rarer causes of collapse include:

- Neurological problems.
- Toxic or allergic reaction to local anaesthetic.
- Use of monopolar diathermy in patients with pacemakers.

The Resuscitation Council UK provides excellent guidelines about the immediate management of the collapsed patient. These are regularly updated and readers are referred to these for more detailed information that is beyond the scope of this text (see www.resus.org.uk/SiteIndx.htm).

> **DON'T FORGET** ▶▶
> The most common problem is a simple faint. It is important to diagnose and treat this promptly to avoid inappropriately aggressive resuscitative measures!

PREVENTION

Serious problems during minor surgery that require resuscitation are fortunately highly uncommon. However, it is very important that everyone knows what to do if things go wrong and a patient collapses. It is vitally important that you have thought through *in advance* how to deal with this situation. The surgeon must be confident that the surgical team know what to do in an emergency.

Planning

Contingency plans for dealing with unexpected collapse should be regularly rehearsed with all members of the clinical team.

Training

You must ensure that you are fully up to date with modern procedures and policies. Make sure that you and your staff attend regular practical courses on cardiopulmonary resuscitation. A summary of the current guidelines on cardiopulmonary resuscitation should be available in all rooms where minor procedures are carried out. Figures 16.1 and 16.2 (next page) show the resuscitation algorithms published by the Resuscitation Council (UK) for basic and in-hospital resuscitation.

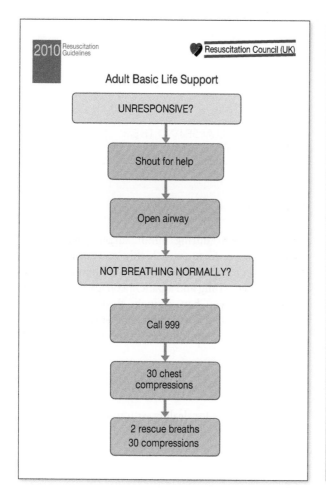

Figure 16.1 Resuscitation Council (UK) 2010 guidelines for adult basic resuscitation. (Used with kind permission from the Resuscitation Council, United Kingdom.)

Figure 16.2 Resuscitation Council (UK) 2010 guidelines for in-hospital resuscitation. (Used with kind permission from the Resuscitation Council, United Kingdom.)

CAUSES OF COLLAPSE AND THEIR MANAGEMENT

Reflex syncope (vasovagal syncope)

The most common cause of loss of consciousness in connection with minor surgery is reflex syncope (neurally mediated syncope, vasovagal syncope), otherwise known as simple fainting. Reflex syncope occurs as a result of simultaneous overstimulation of the parasympathetic system and suppression of the sympathetic system. In minor surgery, this can be triggered by:

- A warm environment (e.g., a poorly ventilated or non-air-conditioned operating room).
- The emotional stress of the procedure (e.g., anxiety, fear).
- Dehydration: Some patients wrongly believe that they should fast before a local anaesthetic procedure.

These triggers lead to cardioinhibitory (bradycardia) and vasodepressor (vasodilatation and hypotension) responses, which in turn lead to cerebral anoxia.

Management

Treatment for vasovagal syncope focuses on the avoidance of triggers, restoration of blood flow to the brain during an impending episode, and measures that interrupt or prevent the pathophysiological mechanism described above.

Avoidance of triggers

Clinical rooms where minor surgery takes place should be well ventilated without compromising confidentiality. Temperature control should be in place, ideally with air-conditioning, as fans can potentially blow dust into the sterile operating field.

Pain can also be the trigger, and the local anaesthetic should be administered by the least painful method (warming up the agent to room temperature, using fine-bore needles, avoiding injecting into inflamed areas, and injecting slowly). Effective anaesthesia should be confirmed before commencing the initial incision.

Remember that accompanying friends or relatives who are adamant that they will watch the surgery, and sometimes even observing medical students, are prone to stress- or fear-induced syncope.

Restoration of cerebral perfusion

Most people experience prodromal symptoms prior to the loss of consciousness, and therefore a quick response may prevent it. Most minor surgery should be carried out with the patient lying down, although it is sometimes more convenient for very minor procedures, for example the diathermy excision of small skin tags around the neck, to be performed with the patient sitting. Getting the patient to lie down and elevating the patient's legs is usually effective in restoring circulation. An operating couch that allows the head to be lowered and the feet to be raised is strongly recommended as this makes the management of reflex syncope much more straightforward.

Anaphylaxis

Anaphylaxis or Type 1 hypersensitivity is an extremely severe, life-threatening systemic allergic response characterised by rapidly developing life-threatening airway and/or breathing and/or circulatory problems usually associated with skin and mucosal changes such as angio-oedema or urticaria. The patient is usually anxious and can experience 'a sense of impending doom'. However, there is a wide range of possible presenting symptoms, and these can be non-specific. It is therefore recognised that the resulting diagnostic problems have, and will inevitably continue to result in, both under- and overtreatment.

Anaphylaxis is most likely if *all* of the following are present:

- Sudden onset and rapid progression of symptoms.
- Life-threatening airway and/or breathing and/or circulatory problems.
- Skin and/or mucosal changes (noting that these changes in isolation do not indicate an anaphylactic reaction).

Oedema of the face, lips, and tongue (angio-oedema) can develop rapidly and be very frightening. A widespread urticarial skin eruption may occur but is not always present. Patients can also have gastrointestinal symptoms, for example abdominal pain, incontinence, or vomiting. Diagnostic difficulties are most common in children, which is one of the reasons why minor surgery is best avoided in children unless the surgical team has particular expertise and knowledge in this area.

In adults, the two most common differential diagnoses are panic attacks and vasovagal attacks. The absence of airway and breathing difficulties and swelling helps to differentiate these from anaphylactic attacks, but patients with a genuine history of anaphylaxis may be prone to panic attacks if they think they may be exposed to an allergen. Vasovagal attacks cause bradycardia as opposed to tachycardia.

Management of anaphylaxis

Adrenaline (epinephrine) is the most important drug in the treatment of anaphylaxis (Figure 16.3, next page). It acts both on alpha and beta receptors to reverse the clinical manifestations of anaphylaxis and also inhibits the release of histamine. Adrenaline should therefore always be available and easily accessible wherever minor surgery is carried out.

There is always conflict caused by the fact that it is more effective the earlier it is given at a time when the diagnosis of anaphylaxis may be difficult, meaning that there are cases when it is given when the diagnosis proves to be incorrect. However, most of the risks associated with adrenaline occur when it is given intravenously. It is essential that it is not administered intravenously as this will not only trigger a feeling of impending doom in the patient, but also produce hypertension, tachycardia, and arrhythmias. It is therefore best given intramuscularly into the anterolateral aspect of the thigh.

The non-breathing, unresponsive patient

Cardiopulmonary resuscitation should be started if a patient becomes unconscious, does not respond, and does not breathe normally. The patient is therefore in either cardiac or respiratory arrest, with the former more likely for adults and the latter more common in children. This is reflected in the small differences in the basic life support (BLS) algorithms for each group. The procedures described in this book may be performed in non-acute settings outside hospitals where access to the equipment and drugs required for advanced life support is unavailable. In this situation, emphasis is on BLS and sending for expert help.

Principles of basic life support

Diagnosis is no longer based on the absence of a carotid pulse, as it has been shown that pulse palpation for 10 seconds is unreliable for determining the presence or absence of an effective circulation. The absence of 'signs of life,' such as response to stimuli, normal breathing (rather than abnormal gasps), or spontaneous movement should trigger cardiopulmonary resuscitation.

In the event of cardiac arrest, the heart may be in a shockable rhythm (e.g., ventricular fibrillation) or a non-shockable rhythm (e.g., asystole). In either case, BLS is effectively a holding procedure and buys time while awaiting either the arrival of a defibrillator or the spontaneous restarting of the heart. It is therefore important to shout for help prior to assessing the patient and to call for a defibrillator immediately the diagnosis of arrest is made, even before the commencement of cardiopulmonary resuscitation.

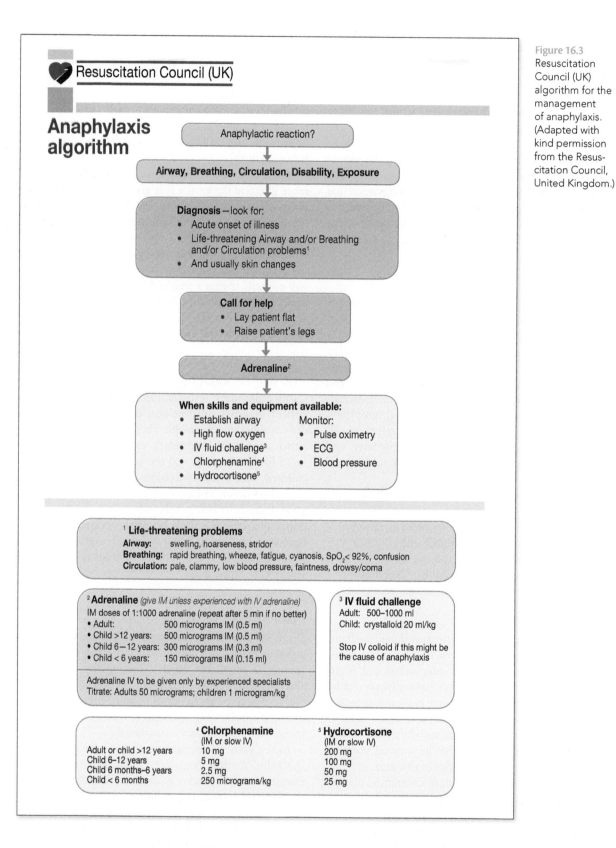

Figure 16.3
Resuscitation
Council (UK)
algorithm for the
management
of anaphylaxis.
(Adapted with
kind permission
from the Resus-
citation Council,
United Kingdom.)

In non-asphyxial cardiac arrest, the blood oxygen saturation remains high for a few minutes. Therefore, chest compressions are much more important than ventilation during the first few minutes of BLS.

Emphasis is placed on good quality chest compressions and minimising the number and duration of gaps during chest compression. Compress the chest to a depth of 5–6 cm and at a rate of 100–120 per minute. It is also advised not to stop to check the victim or discontinue cardiopulmonary resuscitation unless the victim starts to show signs of regaining consciousness and starts to breathe normally.

Local anaesthetic toxicity and its management

Chapter 7 describes local anaesthetic preparations, safe dosages, and signs of local anaesthetic toxicity. The most commonly used local anaesthetic is lidocaine, and early symptoms and signs of overdosage include circumoral tingling, tinnitus, and slight confusion or oddness of speech. The patient will sometimes complain of a metallic taste. By talking to the patient you will notice these signs immediately.

It is obviously essential in this situation to stop giving any further local anaesthetic. If overdosage continues, the patient may develop nystagmus, dysphasia, or muscular fasciculation. In later stages, loss of consciousness supervenes, with fits, cardiac arrhythmias, and respiratory and cardiac arrest. It is very unlikely that this situation will arise with the procedures and quantities of local anaesthetic recommended in this book, but for completeness a management algorithm is included (Figure 16.4).

Figure 16.4
Management of local anaesthetic toxicity: the Association of Anaesthetists of Great Britain & Ireland 2010 Guideline (continued on next page).

AAGBI Safety Guideline
Management of Severe Local Anaesthetic Toxicity

1 Recognition

Signs of severe toxicity:
- Sudden alteration in mental status, severe agitation or loss of consciousness, with or without tonic–clonic convulsions
- Cardiovascular collapse: sinus bradycardia, conduction blocks, asystole and ventricular tachyarrhythmias may all occur
- Local anaesthetic (LA) toxicity may occur some time after an initial injection

2 Immediate management

- Stop injecting the LA
- Call for help
- Maintain the airway and, if necessary, secure it with a tracheal tube
- Give 100% oxygen and ensure adequate lung ventilation (hyperventilation may help by increasing plasma pH in the presence of metabolic acidosis)
- Confirm or establish intravenous access
- Control seizures: give a benzodiazepine, thiopental or propofol in small incremental doses
- Assess cardiovascular status throughout
- Consider drawing blood for analysis, but do not delay definitive treatment to do this

3 Treatment

IN CIRCULATORY ARREST
- Start cardiopulmonary resuscitation (CPR) using standard protocols
- Manage arrhythmias using the same protocols, recognising that arrhythmias may be very refractory to treatment
- Consider the use of cardiopulmonary bypass if available

GIVE INTRAVENOUS LIPID EMULSION
(following the regimen overleaf)
- Continue CPR throughout treatment with lipid emulsion
- Recovery from LA-induced cardiac arrest may take >1 h
- Propofol is not a suitable substitute for lipid emulsion
- Lidocaine should not be used as an anti-arrhythmic therapy

WITHOUT CIRCULATORY ARREST
Use conventional therapies to treat:
- Hypotension
- Bradycardia
- Tachyarrhythmia

CONSIDER INTRAVENOUS LIPID EMULSION
(following the regimen overleaf)
- Propofol is not a suitable substitute for lipid emulsion
- Lidocaine should not be used as an anti-arrhythmic therapy

4 Follow-up

- Arrange safe transfer to a clinical area with appropriate equipment and suitable staff until sustained recovery is achieved
- Exclude pancreatitis by regular clinical review, including daily amylase or lipase assays for two days
- Report cases as follows:
  in the United Kingdom to the National Patient Safety Agency (via www.npsa.nhs.uk)
  in the Republic of Ireland to the Irish Medicines Board (via www.imb.ie)
- If Lipid has been given, please also report its use to the international registry at www.lipidregistry.org. Details may also be posted at www.lipidrescue.org

Your nearest bag of lipid emulsion is kept ....

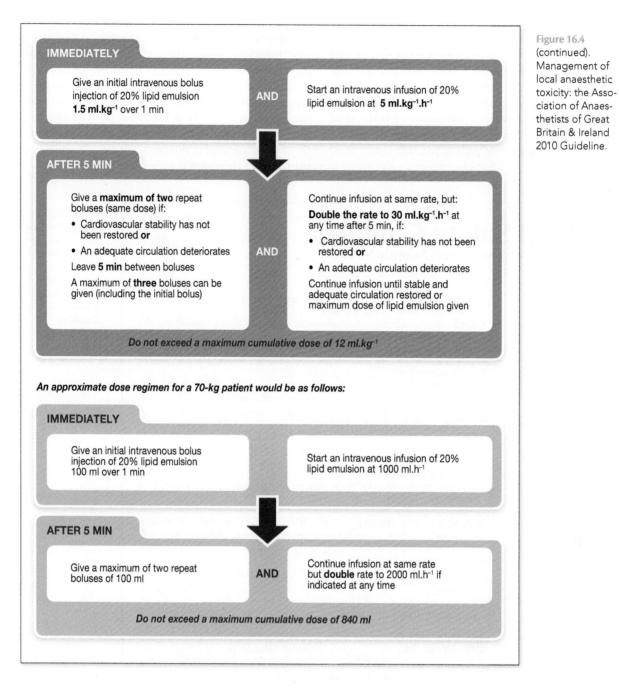

IMMEDIATELY

Give an initial intravenous bolus injection of 20% lipid emulsion **1.5 ml.kg⁻¹** over 1 min

AND

Start an intravenous infusion of 20% lipid emulsion at **5 ml.kg⁻¹.h⁻¹**

AFTER 5 MIN

Give a **maximum of two** repeat boluses (same dose) if:
- Cardiovascular stability has not been restored **or**
- An adequate circulation deteriorates

Leave **5 min** between boluses

A maximum of **three** boluses can be given (including the initial bolus)

AND

Continue infusion at same rate, but:

Double the rate to 30 ml.kg⁻¹.h⁻¹ at any time after 5 min, if:
- Cardiovascular stability has not been restored **or**
- An adequate circulation deteriorates

Continue infusion until stable and adequate circulation restored or maximum dose of lipid emulsion given

Do not exceed a maximum cumulative dose of 12 ml.kg⁻¹

An approximate dose regimen for a 70-kg patient would be as follows:

IMMEDIATELY

Give an initial intravenous bolus injection of 20% lipid emulsion 100 ml over 1 min

Start an intravenous infusion of 20% lipid emulsion at 1000 ml.h⁻¹

AFTER 5 MIN

Give a maximum of two repeat boluses of 100 ml

AND

Continue infusion at same rate but **double** rate to 2000 ml.h⁻¹ if indicated at any time

Do not exceed a maximum cumulative dose of 840 ml

Figure 16.4 (continued). Management of local anaesthetic toxicity: the Association of Anaesthetists of Great Britain & Ireland 2010 Guideline.

Chapter 17

Basic surgical techniques

INTRODUCTION

This chapter describes how to handle correctly some of the core skin surgery instruments, and then goes on to describe the key skills required to perform a straightforward ellipse excision and close the wound with sutures or other skin closures. Levels of difficulty are indicated by scalpel ratings. The more scalpel blades, the more difficult the procedure and the more practical experience will be required to become competent at the technique.

The techniques of shave excision, curettage, and cautery are described in Chapter 19, and excision of cysts and lipomas in Chapter 20. Details of the frequently used and appropriate surgical instruments for skin surgery are included in Chapter 1 along with important information about sterilisation. Operating with the correct instruments, of good quality, makes performing surgery safer and more enjoyable.

HANDLING COMMON SURGICAL INSTRUMENTS

Scalpel

Hold the scalpel (usually a No. 15 blade with size 3 Bard–Parker handle, or a round Beaver handle) like a pen, perpendicular to the skin (Figure 17.1a). This is different from the traditional surgeon's grip (Figure 17.1 b), which is useful for large incisions, but not so useful for most skin surgery incisions.

Attaching the blade to the handle

When operating with a reusable scalpel handle, you will need to attach the disposable blade carefully. This is best achieved by holding the blade at the base of the cutting edge in a pair of curved mosquito forceps (see Video Clip 17.1—http://goo.gl/0UUqf). Do not risk damaging suture forceps for this procedure. To remove the blade, you reverse the procedure, holding the blade at the base, to lever it off the handle. Alternatively use a disposable Swann–Morton blade remover.

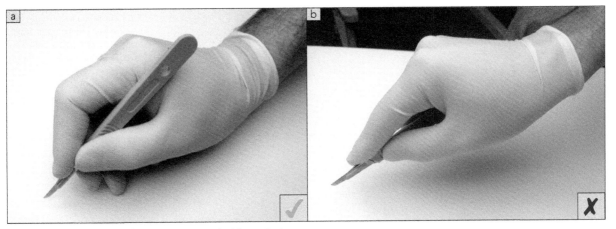

Figure 17.1 (a) Correct and (b) incorrect way to hold a scalpel.

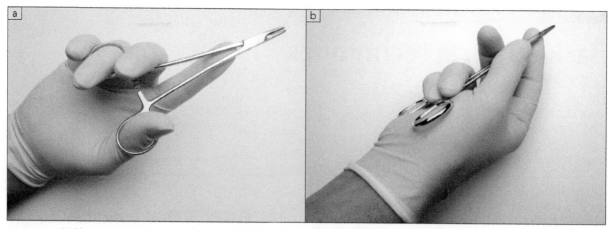

Figure 17.2 (a) The conventional surgeon's grip and (b) the palm grip for holding a suture holder.

Suture holder (needle holder)

Suture holders can be held in a number of ways depending upon the type of suture being undertaken. The traditional surgeon's grip (Figure 17.2a) is less used in skin surgery as it is better suited to inserting sutures into cavities. Instead the 'palm grip' (Figure 17.2b) is often used. The key is that the surgeon should feel comfortable with whichever grip is used.

The advantage of the skin surgeon's palm grip is the ease with which it allows the instrument to rotate through 180° as the curved suture needle is inserted, passed through, and then removed from the skin. Using the palm grip, the needle is easily inserted at 90° to the skin, rotated in through, and then rotated out through the skin at 90°; the importance of this will become clear later in the chapter, when the insertion of sutures is discussed.

Positioning the needle in the suture holder

The needle should be held at the tip (or very close to the tip) of the suture holder, at 90° to it and two-thirds of the way down around the needle, to avoid it bending when used. Suture/needle holders with tungsten carbide jaws (see page 11) have narrow jaws that do not flatten the curved needle, while at the same time ensuring a firm grip on the needle. Figure 17.3a shows the needle held correctly at the tip of the needle holder and at 90° to it, with the needle held no more than two-thirds along its length. Any further and the needle holder would be grasping the hollow, crushable, and bendable section of the needle.

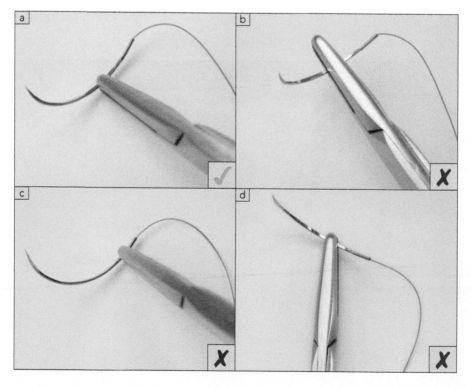

Figure 17.3 Position of the needle in the holder: (a) correct; (b) incorrect— needle holder liable to flatten the needle; (c) incorrect— needle held by the bendable hollow section; (d) incorrect— needle at an angle.

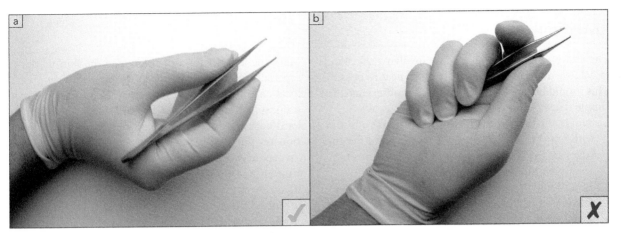

Figure 17.4 Holding forceps (a) correctly and (b) incorrectly.

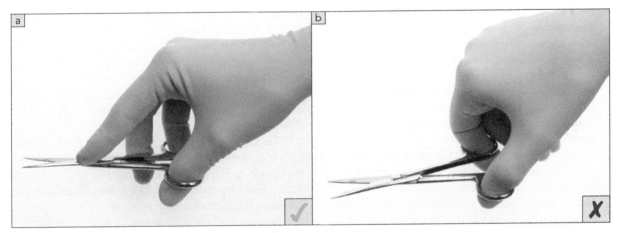

Figure 17.5 (a) Holding scissors correctly and (b) incorrectly.

Forceps

Tissue forceps should be held like the scalpel, in a pen grip, and not in the 'screwdriver' grip used with the needle holder (Figure 17.4). Using them in a screwdriver grip gives rise to excess tissue forces and can result in rotational damage to the fine ends of the forceps.

Scissors

The technique for improved handling of scissors involves using the thumb and middle fingers to operate the scissors and using the index finger to stabilise the scissors over the hinge joint (Figure 17.5a). In addition, it is possible to rotate and hold the scissors 'in reverse' to reduce the risk of injury when not actually cutting. It is then a simple procedure to rotate the scissors back to the cutting position. Figure 17.5b shows the wrong way to hold the scissors.

OPERATING ON THE SKIN: IMPORTANT PRINCIPLES

The aim of any surgical procedure involving the skin is to achieve a scar that is as small and as neat as possible. This should be possible in most cases by observing a few simple rules:

- Skin is a living tissue and must be treated gently and with respect. Good healing will only occur if the cut edges are held during healing in their exact position and under minimal or no tension.
- Skin should be cut with a sharp scalpel rather than scissors, which have a shearing action.
- Tissues should be handled as little as possible, and particularly not with any crushing forceps. Skin hooks should be used to hold or retract skin flaps.
- Deeply placed absorbable sutures should be used to allow closure in layers whenever possible, and their knots tied in the deeper plane.
- With deep and absorbable sutures, the least bulk of suture material should be left in the wound to be absorbed.
- Skin sutures, when used, should be of the minimum calibre required to hold the wound together, and should be removed as soon as wound integrity allows.
- Numerous fine skin sutures that distribute tension evenly are preferable to a few widely spaced large stitches that concentrate skin tension.
- Haemostasis should be achieved with care and, when required, with the avoidance of excessive cautery to the wound. In most minor surgical procedures, haemostasis should not be a problem.
- The surgeon who inserts the sutures should ideally be the person who removes them, or at least supervises their removal. Only by personally examining each wound postoperatively can improvements in technique be achieved.

CUTTING AN ELLIPSE

Marking the ellipse

Mark the lesion with a pen designed for skin marking, especially if the lesion is deep, before infiltrating with local anaesthetic or you may be unable to find it after infiltrating around it (see Chapter 7 for information on local anaesthesia). Always mark out the proposed incision on the skin before cutting anything. Any adjustments can easily be made at this stage before committing yourself to a scar by incising the skin. Bear in mind that if you cover the patient with sterile towels, you will find it more difficult to get your bearings. A sterile or non-sterile skin marker pen can be used according to personal preference.

It is important to ensure the markings do not wash off immediately when the skin is cleaned with antiseptic solution. An aqueous solution is less likely to cause this than an alcohol-based one.

Even if your incision is elliptical, the result will be a linear wound. Consider first in what orientation you want this line, and either mark each end of it on the skin with a dot or draw a line along which the intended scar will run. The apex of each end of the ellipse will lie along this line.

Next mark each side of the lesion with a dot. These two dots will represent the side of the ellipse at the narrowest margin to the lesion. This margin should be no less than 2 mm (dependent upon the lesion). Then draw the ellipse, making sure it encompasses the lesion adequately, taking account of the skin creases.

The ratio of the ellipse will usually be such that the length is three times the width in order to close the wound easily (Figure 17.6a). It is very easy to draw the ellipse too short, resulting in a more spherical or ovoid excision that will tend to stretch during healing (Figure 17.6b). When learning these measurements, it is worth using the scale on the marker pen, or on a ruler to check the 3:1 ratio. Remember that a 10 mm diameter lesion will need an ellipse 14 mm wide, and this in turn means an ellipse 42 mm long.

Once the area has been marked up, infiltrate with local anaesthetic and wait for this to take effect (see Chapter 15).

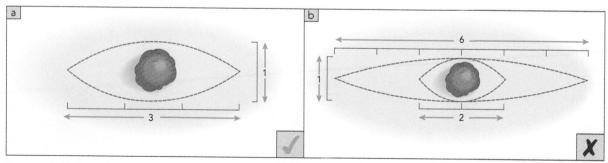

Figure 17.6 (a) Correct proportions—3:1 ratio, and (b) incorrect proportions for an ellipse.

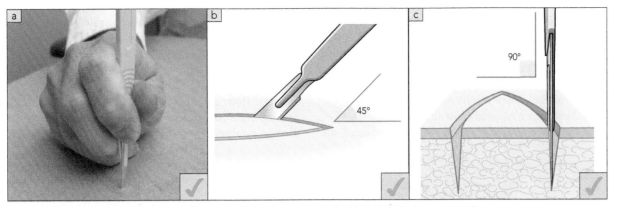

Figure 17.7 Correct incision technique: (a) 'pen' grip; (b) 45° cutting angle; (c) perpendicular wound edge.

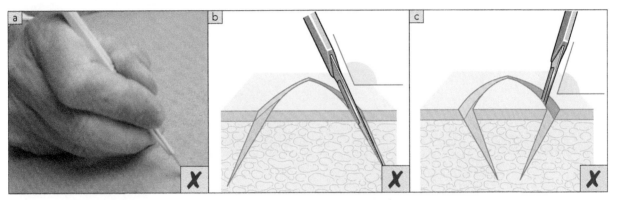

Figure 17.8 Incorrect incision technique: scalpel held at an angle to the perpendicular..

Making the incision

Using the scalpel

Hold the scalpel in a 'pen grip' and not a 'knife grip', perpendicular to the skin, and at a cutting angle of about 45° (Figure 17.7). It is important to remember that your hand will tend to hold the scalpel at an angle to the perpendicular. Check that you resist this tendency (unless following the orientation of hair follicles on hair-bearing skin) (Figure 17.8).

Incise the skin boldly and avoid tentative scratching. The scalpel blade should produce clean, linear incisions (Video Clip 17.2a—http://goo.gl/wZJcs). It must not be used like an artist's pencil to produce a 'feathered' edge (Video Clip 17.2b—http://goo.gl/6xvJ7). By always cutting perpendicular to the skin, you will ensure that the cut edge of the wound remains at the very least perpendicular, and at best slightly undermined (see Figure 17.7c).

Following the skin markings

When cutting into skin, the purpose of skin marking will become apparent. It is for good reason that carpenters state 'Mark twice, cut once.' With the cut lines already marked out, the surgeon is left with the relatively easy task of ensuring that the blade follows the line (Figure 17.9). There is a natural tendency to cut *inside* the marked lines. This tendency should be resisted, as the distance between the lesion and the margin will be reduced and an incomplete excision may result. The blade should follow either the centre or the outside edge of the skin marker. Keep to the marks you have made and do not modify the incision when you start to cut.

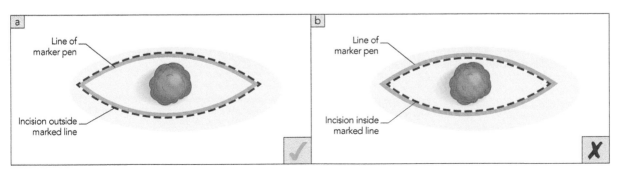

Figure 17.9 Following the skin markings (a) correctly and (b) incorrectly.

Cutting an ellipse

Follow the skin markings with a smooth action from one apex of the ellipse, maintaining skin tension with your other hand, but avoiding cutting toward your own or your assistant's fingers. Stop a millimetre or two from the second apex (Figure 17.10 and Video Clip 17.3a,b,c). Then do the same on the other side of the ellipse, again stopping just short of the end. Then, with the blade rotated through 180° in your hand, and with the sharp edge toward the cut side, starting from the second apex, finish off the ellipse on both sides. By doing this you reduce the chance of creating a 'fishtail'-shaped incision (Figure 17.11a and Video Clip 17.4). You can also avoid the fishtail effect by taking the first cut from each point toward the centre and then joining each edge up in the middle; this technique is also acceptable.

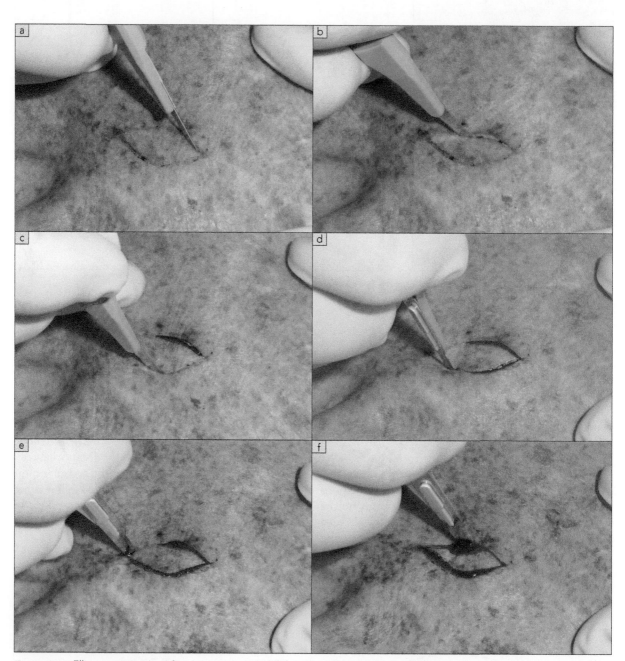

Figure 17.10 Ellipse excision: (a–c) from one apex, and (d–f) from the other apex. See Video Clips 17.3a—http://goo.gl/7B55P; 17.3b—http://goo.gl/OjCQE; 17.3c—http://goo.gl/MUpB0.

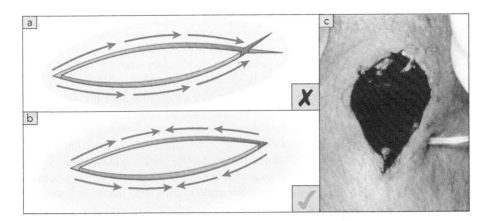

Figure 17.11 Comparison between (a) an incorrect 'fishtail' incision and (b) a correct incision. (c) Both apices have been overcut, creating one fishtail incision. See Video Clip 17.4— http://goo.gl/VUEeA

Depth of the incision

The depth of the incision should be the full thickness of the dermis and almost always to the fat layer (exceptions include the back of the hand and the pretibial area, where fat is absent). If the incision does not reach this depth, closure will be under tension and healing will be affected. Your incision should ideally cut through these layers and down to the fatty layer in one clean cut. This is, however, rarely possible except with very delicate skin, and it is often safer to repeat the incisions, gradually cutting down to the fat layer, rather than to risk cutting too deeply with the first incision. Figure 17.12 illustrates an ellipse excision, down to the fat but avoiding blood vessels.

Removing the lesion

Use a skin hook or fine dissecting forceps to hold up the apex of the specimen at one end, and dissect the lesion out along the fat plane (Figure 17.13 and Video Clip 17.5). Take care to avoid structures running superficially in the fat layer (nerves and blood vessels). With the right level of tension on a skin hook, it is almost possible to lift the specimen off the fat layer, just using the scalpel to lightly facilitate this. This level of tension will also help maintain haemostasis.

Some surgeons advocate cutting the specimen from the fat layer with scissors, others with the scalpel. Either will do. If the margins have been cut down to, but not through, the fat layer, it should be easy to divide the lesion from the fat with the aid of gentle traction on the specimen. The more friable the specimen, the gentler the traction should be to avoid tearing it. Ideally, hold the specimen (using either a skin hook or forceps) by the apex. This will avoid any crush artefact of the lesion.

While cutting through the fat layer, use the skin hook or forceps to reflect the specimen back to enable visualisation of the underlying area. In this way, any important structures can be seen and accidental damage avoided. Where such structures are expected, the technique of hydrodissection may be used (see Chapter 7).

As the specimen is removed, pressure should be applied to the wound to reduce bleeding. Place the specimen in a histology pot clearly labelled with the patient's details, the site of the lesion, and the date. Where multiple specimens are to be removed, use in addition a simple 'a', 'b', 'c' method of labelling, and record this in the patient's records.

Cutting an ellipse

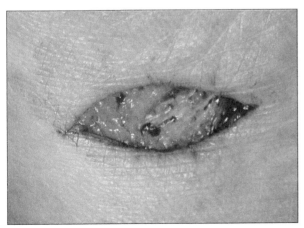

Figure 17.12 Excision down to fat, avoiding the blood vessel. See Video Clip 17.5—http://goo.gl/pTZLy.

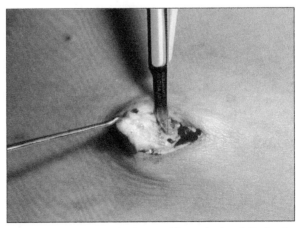

Figure 17.13 Dissecting the lesion with a scalpel and skin hook.

Undermining

Undermining is the technique whereby the surrounding skin is lifted free of the underlying layer prior to wound closure (Figure 17.14 and Video Clip 17.6). This technique may be necessary to reduce the tension caused when the cut edges are brought together for suturing, by allowing the skin edges to move together without compressing deeper planes and the skin to stretch more easily. Undermining is not always required, especially if the existing skin tension is slight, and may be best avoided in areas of anatomical concern (where important structures are located close to the surface). The technique should be undertaken carefully, gently, and usually with blunt dissection, as there is commonly a lack of direct visualisation.

An instrument (ideally blunt-ended, curved iris scissors) is inserted under the edge of the wound, between the dermis and subcutaneous fat. The instrument is inserted closed and parallel to the skin (the aim is not to go deeper, but to follow the existing resection depth) and then opened to bluntly dissect the edges free of the fat.

This process should be undertaken methodically and progressively around the wound edge. In this way, significant structures will be avoided and problems with haemostasis are less likely to arise. The process is facilitated by the use of a skin hook to raise and stabilise the area of skin being undermined. As undermining is more likely to reach the anaesthetised margin, it is advisable to ensure that the patient is asked to report any pain or discomfort while undermining takes place. Undermining should involve the circumference of the wound. Areas of resistance will occasionally need to be cut with the scissors. Ensure, however, you know exactly what you are cutting, and never cut blind.

Once undermining is complete, there should be reduced skin tension when the wound edges are brought together. The wound now requires closure.

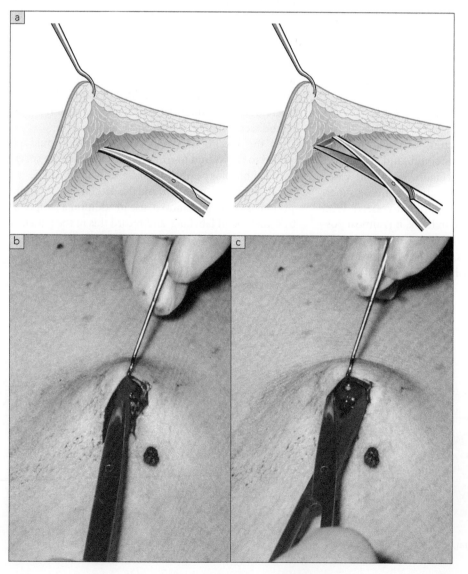

Figure 17.14 (a) Diagrammatic representation of undermining technique. Undermining with scissors (b) closed and (c) open. See Video Clip 17.6—http://goo.gl/b3Rx7z.

SKIN CLOSURE

Whatever suture you use to close the wound, you must be able to tie surgical knots, so the next section considers this. This is then followed by a section on different suturing techniques and finally other types of skin closure.

Knot-tying

Knot-tying is an art form it itself. General surgeons perfect the single-handed knot-tying technique, which is essential within body cavities. But although this is impressive to watch, it is unnecessary and usually inappropriate for skin surgery as the use of suture material will be excessive. More appropriate is the instrument-tied knot. This method of tying conserves the suture and also allows very precise knot tension.

The instrument-tied knot consists of using the needle holder to produce the turns or throws of the knot, and to pull the ends through to tie the knot (Video Clip 17.7—http://goo.gl/glkNr). The act of rotating one end of the suture upon the other is termed a *throw*. The more throws in one direction, the more the knot will tend to hold, but also the greater the resistance there will be to its being tightened. Rotating a second throw in the opposite direction may be sufficient to tie the knot, but for smooth monofilament material several alternating throws may be required.

The first golden rule of knot-tying is to pull most of the suture material through the skin to the side with the needle attached (avoiding the obvious mistake of pulling the end too far). This should make it easier to grab the end of the suture with the needle holder. If the majority of the length of the suture is not pulled through, the likely result is either a large amount of wasted material or the complication of a loop of suture being pulled through as the knot is tied.

During surgery, knot-tying involves two distinct steps. The purpose of the first step is to secure precise approximation of the wound edges by tying either a two-throw or a three-throw knot. The second step is to lock the suture to prevent slippage. In the description that follows, it is assumed that the surgeon is right-handed.

With the needle holder held in the traditional surgeon's grip in the right hand and the needle end (but *not* the needle) of the suture held in the left hand, a number of loops or throws around the needle holder can be made (three throws for monofilament, two throws for braided sutures). This action can take place at a distance from the patient. With plenty of suture material between the left hand and the patient, there is no need to struggle to complete these throws close to the wound. This is best achieved with a combination of the left hand looping the suture around the needle holder with the right hand moving the tip of the needle holder around the left hand.

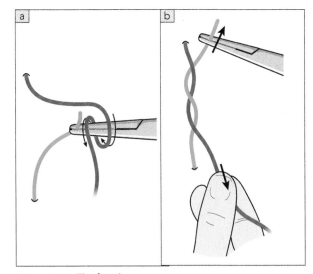

Figure 17.15 The first throw.

Next, the jaws of the needle holder (with the throws of suture material around the arms of the needle holder) are directed down by the right wrist to grasp the free end of the suture, close to the skin (Figure 17.15a). This free end is drawn through the throws of the knot by withdrawing the suture holder in the right hand away from the wound (Figure 17.15b).

The resulting knot now needs to be drawn down to the skin. The trick here is to pull the knot tight by pulling the left hand (the needle end of the suture) away from the patient while at the same time advancing the right hand with the needle holder tip toward the skin. This minimises wastage of the suture material. The aim is to end up with plenty of suture material in your hand and very little wasted at the needle holder tip. If both left and right hands are pulled to form the knot, a large amount of suture material will be wasted. By pulling in the ends in the same orientation as the knot (and perpendicular to the wound), the skin edges can be brought together gently.

When using interrupted sutures, the suturing process should do no more than allow the skin edges to touch; any more tension and postoperative wound swelling (while healing) will cause the sutures to dig into the skin, causing pain and inflammation, and at worst causing the suture to pull through the wound edges.

Once the first throws have been tightened down in contact with the wound, the surgeon will be able to confirm the accuracy of the apposition of the wound edges. If there is excess separation of the wound edges, the two-throw or three-throw knot can be gradually tightened to bring the wound edges closer together. The knotted suture loop should bring together the wound edges without devitalising the tissue encircled by the suture loop.

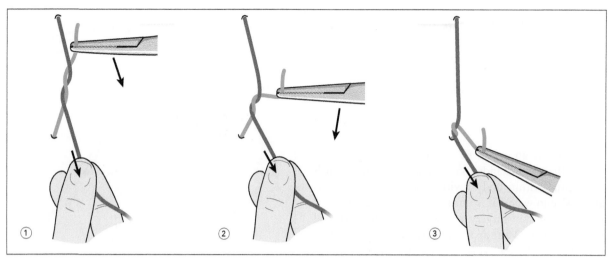

Figure 17.16 Locking the throw.

If the knot slips at this stage, it can be 'locked' by bringing one suture end across the wound, under tension so that both suture ends are together (Figure 17.16). The end that has been pulled over in this procedure is now 'locked' and will remain so unless it is pulled in the opposite direction to which it was locked.

A second throw, performed counter to the first (Figure 17.17), provides a reasonably stable suture, but with monofilament the knot is not complete.

At least one extra throw, in the same direction of rotation as the first, should be performed. This final throw is the one that allows the knot to be pulled tight without fear of tightening the suture loop and crushing skin. The ends of the suture should then be cut to leave sufficient

for any slight knot loosening. Deep-buried sutures will be trimmed very close to the knot, but longer cut ends are necessary for interrupted skin sutures to facilitate both suture location and suture removal in hair-bearing skin.

What precisely do we mean by a throw, and what are the knots?

A single-wrap throw is formed by wrapping the two strands around each other so that the angle of the wrap equals 360° (see Figure 17.15). In a double-wrap throw, the free end of a strand is passed twice, instead of once, around the other strand; the angle of this double-wrap throw is 720° (Figure 17.18). The tying of one or more additional throws completes the knot.

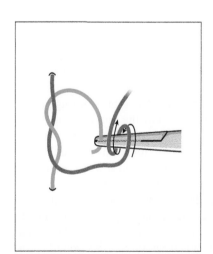

Figure 17.17 The second throw.

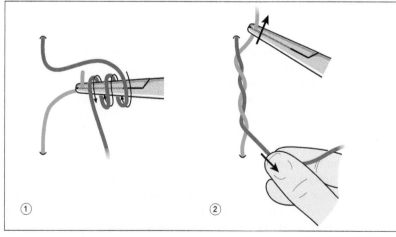

Figure 17.18 Double-wrap throw.

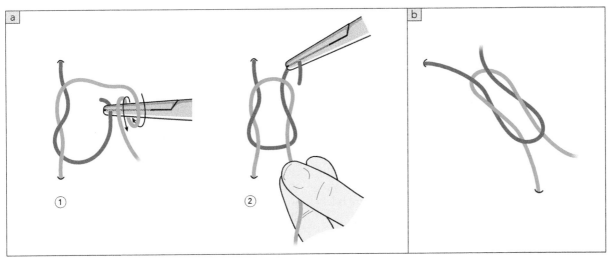

Figure 17.19 (a) Tying a reef knot. (b) A reef knot.

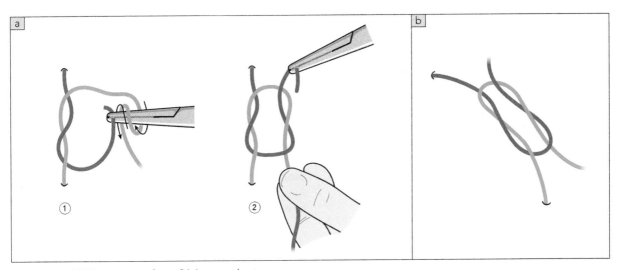

Figure 17.20 (a) Tying a granny knot. (b) A granny knot.

The configuration of the knot can be classified into two general types by the relationship between the knot ends and the loop. When the loop and the end of the two throws exit on the same side of the knot or parallel to each other, the type of knot is judged to be square or reef knot (Figure 17.19). The knot is considered to be a granny knot if the loop and end exit or cross different sides of the knot (Figure 17.20).

A simple code has been devised to describe a knot's configuration. The number of wraps for each throw is indicated by the appropriate number. The relationship between each throw being either crossed (granny) or parallel (reef) is signified by the symbols $\times$ and $=$, respectively. In accordance with this code, a square (reef) knot is designated $1 = 1$ and a granny knot, 1×1. From this it should be clear what is meant by a $2 \times 2 \times 2$ knot without giving the knot a name. All surgical knots can be defined by this international language. For most monofilament sutures, the knot will be $3 = 1 = 1$.

Suturing techniques

This section describes the common suturing techniques. These include interrupted sutures, buried interrupted sutures, mattress sutures, and the continuous subcuticular suture. Whatever the suture type, safe, accurate suturing requires deft handling of the suture holder, delicate handling of the skin, and attention to detail in respect of the knot-tying described above.

> **GOLDEN RULE** ✳
> Always close in layers. Wherever possible, skin wounds should be closed in layers using buried interrupted sutures, followed by either interrupted or subcuticular sutures. This will reduce skin tension and the chance of the wound stretching, or dehiscence.

Skin closure

// Interrupted skin sutures

Needle position in suture holder

As described earlier in the chapter, the needle should be held at the tip of the needle holder and at 90° to it, with the needle no more than two-thirds along its length to avoid grasping the hollow, crushable, and bendable section of the needle (see Figure 17.3a).

Passing the needle and suture through the skin

When suturing through skin, it is important that the needle is inserted at 90° to the skin and subsequently emerges at 90° to the skin. This ensures that any tension is borne by the full thickness of the skin and there is less chance of the suture cutting through the skin.

For all but the smallest of wounds, it is best to undertake each suture in two 'bites' (Figure 17.21 and Video Clip 17.8a,b) as follows:

- Insert the needle through one side of the wound, rotating the suture holder as it passes through the skin, the rotation mirroring the curve of the needle.
- Grab the inserted needle with either the suture holder or your forceps.
- Reposition the needle on the suture holder and then match the size of 'bite' on the other side of the wound with the needle emerging at 90° to the skin (Figure 17.21b,c).

As the needle point emerges through the skin, it will again need to be held by the needle holder or forceps. At all times, avoid holding the needle by the very tip as the tip of the needle is very easily bent or broken. This is why it is often better to insert the suture in two small 'bites' one side at a time than one big 'bite'. The needle needs to be drawn or rotated through the skin in an arc, mirroring its curved profile (Figure 17.21e).

At all costs, avoid pulling the needle straight through the skin surface. At the very least, the needle will bend; at worst, it will break or tear the skin. As the needle exits the skin and the suture material begins to appear, the needle point should almost be touching the insertion point. In this way, the needle has executed an almost perfect circle. Sutures inserted and withdrawn in this method require very little effort to complete. The knot is then thrown (see above), and sufficient tension is applied across the wound to achieve wound edge apposition.

Suture placement

The surgeon repeats the suture process described above along the length of the wound (Figure 17.22). Suture placement should be sufficiently spaced to bring the edges together without the wound gaping in between. Ideally, all the knots should be located to one side of the wound. This ensures that the line of the wound is free from knots, the wound is more easily cleaned, and the sutures are more easily removed. The suture placements shown in Figure 17.23 are incorrect.

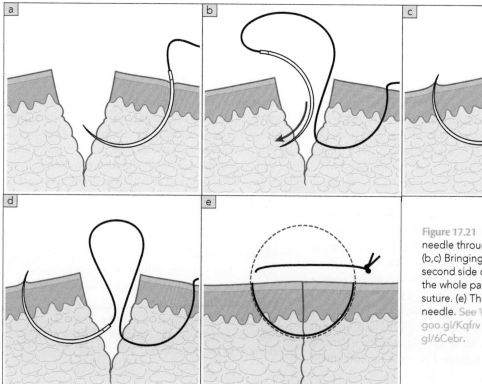

Figure 17.21 (a) Passing the needle through the first skin edge. (b,c) Bringing the needle through the second side of the wound. (d) Showing the whole path of the needle and the suture. (e) The circular arc of the needle. See Video Clips 17.8a—http://goo.gl/Kqfrv and 17.8b— http://goo.gl/6Cebr.

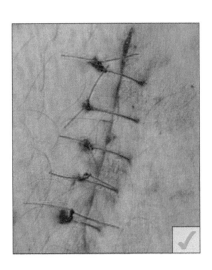

Figure 17.22 Correct placement of sutures.

Progressive halving

Some surgeons advocate placing the first suture in the centre of the wound and then inserting subsequent sutures equidistant on each side, so-called 'progressive halving' (Figure 17.24 and Video Clip 17.9), the rationale being to ensure that the wound closes symmetrically. The drawbacks are that this places the first suture under the greatest of tension, it can make the first knot difficult to tie, and it is more likely to cause the suture to tear through the skin. A skilled skin surgeon should be able to judge suture placement to avoid unequal closure. Progressive halving is of most use in very small procedures, but in larger wounds, it is usually better to start suturing at one end and work along the wound, placing sutures equally to avoid excessive skin tension.

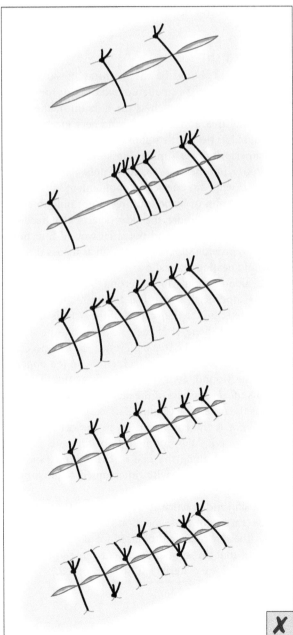

Figure 17.23 Incorrect suture placement.

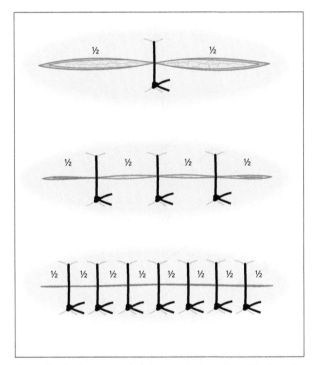

Figure 17.24 Progressive halving. See Video Clip 17.9—http://goo.gl/ZDzp5.

Dog ears

A 'dog ear' occurs either when the sutured edges are of different lengths or when the surgeon closes an ellipse of significantly less than 3:1 length-to-width ratio. Minor differences in wound edge length can usually be accommodated without causing a dog ear (see Chapter 25 for more information on crescentic excisions). The skill of closing such a wound is to space out the sutures so that a dog ear does not occur.

Some surgeons advocate cutting a lesion out with a circular excision, then judging where the least skin tension exists (by looking at the shape of the wound) and then closing the centre of the wound to follow that orientation, followed by cutting out the two dog ears that are created. Dog ears may therefore occur by design, as a result of different tensions between the sides of the wound or as a consequence of suture placement. It is easier to remove a dog ear that forms at the end of a wound than one that forms in the middle (a good reason for closing a wound by suturing from one apex to the other, and not from both apices to the middle).

The technique used to remove the defect is simple: the incision is extended to remove the raised dog ear of skin. In order to do this, a fine skin hook should be used to pull the raised 'tented' section of skin across and down to one side, against the normal skin. A cut is then made along the base of the 'tent'. The cut material is then lifted up and the whole of the flap of skin pulled across to the other side; the remaining 'base of the tent' is cut off in a similar way, leaving a small straight incision to suture (Figure 17.25).

When removing the dog ear, care needs to be taken to avoid either cutting outward beyond the new apex (creating a 'fishtail' scar) or cutting inward and through a suture (see Video Clip 17.10—http://goo.gl/HYYsC).

/// Buried sutures

Buried sutures should be the mainstay of skilled skin surgery for all but the smallest of wounds, or for certain anatomical locations (such as the dorsum of the hand, the pretibial area, and some head and neck locations). To date, there has been little published evidence to support their superiority over simple skin sutures (Al-Abdullah *et al.*, 2007), but there is a wealth of personal experience, especially with the newer monofilament absorbable sutures. The aim of buried sutures is not only to eliminate dead spaces under the skin (spaces that facilitate postoperative bleeding and potential wound infection), but to also provide support to the skin as it goes through the wound healing phases.

The aide-memoire for inserting buried sutures is: 'deep to superficial; superficial to deep'. The needle is first inserted into the *deep* aspect of the dermis and exits *superficially* at the level of the epidermis on one side of the wound (Figure 17.26 a,d). From here, the needle is inserted *superficially* into the epidermis on the opposite side of the wound, at the same depth as the first side, and exits the *deep* aspect of the dermis, again at the same depth as the other side (Figure 17.26b,e).

The knot is thereby tied deep to the dermis, i.e., it is a buried knot. With a buried knot the ends need to be pulled tight along the line of the wound (and not across the wound as with interrupted skin sutures; Figure 17.26g).

With skill and practice, it is possible to close nearly all wounds (except for those mentioned before) with buried sutures, thereby reducing the need for skin sutures. It is important that the knot ends are cut short to minimise the bulk of suture material left to be absorbed.

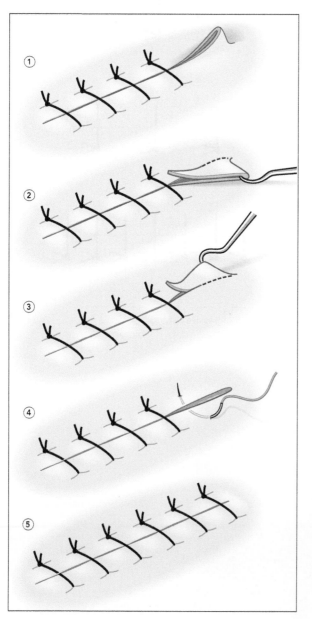

Figure 17.25 Diagrammatic representation of correcting a dog ear.

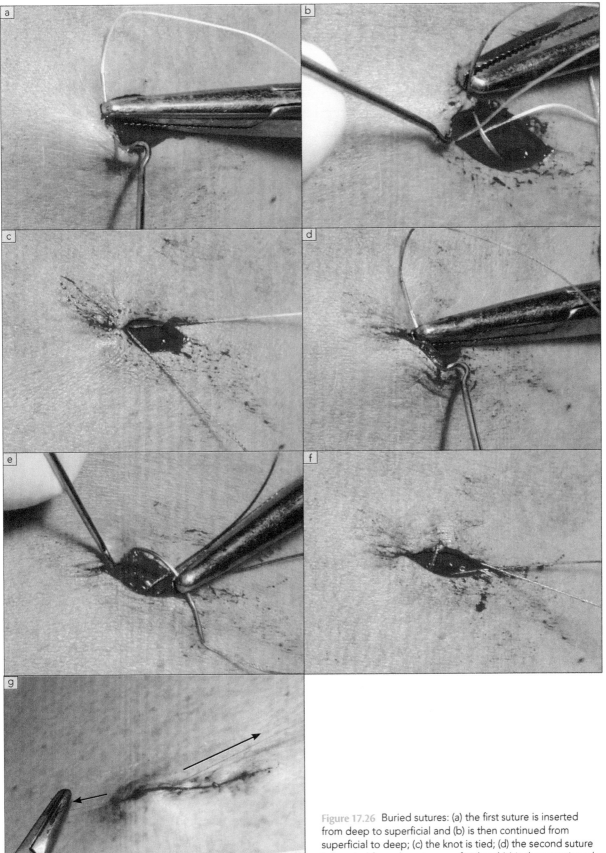

Figure 17.26 Buried sutures: (a) the first suture is inserted from deep to superficial and (b) is then continued from superficial to deep; (c) the knot is tied; (d) the second suture is inserted from deep to superficial and (e) is then continued from superficial to deep; (f) the second suture before knot-tying; (g) tightening a buried knot.

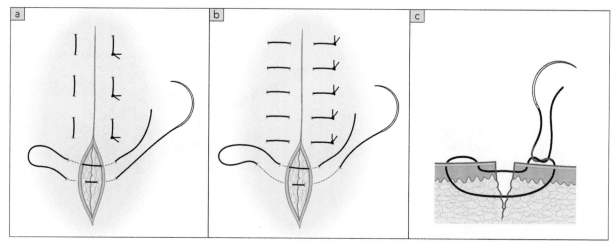

Figure 17.27 Diagrammatic representation of mattress sutures: (a) horizontal; (b) vertical; (c) cross-section of a vertical mattress suture.

Mattress sutures

This form of suture utilises a 'loop' of skin on each side of the wound to achieve greater tensile strength and also to help eliminate dead spaces (Figure 17.27). Mattress sutures may be horizontal or, more commonly, vertical. Although this is a useful suture technique to be able to perform, the cosmetic outcome is not usually as good as for other types of sutures, so these sutures are less widely used than the others described in this text.

// Horizontal mattress sutures

The horizontal mattress suture is effectively two linked interrupted skin sutures (Figure 17.28). The first part is exactly like an interrupted suture, but instead of throwing a knot, the needle is reinserted at a suitable distance from the first exit point and exits at an equal distance on the other side of the wound. The strength is gained from spreading the tension across the skin between the two sutures. This can be useful where there is little dermal thickness (e.g., the shin).

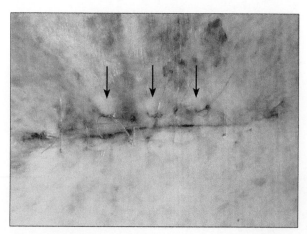

Figure 17.28 Horizontal mattress sutures (arrowed) with alternate skin sutures.

// Vertical mattress sutures

The initial 'bite' taken by the needle through the skin is larger than that used for a simple interrupted skin suture. The needle is inserted further from the incision edge, and the depth of the insertion is greater. The needle is withdrawn from the depth of the wound before an identical, large 'bite' is taken into the opposite side. After this, the direction of needle travel is reversed, and a traditional interrupted skin suture is inserted with smaller 'bites,' but in line with the deeper 'bites'. The ends are then tied under tension to bring the wound edges together (Figure 17.29 and Video Clip 17.11).

Any skin tension is taken up between the deeper and superficial 'bites' rather than between the superficial ones and the wound edges. This reduces the likelihood of the suture tearing through the skin, increases the amount of tension that can be used to bring edges together (for difficult to close wounds), and helps eliminate dead space.

So why isn't this closure used for all skin wounds? First, it doubles the number of skin penetrations by the suture material, thereby potentially doubling the number of puncture scars and entry points for infection. Second, as the edges come together and the knot is tensioned, the wound takes on a marked 'everted' appearance, with a noticeable ridge (which may take a little while to subside after the sutures have been removed; Figure 17.28h). Although experience shows that this everted wound produces a wound of great strength, it can also appear quite disfiguring to the patient. Patients need to be reassured that the wound will flatten as it heals.

Third, mattress sutures need to be removed, and when they are removed both superficial and deep wound support is removed. As buried sutures can take the place of a mattress skin suture in many locations, and provide continued wound support after any skin sutures have been removed, they are usually the favoured skin closure.

For all these reasons, mattress sutures are often best reserved for those areas where their cosmetic appearance is less visible, or where buried sutures can be difficult to insert (e.g., the scalp).

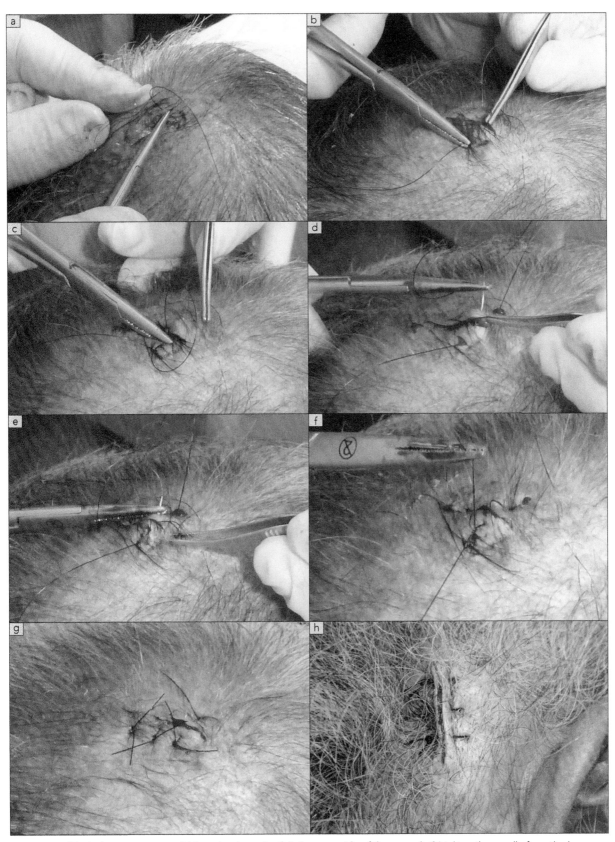

Figure 17.29 Vertical mattress suture: (a) inserting large 1st 'bite' on one side of the wound; (b) taking the needle from the large 1st bite; (c) inserting equally large bite on the other side of the wound; (d) taking the needle from other-side large bite; (e) inserted needle for smaller second bite; (f) tying the knot; (g) three completed mattress sutures; (h) everted edge of mattress suture wound. See Video Clip 17.11—http://goo.gl/3XAN0.

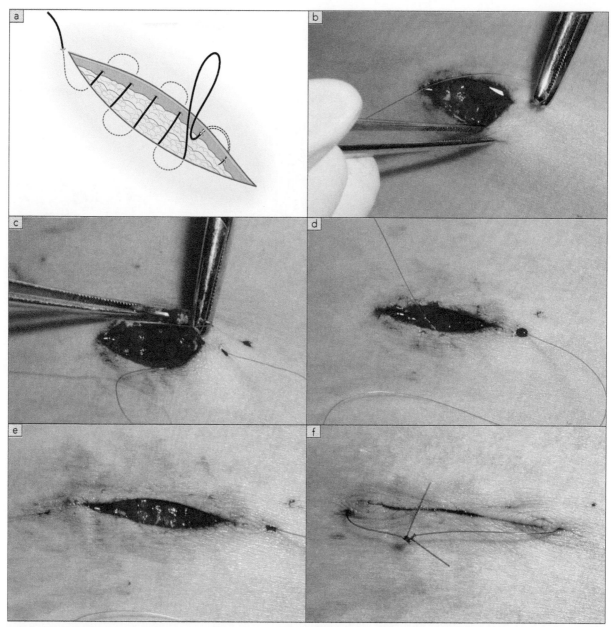

Figure 17.30 (a) Diagram of subcuticular suture insertion. (b–f) Inserting a subcuticular suture. See Video Clips 17.12a—http://goo.gl/ku2TD and 17.12b—http://goo.gl/UkmzJ.

⫶⫶⫶ – ⫶⫶⫶⫶ Continuous subcuticular sutures

This form of skin closure will be familiar to many hospital doctors: large incisions can be closed with a running, subcuticular suture of nylon utilising a straight needle. Although the principle is the same for skin surgery, the smaller incisions require the use of curved rather than straight needles. This form of closure is only suitable where there is little skin tension, otherwise the suture risks being exposed by wound edge separation.

In its simplest form, the suture needle is inserted through skin just distant to one of the apices of the wound. The needle exits, within the epidermis of the wound, close to the apex. From here, it is inserted horizontally into the opposite wound edge and then out again (Figure 17.30 and Video Clip 17.12a,b).

The exit point on one side corresponds to the next insertion point on the other side. The wound is thus closed with a number of S-shaped loops from side to side. When the second apex is reached, the suture needle exits the skin at a distance similar to the distance of the entry point from the first apex. The ends of the suture can then be tied together. An alternative to tied ends is the use of small crimped metal clips to hold the suture ends.

Once the wound has gained strength (7–10 days), the suture can be cut and withdrawn, although on longer wounds this can be problematic, due to friction. The tip here is to allow one S-shaped suture loop through the skin half way, enabling the resultant suture to be cut in two and withdrawn from each side when it is time for removal.

Additional tapes (such as Steri-Strips™) can be applied across the wound. A variation on this subcuticu lar suture is to use absorbable material, which allows the suture to remain *in situ*. If the ends are brought out through the skin and tied, they will need to be trimmed under tension (after the same time interval that the non-absorbable equivalent is pulled out and removed).

A final variation on this theme is to use an entirely buried absorbable suture in two layers. The first layer closes the wound with buried, interrupted, absorbable sutures. As the final suture (at one apex of the wound) is tied, only the loose end is cut. The still attached suture needle is then inserted from the knot in the deep layer up to the epidermis close to the apex. From here, a running subcuticular suture is completed as normal. The final end of the suture can then be trimmed, under tension, so that the whole suture remains buried.

If there is concern that the wound might open slightly, thereby exposing the suture material, the needle can be taken out through the skin and then reversed and reinserted back on itself (effectively producing a loop under the skin) prior to exiting the skin one last time. After trimming the suture, it will be able to provide some extra tensile support to the wound through this doubled-back path. This double-layered closure with absorbable sutures is particularly useful where the wound is likely to stretch and the dermis is sufficiently thick, for example on the back.

The main drawback with a continuous subcuticular suture wound closure is that it effectively seals the wound edges together. Whereas blood or serous fluid can leak out between interrupted sutures, this is not possible with a continuous subcuticular suture. Therefore avoid using this closure when bleeding may be more likely to occur, or ensure that adequate pressure bandaging is used postoperatively.

Other skin closures
Skin adhesives
Several adhesives have been developed for wound closure. One substance, cyanoacrylate, has been used for over 25 years. Although it can be useful for allowing wound edges to be held together, the material will not hold wound edges that are under tension. It is therefore best for incisions, lacerations, or where buried sutures have been used (Figure 17.31).

Subcutaneous (buried) sutures should be used to take the tension off the skin edges prior to applying the cyanoacrylate. Subcutaneous suture placement will aid in everting the skin edges and minimise the chances of deposition of cyanoacrylate into the subcutaneous tissues. Some cyanoacrylate glues can induce a substantial inflammatory reaction if applied subcutaneously. If used superficially on the epidermal surface, little problem with inflammation occurs. Indeed, cyanoacrylate used to be used as a barrier

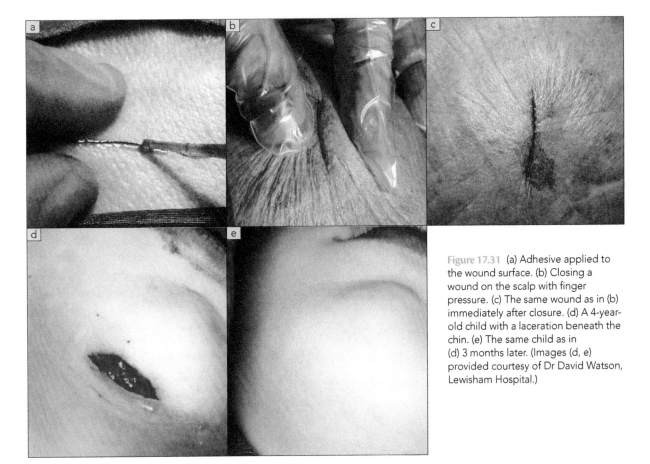

Figure 17.31 (a) Adhesive applied to the wound surface. (b) Closing a wound on the scalp with finger pressure. (c) The same wound as in (b) immediately after closure. (d) A 4-year-old child with a laceration beneath the chin. (e) The same child as in (d) 3 months later. (Images (d, e) provided courtesy of Dr David Watson, Lewisham Hospital.)

against common bacteria, including certain staphylococci, pseudomonads, and *Escherichia coli*.

Fibrin-based tissue adhesives can be created from autologous sources or pooled blood. They are typically used for haemostasis and can seal tissues. Although they do not have adequate tensile strength to close the skin, fibrin tissue adhesives can be used to fix skin grafts or seal cerebrospinal fluid leaks.

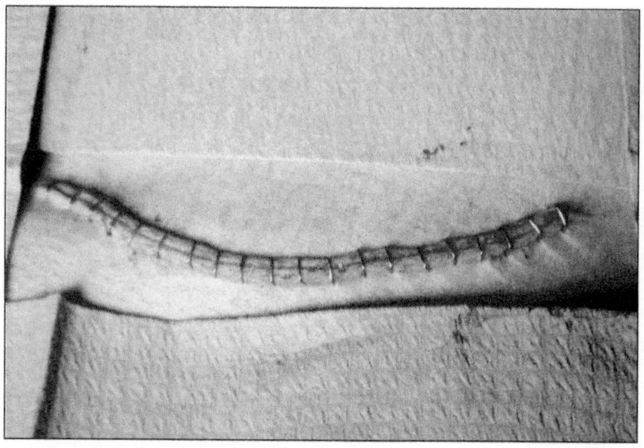

Staples

Staples provide a quick method of wound closure (Figure 17.32), and studies have shown decreased wound infection rates with them. Staples are composed of stainless steel, which is less reactive than some traditional suture materials. The act of stapling requires minimal skin penetration so potentially fewer microorganisms are carried through the skin. Staples are more expensive than traditional sutures and also require great care in placement, especially in ensuring the eversion of wound edges. With proper placement, the resultant scar is cosmetically equivalent to that of other closure techniques.

However, the removal of staples, like skin sutures, leads to a loss of all wound support, and because of their bulk they are less suitable for those areas where buried sutures and closure by layers is difficult (the scalp, pretibial region, and some facial areas). In addition, they cannot be used to bring together wound edges in the same way that a tightened skin suture can. For these reasons, their use is almost entirely limited to closing surgical incisions rather than excisions.

Tape

Closure using adhesive tapes was first described in France in the 1500s, when Pare devised strips of sticking plaster that were sewn together for facial wounds. This method allowed the wound edges to be joined and splinted together. The porous self-adhesive sterile paper tapes (e.g., Steri-Strips™; Figure 17.33) used today are reminiscent of these earlier splints. They can be used to ensure proper wound apposition and to provide additional wound reinforcement. These tapes can be used in addition to skin sutures or with deep sutures, and instead of skin sutures or even alone where skin tension is minimal (e.g., incisions and lacerations).

Skin adhesives (e.g., OpSite® spray or tincture of Benzoin; Figure 17.34) aid tape adherence.

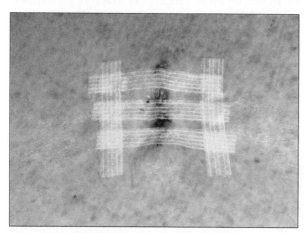

Figure 17.32 Wound closed with staples.

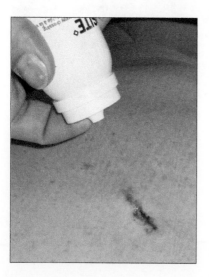

Figure 17.33 Wound (closed with buried sutures only) supported by Steri-Strips™.

Figure 17.34 OpSite® spray used prior to tape support.

REFERENCES

Al-Abdullah T, Plint AC, Fergusson D (2007) Absorbable versus nonabsorbable sutures in the management of traumatic lacerations and surgical wounds: A meta-analysis. *Pediatric Emergency Care* 23: 339–44. See also: www.crd.york.ac.uk/crdweb/ShowRecord.asp?LinkFrom=OAI&ID=12007001972 (accessed July 2012).

LINKS TO VIDEO CLIPS

VC 17.1   VC 17.2a   VC 17.2b

VC 17.3a   VC 17.3b   VC 17.3c

VC 17.4   VC 17.5   VC 17.6

VC 17.7   VC 17.8a   VC 17.8b

VC 17.9   VC 17.10   VC 17.11

VC 17.12a   VC 17.12b

VC 17.1: Attaching the scalpel blade
http://goo.gl/0UUqf

VC 17. 2a,b: Using the scalpel
http://goo.gl/wZJcs
http://goo.gl/6xvJ7

VC 17.3a,b,c: Ellipse excision
http://goo.gl/7B55P
http://goo.gl/OjCQE
http://goo.gl/MUpB0

VC 17.4: Fishtail incision
http://goo.gl/VUEeA

VC 17.5: Excision down to fat
http://goo.gl/pTZLy

VC 17.6: Undermining
http://goo.gl/b3Rx7z

VC 17.7: Knot-tying
http://goo.gl/glkNr

VC 17.8a,b: Interrupted sutures
http://goo.gl/Kqfrv
http://goo.gl/6Cebr

VC 17.9: Progressive halving
http://goo.gl/ZDzp5

VC 17.10: Dog ears
http://goo.gl/HYYsC

VC 17.11: Vertical mattress suture
http://goo.gl/3XAN0

VC 17.12a,b: Subcuticular suture
http://goo.gl/ku2TD
17.12b—http://goo.gl/UkmzJ

Chapter 18

Haemostasis

INTRODUCTION

The equipment required to effectively manage haemostasis is discussed in Chapter 1. Medications that can lead to increased bleeding (such as warfarin, aspirin, and antiplatelet drugs), and their management in relation to minor surgery, are discussed in Chapter 5. Chapter 6 considers the anatomical hazards that may lead to haemorrhage. This chapter starts by reminding the surgeon about surgical skills that are important to reduce unnecessary bleeding and then describes how to establish haemostasis during the surgical procedure using common techniques such as pressure, electrocautery, diathermy, and chemical cautery.

Haemorrhage during surgery can cause anxiety for both the patient and the surgical team. It is important for the surgeon to demonstrate a confident, relaxed manner to keep the patient relaxed. A relaxed patient is likely to have a more normal blood pressure, and this in itself can reduce bleeding.

SURGICAL TECHNIQUE TO REDUCE BLEEDING

The surgeon must be aware of the surface anatomy and any significant underlying vessels (see Chapter 6) and take care with the initial incision. In particular, it is important to make an incision to reach the subcutaneous fat, but being careful to avoid incising below this depth.

Avoiding underlying structures

The skin should be handled carefully using skin hooks or other retractors to lift the skin away from any underlying vessels (Figure 18.1). Elevating the skin not only lifts the specimen away from the underlying vessels, but also improves visibility, enabling the surgeon to avoid inadvertently lacerating the blood vessels. If a blood vessel does need to be cut, it can be clamped with artery forceps or sealed with diathermy first. If necessary, an absorbable ligature can be tied.

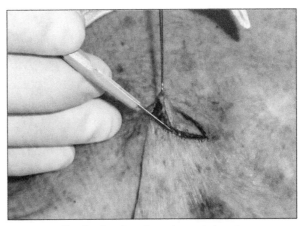

Figure 18.1 Skin hook aiding dissection and elevation.

Avoidance of underlying structures may be facilitated by the technique of hydrodissection. In this, a reasonable volume of anaesthetic with or without normal saline is injected under the lesion. The volume effect helps lift the lesion clear of the underlying structures. This technique is particularly useful over the temporal artery and around the inner canthus of the eye. If there are concerns about the anaesthetic volume, normal saline can be used after the anaesthetic. The volume of fluid used also creates a pressure effect, further reducing bleeding. See Chapter 7 for further information about this technique.

GOLDEN RULES ✳

Surgical technique and reducing the likelihood of bleeding:

- Be aware of the surface anatomy and any underlying major vessels (see Chapter 6).
- Take care with the initial incision.
- Handle the skin carefully, and expose any underlying structures.

Blunt dissection

If blunt dissection is required for the removal of large lesions (including epidermoid cysts) and to undermine the edge of excisions to aid closure, cutting 'blind' should be avoided. Dissecting scissors or forceps should be inserted closed and then opened to release tissues by blunt dissection (see Figure 17.14). The temptation to reverse this action and to cut should be resisted as it is too easy to cut through a blood vessel. If the surgeon does transect a vessel while undermining the edge of an excision, it can be difficult to locate and stop the bleeding.

Punch biopsy

Punch biopsies, although considered a very 'minor' procedure, can cause significant bleeding for the following reasons (Figure18.2):

- The punch can cause laceration of underlying blood vessels.
- The shape of the punch biopsy can interfere with normal tissue retraction, leading to reduced constriction of small blood vessels.
- The punch biopsy incision is often too small to allow individual bleeding points to be identified.

To achieve haemostasis, it may be necessary to insert one or more sutures of adequate calibre and depth of 'bite'.

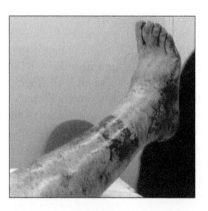

Figure 18.2 Bleeding post punch biopsy of the shin; the patient had walked home when this occurred.

PRESSURE/ELEVATION

Haemorrhage can be spurting, alarming and arterial, or it can be more oozing of relatively oxygenated capillary blood or deoxygenated venous blood. All bleeding will be reduced by correctly applied pressure; in addition, venous oozing is often reduced or even halted by the simple manoeuvre of elevating the bleeding point (most easily accomplished with a limb [Figure 18.2]). Once venous bleeding has stopped, the operating area will be much easier to visualise, so closure is greatly facilitated.

A well-trained assistant can greatly help safe surgery by applying pressure, and keeping it applied whenever the surgeon is not actively working on the operating site. Any pressure applied needs to be maintained for long enough to allow the clotting process and platelet aggregation to take place—early release of pressure is likely to disrupt the clotting process and prolong bleeding. Dabbing the wound with a gauze swab will greatly increase bleeding by disrupting clot formation and is to be avoided.

If the operation site is a limb, elevation of the limb will reduce arterial and venous bleeding and facilitate surgery. However, if the limb is normally dependent (e.g., the lower leg), it is important that adequate pressure is applied to the wound after closure to stop postoperative bleeding. After that, it is important to check the wound does not bleed after the patient stands up.

LIGATION

With the advent of bipolar diathermy, it is unusual to need to ligate bleeding vessels, but this remains a useful technique for difficult circumstances or situations where diathermy is not available.

In order to ligate a bleeding vessel, it is first important to be able to apply small artery forceps to the bleeding vessel (Figure 18.3 and Video Clip 18.1a,b). Once this has been achieved, the vessel can be tied with either an instrument-tied suture or with a surgeon's knot, the

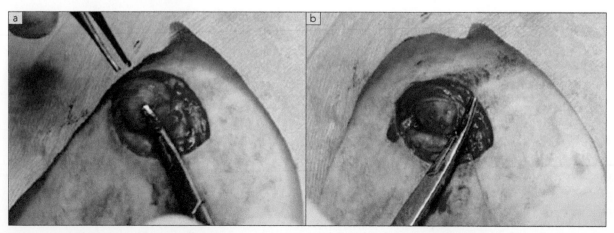

Figure 18.3 (a) Clamping and (b) tying off a bleeding vessel. See Video Clips 18.1a: http://goo.gl/EyFVa and 18.1b: http://goo.gl/c3JV9.

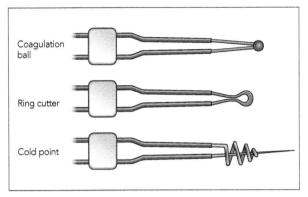

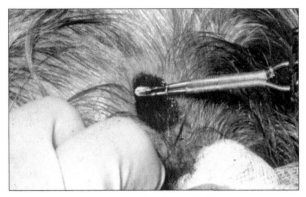

Figure 18.4 Electrocautery tips.

Figure 18.5 Electrocautery with a flat tip for haemostasis. See Video Clip 18.2: http://goo.gl/Vw5gs.

suture being slipped past the forceps and onto the vessel prior to tying. It is important to remember that both ends of a lacerated vessel will need ligation. The material used to ligate the vessel needs to be absorbable, either monofilament or braided.

ELECTROCAUTERY

Electrocautery is still widely used to establish haemostasis in minor surgical procedures. A red-hot platinum wire is used to coagulate small blood vessels or to cut through tissue. It differs from diathermy (see 'Diathermy') in that it works solely by heat. More information about the equipment and method of action of electrocautery is contained in Chapter 1. The ball-end tip is most commonly used for haemostasis (Figure 18.4). This tip stops bleeding without cutting through the tissues.

Technique
In general, the best temperature is when the wire is a dull red colour. If the wire is too hot, it cuts through tissue without coagulating and causes excessive local tissue destruction; if it is not hot enough, it sticks to the tissues

(Figure 18.5 and Video Clip 18.2). With mains-powered electrocautery, you will need to adjust the power (via a simple rheostat) to produce the right amount of heat.

It is important to remember that the heat produced by electrocautery destroys tissue more widely than you can see. Consequently, if a histological specimen is required, you should take a biopsy before using electrocautery. Never use spirit-based skin cleaning solutions with electrocautery as these may ignite and burn the patient.

DIATHERMY

Diathermy is another technique used for haemostasis (Figure 18.6). It uses electricity rather than just heat to produce its effects. Surgeons will use either *bipolar* or *unipolar* diathermy (see Chapter 1). For minor surgery, the Birtcher hyfrecator is often used to coagulate tissues in a similar way to electrocautery. A sharp tip is usually used for single vessels, and a blunt one for general cautery. The instrument handle should be protected by single-use sterile sheaths. Surgeons should familiarise themselves with the equipment and the settings on the machine by referring to the manufacturer's information.

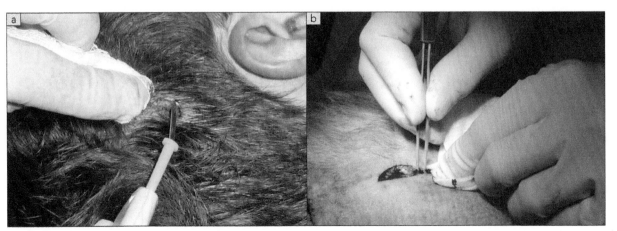

Figure 18.6 (a) Unipolar diathermy (hyfrecator) in use on a shaved lesion from the scalp, producing fulguration. (b) Bipolar diathermy used to achieve haemostasis during an excision.

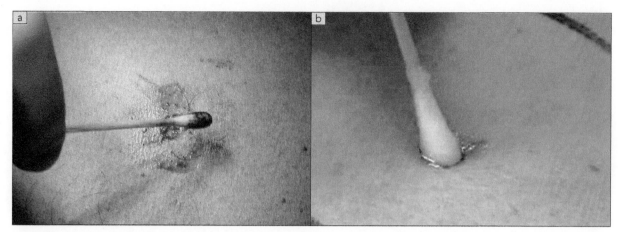

Figure 18.7 (a) Driclor® rolled (with a cotton bud) onto a shaved lesion. (b) Applying Driclor® with a cotton bud held stationary over a smaller lesion. See Video Clip 18.3: http://goo.gl/JsuqO.

CHEMICAL CAUTERY

There is a limited role for chemical cautery, but it can be used as an adjunct to diathermy or cautery. For anything other than a very minor procedure, reliance on chemical cautery alone would be inappropriate. Chemical cautery can reduce bleeding by tissue constriction (styptics) or platelet aggregation.

Styptics

These cause tissue constriction, the most commonly used chemicals being aluminium chloride and silver nitrate. Styptics are most useful when applied to an area that has been curetted or shaved, where there are no large bleeding vessels, and where there is a surface over which the chemical can work.

Technique

Aluminium chloride is found within the antiperspirant product Driclor® and is most simply applied by rolling a cotton bud soaked in the solution over the bleeding area (Figure 18.7 and Video Clip 18.3). Silver nitrate sticks can be used in a similar way and are probably more effective. As well as causing tissue constriction, silver nitrate causes chemical burning and tissue damage. Silver salts can tattoo the skin so their use should be avoided over the face and in cosmetically important areas.

Platelet aggregators

Microfibrillar collagen haemostat and chitosan

Microfibrillar collagen haemostat is a topical agent that has been shown to attract platelets and facilitate clot formation, thereby reducing bleeding. It is derived from bovine collagen and activates the intrinsic pathway of the coagulation cascade. Chitosan is a natural compound that works in a similar way but is in addition not impaired by anticoagulants and inhibits bacterial colonisation. Although the use of these agents is well established in many military and trauma units, they are not commonly used in minor surgery facilities.

Alginate dressings

Alginate dressings (Sorbsan®, Kaltostat®) are widely used in the United Kingdom for haemostasis as platelet aggregators. However, evidence of their efficacy on acute wounds is limited. There is controversy over the activity of alginate dressings to promote haemostasis through platelet aggregation. Alginates containing zinc ions are probably the most effective.

LINKS TO VIDEO CLIPS

VC 18.1a

VC 18.1b

VC 18.2

VC 18.3

VC 18.1a and b: Ligation
http://goo.gl/EyFVa; http://goo.gl/c3JV9

VC 18.2: Electrocautery
http://goo.gl/Vw5gs

VC 18. 3: Chemical cautery
http://goo.gl/JsuqO

Chapter 19

Dermatological techniques and tips

INTRODUCTION

This chapter is divided into two sections. The first part describes specific dermatological techniques that require local anaesthetic but do not, for the most part, require the use of sutures. They are relatively simple techniques that are easily learned and can provide a good cosmetic outcome. Chapter 1 discusses the equipment needed for these procedures.

Levels of difficulty are indicated by scalpel ratings. The more scalpel blades, the more difficult the procedure and the more practical experience will be required to become competent at the technique.

At the end of this chapter, there is a short section with tips about the surgical management of some of the skin lesions described in Chapter 9.

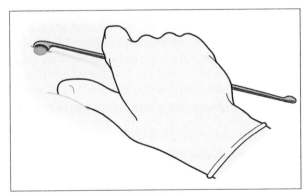

Figure 19.1 Curettage: scraping technique.

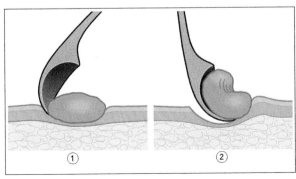

Figure 19.2 Curettage: scooping technique.

SPECIFIC DERMATOLOGICAL TECHNIQUES

// Curettage

Curettage is a very useful technique, performed under local anaesthesia, that allows some benign lesions to be removed and sent for histological examination. Because it involves the removal of very superficial tissue, it gives excellent cosmetic results in selected patients. In particular, if choosing a surgical treatment for seborrhoeic keratoses, it is the treatment of choice.

The technique is performed after infiltration of local anaesthesia into the area of the lesion. During the procedure, the curette either scrapes a surface lesion off the skin or hugs a deeper lesion, developing a plane of cleavage around it. The advantage of the technique is that it causes minimal scarring. The disadvantage is that, unlike an excision, you cannot remove a margin of normal tissue. It is therefore unsuitable for dealing with malignant lesions unless you have special experience.

Curettage combined with electrocautery is used by many dermatologists for the treatment of basal cell carcinomas, but the precise details of the technique are very important. An experienced operator is able to delineate the edge of the tumour by changes in skin structure between the normal and the neoplastic tissue. Unless you have specialist dermatological knowledge, it is recommended that you use the curette only if you are confident that the lesion is benign.

Technique

The key point of curettage is to identify a plane of cleavage and then either scrape or scoop the lesion off the skin and separate it from the surrounding tissue (Figures 19.1 and 19.2). The curette may be a single-use loop curette or a reusable Volkmann spoon (see Chapter 1 for more information). Single-use curettes have a scalpel-sharp usable side and a blunt side.

The more perpendicular the loop curette is to the skin, the more likely it is to cut into the skin rather than scrape the lesion off. An angle of no more than about 30–45° to the skin is effective for scraping—above this angle and the technique becomes a scoop. Put simply,

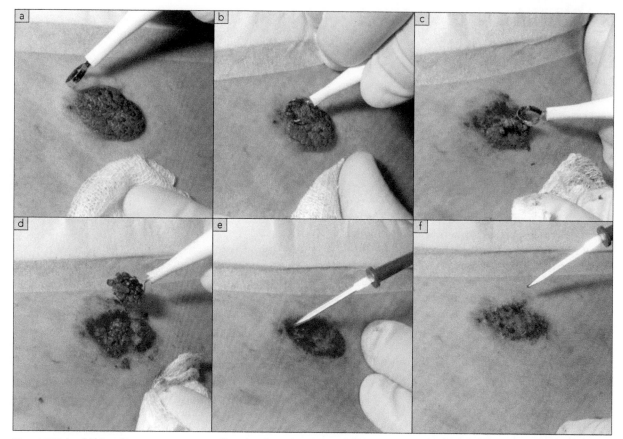

Figure 19.3 (a–d) Using the curette to scrape off a seborrhoeic keratosis. (e,f) Using unipolar diathermy to achieve haemostasis. See Video Clips 19.1a—http://goo.gl/Wvzg3; 19.1b—http://goo.gl/Bt26l; 19.1c—http://goo.gl/ZvN4E.

when scraping off a lesion, the curette is held fairly flat to the surface of the skin. When scooping out a lesion, the curette is held much more vertically and digs more deeply to scoop the lesion out. It is usually best to work around the edge of the lesion, towards the centre, to avoid the chance of the curette slipping into the surrounding normal skin. The scraping technique is more commonly used than scooping.

> **DON'T FORGET ▶▶**
> Ellipse excision of a seborrhoeic keratosis is inappropriate, as it leaves an unnecessary scar.

Scraping

This is the ideal technique for removing seborrhoeic keratoses. These are only lightly attached to the skin as if by a thin layer of glue and may be easily removed by firm scraping using a sideways movement of the curette (Figure 19.3 and Video Clip 19.1a,b,c). The curettings obtained should, even though fragmented, always be sent for histological examination.

The procedure leaves a raw area oozing tiny spots of blood. The bleeding may be stopped by direct pressure, by electrocautery, diathermy (Figure 19.3e,f), or by application of a cotton bud soaked in Driclor® (25% aluminium chloride in 70% isopropyl alcohol). After a few days, this superficial wound will have healed completely, often with minimal scarring. Remember, however, that hyper- and hypopigmented scars may occur, particularly in darker-skinned individuals. Similarly, curettage in some anatomical areas and skin types may be complicated by hypertrophic scarring. The more aggressive the curettage and electrocautery, the more likely it is to lead to permanent scarring.

Scooping

This alternative technique is not as frequently used but can be useful for removing pyogenic granulomas. The curette is held at right angles to the surface at the junction of the lesion and the normal skin. Using firm downwards pressure, develop a plane of cleavage and scoop out the lesion from below (Video Clip 19.2—http://goo.gl/5k8pf; see also Figure 19.2). There may be profuse bleeding from the resulting hole, which should be dealt with by direct pressure, electrocautery, diathermy, or occasionally a suture.

// Shave excision

Shave excision involves slicing off a lesion with a flat blade. It is a highly effective treatment for compound melanocytic naevi, the fleshy lesions that often occur on the face, especially the cheek and lip (see Chapter 9). The attachment and depth of these lesions means that they should not be curetted. The technique produces an excellent cosmetic result, avoiding the need for sutures, and deserves to be more widely used than it is.

Because shave excision does not always completely remove the lesion, the histopathologist will be unable to report on the depth or the completeness of the excision. *The technique should therefore only be used if you are confident that the lesion is benign.*

You should warn patients that, after the procedure, they will be left with a flat or depressed wound the same size as the lesion. However, you can reassure them that this will heal rapidly, the depression will reduce or resolve completely, and the eventual results are usually excellent. Remember that repigmentation can take place, that the lesion may recur, and that any hairs previously present in the lesion may grow back again. In particular, repigmentation in the scar site may be irregular and alarming; this is called a 'pseudo-melanoma' appearance.

Technique

Infiltrate the area carefully with local anaesthetic; too large a volume under the lesion will tend to create a more depressed scar. A useful tip is to infiltrate the anaesthetic slowly into the lesion itself until blanching is noted around the base of the lesion. Next, either grasp the lesion with toothed forceps or transfix it with the injecting needle. Take care not to crush the lesion as this will make histological analysis difficult. Then hold either a scalpel blade (No. 11, 15, 20, or 22) horizontally, or use a purpose-designed DermaBlade®, and slice off the lesion with a gentle but steady to-and-fro motion (Figures 19.4 and 19.5 and Video Clips 19.3a,b); also see Chapter 26, Radiosurgery for blade-free shave excision.

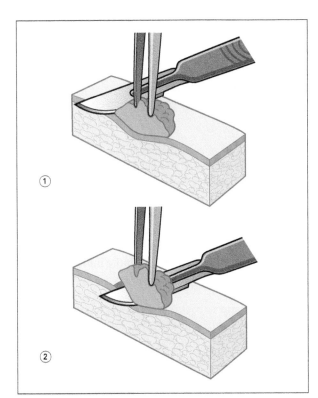

Figure 19.4 Diagrammatic representation of shave excision.

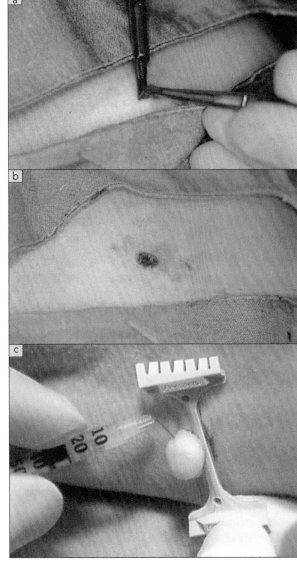

Figure 19.5 (a) Shaving through the base of the lesion with a No.15 blade. (b) Wound following shave excision and cautery. (c) Removing a lesion with a Dermablade. See Video Clips 19.3a—http://goo.gl/Kw6er and 19.3b—http://goo.gl/PNN4a.

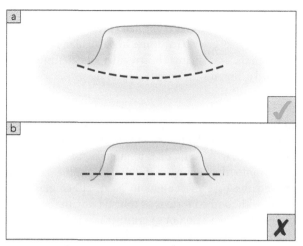

Figure 19.6 Shave excision technique: (a) correct and (b) incorrect. See Video Clips 19.4a—http://goo.gl/WI1tM and 19.4b—http://goo.gl/DjYat.

Make the incision in such a way that the lesion is cut off flush with the skin, or even slightly deeper (Figure 19.6 and Video Clips 19.4a,b). A residual rim of lesion standing proud produces a conspicuous raised scar that casts a shadow. A flat or slightly concave scar may, on the other hand, be easily concealed with make-up.

Bleeding can usually be controlled by pressure or aluminium chloride (see Chapter 18). An alternative is to use the ball end of the electrocautery device. If you are using the electrocautery device near the nose, remember to warn the patient of the smell of singeing flesh. Reassure the patient that the black charred spot seen in the mirror will heal quickly.

Snip excision

This is a quick, easy way to remove skin tags, which are common on the neck, in the flexures, and around the eyes.

Small tags

If the tags are very small, a local anaesthetic is unnecessary—the injection would itself be more painful than cutting the tags. The tag is held firmly in a pair of forceps and snipped off at the base with a pair of sharp scissors. Haemostasis is not usually a problem. Patients can be shown how to perform the procedure themselves if small tags recur.

Larger tags

For removal of larger skin tags, local anaesthetic should be used. Again, the tag is held firmly in the forceps and cut off at the base with scissors (Figure 19.7a and Video Clips 19.5a,b,c). Larger skin tags have a better developed blood supply, so cautery of the base, with electrocautery, diathermy, or aluminium chloride, may be required for haemostasis. Alternatively, an electrocautery cutting tip (ring cutter) can be used, which cauterises as it cuts (Figure 19.7b).

Very large tags may leave a large defect, and here one or more skin sutures can be used to achieve both haemostasis and a good cosmetic result.

Punch biopsy

A punch biopsy is a useful technique to obtain a full-thickness skin specimen, usually for diagnostic purposes, from an inflammatory dermatosis or a skin tumour (but never a suspicious melanocytic lesion). The single-use biopsy punch has a circular blade attached to a pencil-like handle. Various diameters are available. The most useful is the 4 mm punch biopsy; any smaller makes histology difficult. See Chapter 1 for more information.

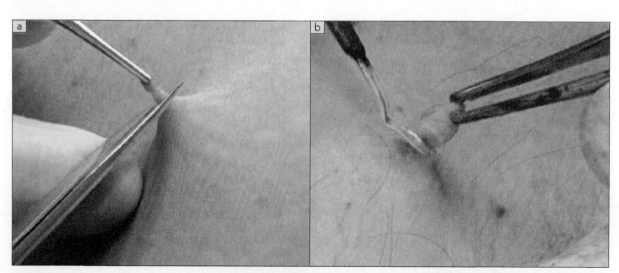

Figure 19.7 (a) Snip excision of a skin tag using scissors. (b) Cautery excision of a skin tag. See Video Clips 19.5a—http://goo.gl/U4u0E, 19.5b—http://goo.gl/O707s, and 19.5c—http://goo.gl/1eU50.

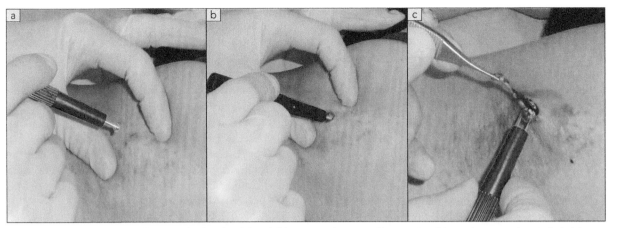

Figure 19.8 Punch biopsy: (a) skin stretched and stabilised; (b) Visi-punch inserted by rotation; (c) punch removed, sample held gently in forceps.

Technique

Choose the site carefully. Ideally, you should stretch the skin at right angles to the lines of least skin tension, so that the wound will take an elliptical shape once the tension is reduced (Figure 19.8a). This means that if a suture is required to close the wound, a better cosmetic outcome will be achieved.

After infiltrating the area with local anaesthetic, hold the punch biopsy vertically over the skin and then press the punch through the epidermis and dermis into subcutaneous fat, rotating it as you push through the skin and into the subcutaneous tissues (Figure 19.8b). It is essential that you take into account the thickness of both the dermis and any subcutaneous fat when pushing the punch biopsy through the skin. Hydrodissection with anaesthetic, or 'pinching' and lifting the skin with the other hand, helps avoid damaging structures below a thin dermis. The punch should just cut through the dermis but no further unless indicated. Carefully lift the specimen up, and cut it at the base through the dermis (Figure 19.8c). Careful handling is essential to avoid a crush artefact. If possible, it is better to lift the specimen with a needle rather than forceps.

It may be possible to establish haemostasis using pressure or diathermy, but it is sometimes necessary to insert a suture or two, depending upon the size of the punch biopsy. Larger punches (6–8 mm) are sometimes used to excise small lesions, but their circular shape is likely to lead to 'dog ear' defects when sutured (see Chapter 17). (See Chapter 18 for more on particular problems of haemostasis and punch biopsy.)

// Cryotherapy

Background

Cryotherapy is the therapeutic use of cold to destroy tissue. It works by producing ice crystals in the intracellular and extracellular fluids. Freezing followed by thawing causes intracellular damage, which leads to tissue necrosis. Liquid nitrogen is the most widely used agent and is by far the best. Other agents such as carbon dioxide snow are now only of historical interest.

Liquid nitrogen has a boiling point of −196°C. It is non-toxic and non-inflammable but can nevertheless be dangerous and should be treated with great respect. It can be used in several ways to apply cold with precision and control.

Cryotherapy is simple to perform and does not usually require local anaesthesia. This apparent simplicity can, however, be deceptive, and it is essential to master the details of the technique in order to use it successfully. Freezing for too short a time is ineffective, while freezing for too long can cause serious damage to the surrounding tissue.

A major disadvantage is that cryotherapy does not *remove* tissue, so you cannot confirm the diagnosis histologically. This means that you must be absolutely certain of the diagnosis before considering this technique.

The ease and apparent harmlessness of the technique can make it seem attractive, and cryotherapy has been advocated for treating a tremendous range of lesions, including some skin malignancies. This is a dangerous practice. Unless you have special experience in this field, it is safest to confine your use of cryotherapy to treating viral warts, solar keratoses, and seborrhoeic keratoses.

> **GOLDEN RULE** ✳
> Never embark on treatment with cryotherapy unless you are confident of the diagnosis and sure that it is appropriate treatment.

Indications
Viral warts

Cryotherapy is still used for treating viral warts, although there is limited evidence to support the efficacy of treatment. It is probable that cryotherapy leads to destruction of the hyperkeratotic tissue produced by the wart, rather than destroying the papillomavirus that causes the wart. Further details about the management of viral warts are included in Chapter 9. Remember that cryotherapy is painful and should be avoided in children.

Solar keratoses

Cryotherapy is an appropriate treatment for localised, thin solar keratoses, *provided that the diagnosis is not in doubt*. See Chapter 9 for further information about the management of solar keratoses.

Seborrhoeic keratoses

Cryotherapy can be used for seborrhoeic keratoses provided that the diagnosis is not in doubt. See Chapter 9 for further information about management of these lesions.

Equipment
Liquid nitrogen

Liquid nitrogen may be bought in bulk and stored in a large Dewar flask, where it will last for up to 3 months. It may be possible to arrange to obtain a supply from the local hospital of only small amounts when needed. Because the boiling point of liquid nitrogen is so low, it continually evaporates and needs to be kept in a specially designed insulated container. A litre of liquid nitrogen in such a container will last for about a day. You should wear gloves and goggles when transferring liquid nitrogen from one container to another.

You must also have a special vented flask to transport liquid nitrogen. This should be kept upright at all times and the vent kept clear. If you are driving with the flask in the car, you should ensure that the vehicle is well ventilated. You should be aware of Health and Safety and Control of Substances Hazardous to Health (COSHH) guidance in the United Kingdom in relation to the storage and transport of liquid nitrogen.

Cryospray equipment consists of a double-insulated metal flask with a screw-top (Figure 19.9). This is fitted with a trigger device and a choice of metal nozzles with differently sized apertures. This allows the controlled delivery of a fine spray of liquid nitrogen that can be precisely aimed.

The cryospray avoids any risk of contamination since the instrument does not touch the patient's skin. It is easy to use and a short period of practice using simulated tissue or an orange will enable you to master the technique.

Technique
Cotton bud

Cotton buds are dipped into a flask of liquid nitrogen and applied to the lesion. This is the simplest technique and is widely used, but it is not as effective as the cryospray. Commercially available cotton buds are too loosely packed to be satisfactory. Make your own by twisting a wisp of cotton wool around the end of an orange stick.

Although freezing destroys wart-infected tissue, the virus itself is not destroyed by the procedure—never dip a used cotton bud into the liquid nitrogen flask or you may cause cross-infection.

Cryospray

Select a suitable nozzle size and direct a fine jet of liquid nitrogen onto the lesion from a distance of about 1 cm. After a short time, the lesion will freeze and turn white (Figure 19.10).

Start counting the freeze time from this point, and continue spraying for between 5 and 10 seconds. Time this carefully, and record the freeze time in the procedure notes. Recommended freeze times are as follows:

- *Common warts*: 10 seconds.
- *Solar keratoses*: 5 seconds.
- *Seborrhoeic keratoses*: 5 seconds. Large, raised, basal cell papillomas may need longer.

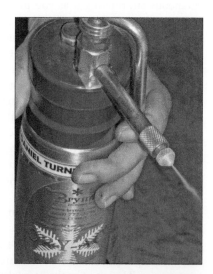

Figure 19.9
Liquid nitrogen cryospray.

Figure 19.10
Liquid nitrogen cryotherapy.

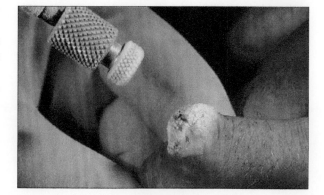

Freeze/thaw cycles

There is evidence that two freeze/thaw cycles are more efficient than a single application. Treat the lesion with liquid nitrogen until it goes white and then stop the treatment and allow the area to return to its normal colour before repeating the cycle.

Complications

Cryotherapy is safe if used correctly, but because it appears so simple it is easy to overlook its dangers. Applying it for too long can cause devastating results. A maximum freeze time of 10 seconds is recommended for most lesions.

Pain and blistering

Although cryotherapy itself does not require local anaesthesia, it can cause severe pain after the procedure. It is most important to explain to the patient the likely effects of treatment, which may be described as a 'freeze burn'. An information leaflet should be supplied. Explain that pain, inflammation, redness, and blister formation are to be expected over the next few days. The blister, which is often haemorrhagic, can be punctured to make it more comfortable. It is probably not necessary to induce blister formation in order to treat viral warts.

There are no hard-and-fast rules about the application of dressings to areas treated with cryotherapy. Advise the patient to dress the lesion as they would a similar wound elsewhere on the body.

Scarring

Scarring may occur if freeze times are prolonged. The nail bed is particularly liable to damage when resistant periungual warts are being treated. This can cause distortion of the nail.

Nerve damage

Paraesthesia and anaesthesia can result from prolonged freezing near peripheral nerves. This is often temporary but may be permanent.

Depigmentation

Changes in pigmentation after cryotherapy are an important complication. Temporary post-inflammatory hypopigmentation is common, but hyperpigmentation may also occur, and these changes are sometimes permanent. Darker skinned people are at particular risk, and the possibility of pigment changes should always be explained before undertaking the procedure.

Tendon rupture

Tendon rupture has been reported after prolonged treatment of warts on the hands. The extensor tendons in particular lie perilously close to the skin. Take particular care when treating warts on the sides of the fingers.

Outcome
Viral warts

Most warts require more than one treatment. The cure rate is probably related to the number of treatments rather than the interval between them. More rapid cure may be achieved by shortening the time between treatments to weekly or fortnightly. When treating warts more frequently, avoid re-treating a wart that is still blistered.

Cryotherapy may not necessarily cure viral warts. Studies have shown that many warts that fail to resolve spontaneously within 3 months or fail to respond to wart paints also fail to respond to cryotherapy. After 12 treatments, cure rates are around 40–50%. Repeated freezing of unresponsive warts is rarely of value.

Combination therapy using a topical salicylic acid preparation (wart paint) between cryotherapy treatments has been shown to be more effective than cryotherapy alone. However, in the first few days after cryotherapy, the site may be too sore to apply wart paint. The patient should be advised to restart application of the wart paint as soon as the inflammatory response from the cryotherapy has settled. Infiltrating local anaesthetic (lidocaine) under the viral wart can significantly reduce the pain of cryotherapy, potentially allowing more extensive treatment.

Solar keratoses and seborrhoeic keratoses

Similar principles apply to treating solar keratoses and seborrhoeic keratoses. A freeze time of 5 seconds is recommended, and more than one treatment is often necessary. Large or raised seborrhoeic keratoses may need up to 10 seconds. The interval between treatments should be 3–4 weeks. If the lesion is on the face, ensure that the nuisance of post-treatment inflammation and blistering will not happen at a socially inconvenient time. Very localised application can be achieved by aiming the liquid nitrogen jet down a funnel onto the skin. An auroscope tip pressed to the skin makes a convenient funnel.

SURGICAL MANAGEMENT OF SOME SPECIFIC SKIN LESIONS

Chapter 9 describes the natural history, presenting features, and suggested management of most of the common skin lesions that are likely to be encountered. This section offers some specific practical advice about the surgical management of a few of these.

Pyogenic granuloma

These lesions are due to vascular proliferation, and in some situations surgical excision will be accompanied by profuse bleeding. In addition, they often occur on the digits, where anaesthesia without adrenaline (epinephrine) increases the likelihood of bleeding. So although these lesions can often be successfully treated with curettage and cautery, the surgeon should be prepared to close the wound site with sutures if necessary and warn the patient prior to the procedure that this may be necessary (Figure 19.11).

As the differential diagnosis of a pyogenic granuloma includes amelanotic malignant melanoma, it is sometimes better, if there is any doubt, to remove the lesion by a formal excision (Figure 19.12).

Consideration should also be given to cosmetic result and healing when deciding whether to use curettage and cautery or ellipse excision. On the lower lip, for example, a better cosmetic outcome might be achieved by ellipse excision (Figure 19.13).

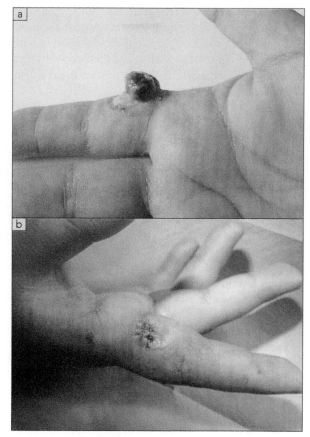

Figure 19.11 (a) Pyogenic granuloma on a digit, which required (b) suturing of the base.

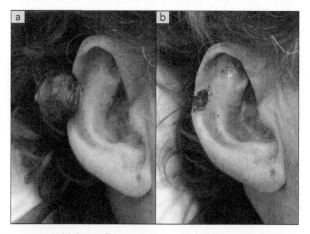

Figure 19.12 (a) A rapidly growing vascular lesion curetted as a presumed pyogenic granuloma, but which was histologically shown to be a malignant melanoma. (b) The site after cautery.

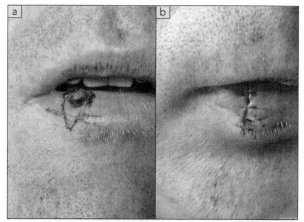

Figure 19.13 Pyogenic granuloma on the lower lip removed by ellipse excision.

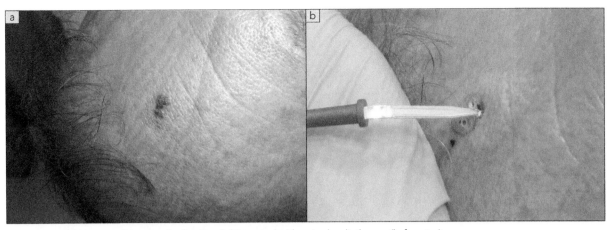

Figure 19.14 (a) Haemangioma on the forehead, (b) treated with unipolar diathermy (hyfrecator).

Haemangioma

The majority of haemangiomas are less dramatic in their growth and presentation than pyogenic granulomas; they may be bright red and arterial or purplish and venous. The latter are particularly common on the lips. Treatment is indicated for those haemangiomas which cause symptoms or disfigurement. Small arterial haemangiomas may be treated with diathermy (Figure 19.14), laser (if available), or, if they are small, punch biopsy excision (especially cherry haemangiomas).

Small venous lakes on the lips may respond well to diathermy, but excision is often required. The surgeon should ensure the vermilion border is marked on each side of the ellipse and that these two marks line up exactly during closure (see Figure 19.13b).

Keratoacanthoma

Remember that these lesions share the histological appearance of a well-differentiated squamous cell skin cancer (although they grow much more rapidly), so they may be better treated by formal excision if this is possible (Figure 19.15). This ensures that the whole lesion is completely removed if there is any subsequent doubt about whether the lesion was a squamous cell carcinoma rather than a keratoacanthoma.

If the lesion is to be curetted, which is a reasonable choice in patients who are elderly and frail where the history suggests keratoacanthoma, it is important to take a full-thickness wedge biopsy first, so that the histopathologist can assess whether the lesion might be a squamous cell carcinoma. Be sure to record on the request form how quickly the lesion developed.

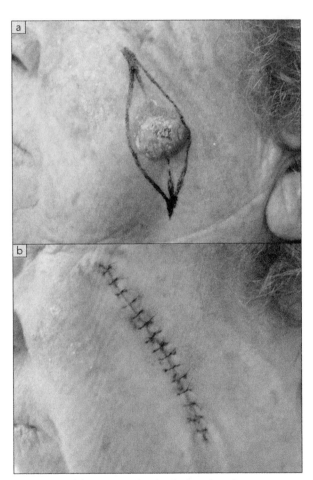

Figure 19.15 (a) Lesion on the cheek, thought to be a keratoacanthoma, (b) formally excised.

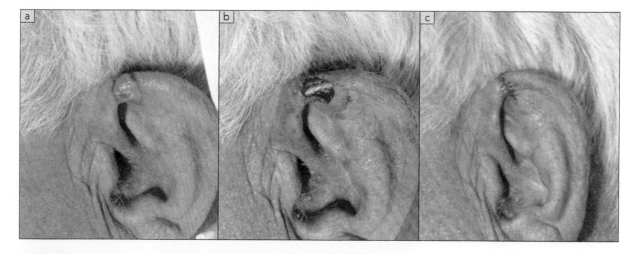

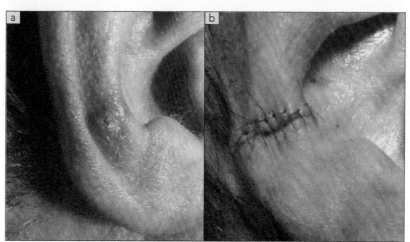

Figure 19.16 Chondrodermatitis nodularis helicis on the helix, (a) before, (b) during, and (c) after surgical excision.

Figure 19.17 (a) Chondrodermatitis nodularis helicis on the antihelix, (b) excised and sutured.

Chondrodermatitis nodularis helicis

Chondrodermatitis nodularis helicis (CDNH) presents as a tender nodule(s) over the helix or antihelix of the ear (Figures 19.16 and 19.17). As the pathology involves the cartilage, it is very important to remove the underlying cartilage, otherwise the condition recurs. The simplest surgical treatment therefore involves removing a wedge of ear along with a smooth sliver of the underlying cartilage (which often has a different, soft consistency in CDNH). Ensure no sharp edges of cartilage remain.

Cutaneous horn

As discussed in Chapter 9, a cutaneous horn is a manifestation of dyskeratosis and is a clinical rather than a pathological diagnosis. On the helix, squamous cell carcinoma can present as a cutaneous horn. It is therefore essential to remove this type of lesion as a primary procedure, where possible (Figure 19.18). On the ear, if a squamous cell carcinoma is suspected, it may be better to refer to a plastic surgeon in order to achieve adequate clearance. Do not forget to palpate for any draining lymph node enlargement as part of your assessment. Elsewhere, a cutaneous horn should be excised with at least a 2 mm margin from the edge of the base.

Figure 19.18 Cutaneous horn on the helix (a) before and (b) after surgical wedge excision. Note the evidence of sun damage (solar keratosis on the antihelix).

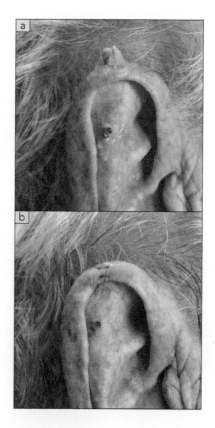

Neurofibroma

Multiple pedunculated skin tumours, or subcutaneous nodules, should raise the suspicion of neurofibromatosis, and the clinician should be familiar with the presentation and complications of type I neurofibromatosis (Figure 19.19). Pedunculated neurofibromas can be removed for cosmetic reasons or if they are catching and irritating; however, those with type I neurofibromatosis usually have such a multitude of growths that this is beyond the realm of primary care surgery.

Pedunculated tumours should be treated with shave excision, and the base can be treated with diathermy or closed with interrupted skin sutures. Those situated subcutaneously should be left or referred for imaging as surgery may result in loss of nerve function.

Dermatofibroma

As discussed in Chapter 9, these firm, nodular lesions are found typically on the limbs, particularly the lower limbs of women. The only treatment is formal surgical excision so the resultant scar must be an improvement on the dermatofibroma to justify excision (unless there is diagnostic uncertainty). Try to limit excision to those lesions which cause problems due to catching or skin irritation.

A narrow elliptical excision should be undertaken, following the relaxed skin tension lines. Closure should aim to produce a flat scar that does not stretch. Therefore buried, absorbable monofilament sutures, such as PDS II, should be considered, followed by support with adhesive strips such as Steri-Strips™.

Where these lesions occur over the tip of the shoulder, an area liable to keloid scarring, the author has found it beneficial to follow initial wound healing with the use of silicone dressings for 2 months.

Cylindroma

This is a rare tumour, also benign, occurring commonly on the scalp. It may initially be mistaken for a pilar cyst until excision is attempted, when a firm, granular, adherent lesion is found. Treatment is by formal, surgical excision.

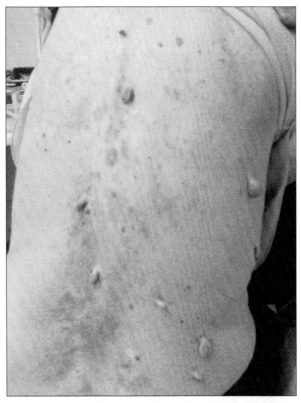

Figure 19.19 Neurofibromas on the back, suitable for simple excision.

Surgical management of some specific skin lesions

LINKS TO VIDEO CLIPS

VC 19.1a	VC 19.1b	VC 19.1c
VC 19.2	VC 19.3a	VC 19.3b
VC 19.4a	VC 19.4b	VC 19.5a
VC 19.5b	VC 19.5c	

VC 19.1a,b,c: Curettage: scraping technique and electrocautery
http://goo.gl/Wvzg3
http://goo.gl/Bt26I
http://goo.gl/ZvN4E

VC 19. 2: Curettage: scooping technique
http://goo.gl/5k8pf

VC 19.3a,b: Shave excision
http://goo.gl/Kw6er
http://goo.gl/PNN4a

VC 19.4a,b: Shave excision
http://goo.gl/WI1tM
http://goo.gl/DjYat

VC 19.5a,b,c: Snip excision
http://goo.gl/U4u0E
http://goo.gl/O707s
http://goo.gl/1eU50

Dermatological techniques and tips

PART 4

Additional surgical skills and procedures

Chapter 20

Other surgical procedures: cysts and lipomas

INTRODUCTION

Information about common different cysts and lipomas is included in Chapter 9. This chapter considers the management of epidermoid, mucous, acne, and meibomian cysts and lipomas. For the most part, surgical management is discussed in detail, but non-surgical options, when appropriate, are described.

Levels of difficulty are indicated by scalpel ratings. The more scalpel blades, the more experience will be required to become competent at the technique.

MANAGEMENT OF EPIDERMOID, PILAR, AND ACNE CYSTS

Chapter 9 describes the different types of cyst you are likely to encounter, epidermoid and pilar cysts being the most common. Their surgical management will vary depending on the size of the lesion, whether there has been any previous infection, and the type of cyst.

Indications for surgery

In many situations, there is no medical need to remove a cyst as it will usually be benign. In particular, small, inconsequential cysts are better left alone as long as the diagnosis is clear. There are, however, some common indications for the surgical removal of a cyst, as described below.

- **Size:**
  - Large cysts can give rise to direct and indirect pressure effects, causing discomfort.
  - Cosmetic disfigurement may result.

- **Contents:**
  - Cysts can discharge an offensive (rancid oil) cheesy material.
  - Rupture of the cyst results in an intense local reaction.
- **Infection:**
  - The cyst may become infected, and this can cause abscess formation that may require incision and drainage. The resultant scarred cyst is often deeply adherent to the surrounding tissues.
- **Malignant transformation:**
  - This is incredibly rare and is not therefore an indication for all cysts to be removed. Some 2% of pilar cysts are reported as developing proliferating pilar tumours; these are not, however, truly malignant, and they are better described as pseudocarcinomatous.

Surgical procedures: overview

The technique for removal depends upon:
- Size.
- Previous infection, inflammation, or surgery.
- Location.

There are three main surgical techniques. The conventional technique for the excision of cysts larger than 5 mm involves a surgical excision through the skin to expose and remove the cyst. For smaller lesions, the cyst can be removed using the so-called 'minimal excision technique' or through a punch biopsy wound.

Whichever technique is used, the aim should be to remove the cyst wall in its entirety as failure to do this will lead to recurrence. For this reason, the open technique, whereby complete removal can be ensured, is recommended and the cyst should ideally be removed whole and unpunctured. Although pilar cysts do not usually demonstrate a punctum, nearly all others do if the surface is inspected carefully. If possible, the cyst should be removed with the punctum.

Surgical excision

Before you start

The circumference of the cyst should be gently palpated and marked out with a surgical pen (Figure 20.1 and Video Clip 20.1). The incision line should be marked out in alignment with the relaxed skin tension lines. Local anaesthetic should be injected around the cyst, taking care to avoid injecting into the cyst itself, as it may rupture.

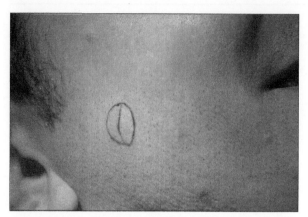

Figure 20.1 Cyst marked around the periphery and along the incision line prior to surgery. See Video Clip 20.1: http://goo.gl/iRBGb.

Remember to take into consideration the location of the cyst and in particular the possibility that its deep margin may reach anatomically important structures (e.g., the parotid gland salivary duct if situated on the cheek). To facilitate removal of the cyst by careful dissection, be sure that the operating site is easily accessible. This is particularly important with larger cysts.

//// Surgical excision of cysts >5 mm diameter, with no previous infection or surgery

These are the most straightforward cysts to remove, and the procedure involves exposing the cyst and carefully dissecting it out complete. Figure 20.2 and Video Clip 20.2 show the procedure diagrammatically, and Figure 20.3 details the excision of an epidermoid cyst on the neck.

Marking the skin

Design your ellipse after demarcating the cyst as outlined above. If a punctum is present, it is best to include this in the ellipse of skin, which should follow the relaxed skin tension lines. Where the skin over the cyst has been noticeably distended, it is also important to widen the incision to remove some of the overlying skin, even if no punctum is visible. Skin marking is shown in Figure 20.1.

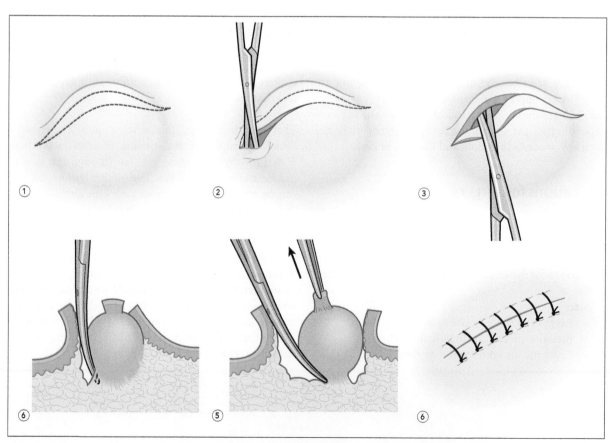

Figure 20.2 Diagram of excision of an epidermoid cyst. See Video Clip 20.2 : http://goo.gl/qn8OM.

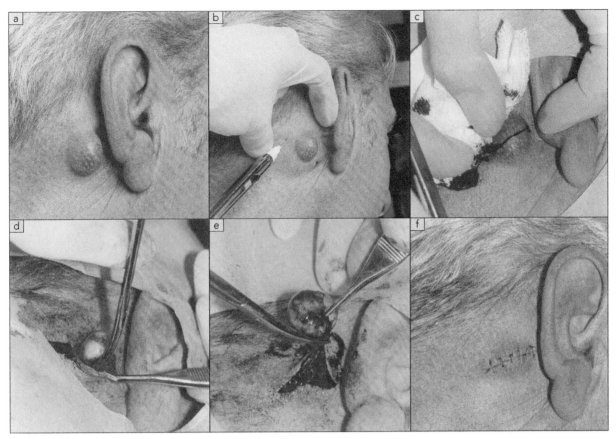

Figure 20.3 Excision of an epidermoid cyst on the neck.

Infiltrating with local anaesthetic

The majority of cysts can be removed painlessly with the circumferential injection of anaesthetic (Figure 20.4). If possible, a small amount of anaesthetic should be injected carefully around the deep aspect of the cyst, avoiding penetrating or bursting the cyst. Some surgeons use the volume of anaesthetic to hydrodissect the cyst wall away from the skin, but once again care should be taken to avoid injecting into the cyst and rupturing it.

Making the incision

Carefully incise along the skin marking over the top of the cyst (Figure 20.5). If it is a large or very superficial cyst, it will need a very shallow incision through the epidermis to avoid encountering the cyst wall. It is important not to rush this process. Time spent here avoiding cutting through the cyst wall will greatly facilitate the removal of the cyst in its entirety.

The length of the incision should equal the diameter of the cyst. It is a mistake to try to remove a cyst through a small incision, as this will only make it more difficult to remove the whole cyst.

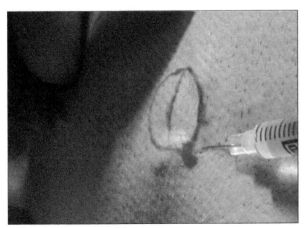

Figure 20.4 Injecting local anaesthetic around the cyst.

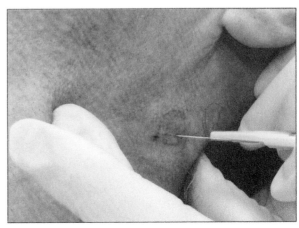

Figure 20.5 Making the incision.

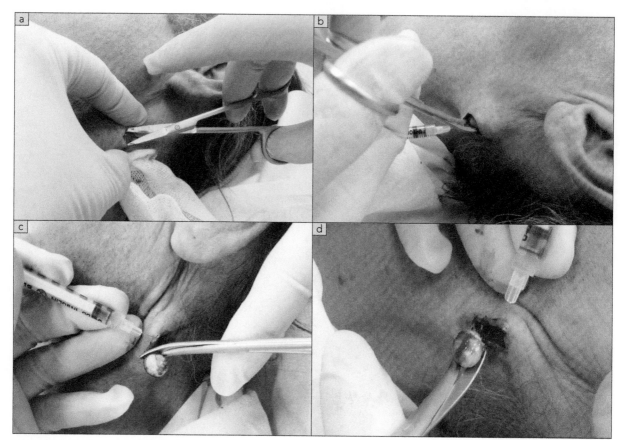

Figure 20.6 Dissecting out and carefully removing the cyst in its entirety. See Video Clip 20.3: http://goo.gl/U6Kel; http://goo.gl/NhgY2; http://goo.gl/o4axP; http://goo.gl/DDLCk.

Removing the cyst

Reaching the cyst wall can be achieved by gently cutting with the scalpel or blunt dissecting with fine, sharp iris scissors, gradually parting the layers until the cyst wall is visible. Using a scalpel, however, risks cutting into and bursting the cyst. Where an ellipse incision has been made, it may help to free one apex and, with a skin hook, lift this and then open up an area underneath it to allow gentle blunt dissection to locate the cyst. Care taken at this stage to identify the cyst wall will pay dividends as far as ease and completeness of removal is concerned.

Where an ellipse of skin with the punctum is also being removed, this should remain attached to the cyst and be used to help hold and lift the cyst. Excess traction will tend to tear the cyst wall. Try to avoid grabbing the cyst with forceps as the cyst walls tend to be very thin and will tear.

Once the cyst wall has been identified, switch to using fine, blunt, curved strabismus scissors (or similar scissors) and use these to dissect around the cyst and separate it from the surrounding tissues. Do this gently and systematically and it will literally 'shell out like a pea'. The cyst will sometimes be tethered at the base so it is important to mobilise the cyst all around and down to the base, gradually parting any adherent tissue.

It is not disastrous if the cyst is ruptured as long as it is still possible to remove the whole of the cyst wall and its contents. The contents are highly irritant to the surrounding skin, and any cyst wall left behind may enable a recurrent cyst to form.

Figures 20.6, 20.7, and 20.8 (and Video Clip 20.3) show cyst removal.

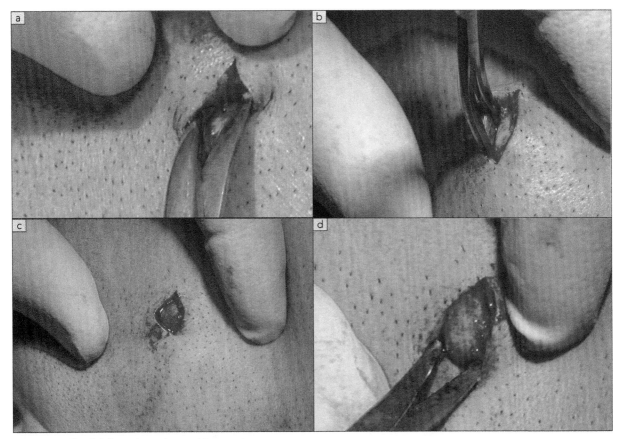

Figure 20.7 Careful dissection using strabismus scissors.

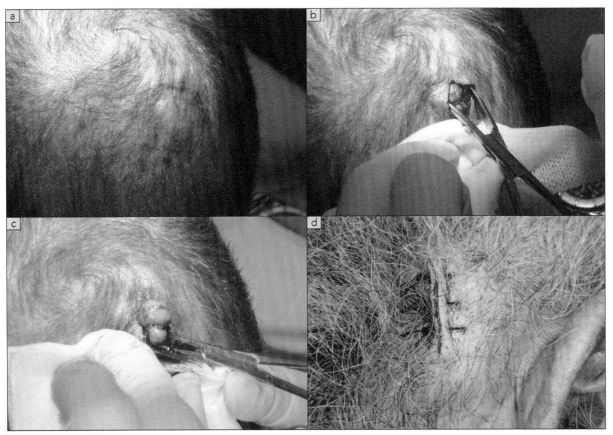

Figure 20.8 Marking (a) and excision (b, c) of a pilar cyst. (d) Sometimes a mattress suture will be required for closure.

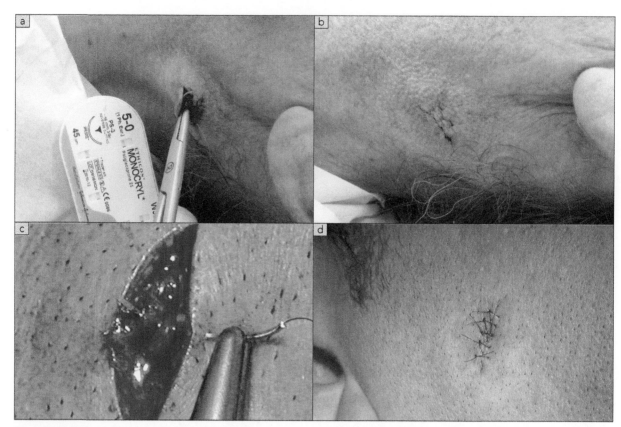

Figure 20.9 Closure after excision of an epidermoid cyst with (a,b) buried monofilament absorbable sutures, and (c,d) non-absorbable monofilament skin sutures.

Closure

Remember that, after the cyst has been removed, you will have created a cavity, and if this cavity is not obliterated it is likely to fill with blood and may become subsequently infected. It is recommended that any thin, redundant skin is excised and the edges of the wound approximated. Deep absorbable sutures can be inserted under the surface and used to help close the cavity (Figure 20.9). Alternatively, mattress sutures can be used for closure (Figure 20.8d) but may not give such a good cosmetic outcome. For smaller cysts, conventional sutures may be effective using larger than usual 'bites' with the needle.

Cysts behind the ear

Cysts at the base of the ear often cause distension of the skin, which needs to be resected to effect closure (Figure 20.10). Care needs to be taken in the postauricular area as 'cysts' here can be enlarged lymph nodes, as shown in Figure 20.11. Here, the cystic lesion is in fact a lymph node full of metastatic squamous cell carcinoma from a previously excised ear primary (the scar can be seen on the helix).

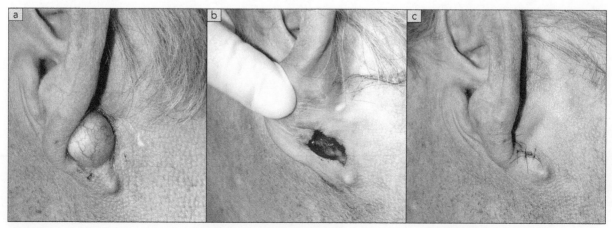

Figure 20.10 Excision of a cyst near the earlobe.

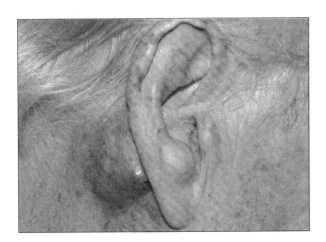

Figure 20.11
Postauricular lymph node from squamous cell carcinoma.

Surgical excision of small cysts less than 5 mm in diameter

Unless they are very superficial, small cysts can be difficult to locate, so it is important to be clear about the indications for surgical excision. Small cysts, especially on the face, are best removed by one of two methods described here.

/// Minimal excision technique

The cyst periphery is marked and infiltrated with local anaesthetic. Introduce a No. 15 scalpel blade into the skin with a 'stab' action down directly into the cyst, and then express the contents. The back of the cyst wall should then be grabbed with fine artery forceps and pulled inside out from the wound, ensuring that the whole cyst wall is removed. The wound can then be closed either with a single suture, skin glue, or a Steri-Strip™. The risk is that some of the cyst wall will be left and the cyst will reform within an area of scarring.

/// Punch biopsy

The cyst is marked and the area anaesthetised as previously described. Using a punch biopsy of an appropriate size (3–4 mm), the whole cyst is removed. The wound is then closed with one or two fine skin sutures. This is a very simple and quick technique. With care, the punch biopsy can be used to cut down to but not through the cyst wall. The cyst can then be extracted or expressed through the biopsy hole.

/// Milia

Milia are tiny keratin-filled cysts that can usually be removed without anaesthetic. The skin surface overlying the milia can be 'nicked' with the sharp bevelled end of a green or white needle. The contents can then be gently expressed with forceps or gloved hands. Any remaining cyst can be hooked out with the tip of the needle or very fine tissue forceps. Pressure applied for a couple of minutes produces haemostasis.

An alternative technique is to use a unipolar diathermy with a sharp tip, set at about 3–4 W. This can be used to diathermy the cyst. The contents usually rupture onto the skin surface. A fine pair of forceps can then be used to express the remains.

> **GOLDEN RULES** ✳
> - Be sure of the diagnosis before you operate.
> - If unsure: delay, refer, or arrange imaging.
> - Ultrasound can help with identifying and delineating lumps and bumps.

Managing a cyst that is or has been infected or is scarred

Infected cysts

Actively infected cysts should be treated like an abscess, with any pus being released by an incision cut through the most thinned and tense section of skin. The inflammation and acidotic state of the tissues renders local anaesthetics ineffective so cryoanaesthesia may be useful (see Chapter 15). The lesion is sometimes so tense that anaesthetic may be unnecessary.

//// Previously infected cysts

Only perform surgery on previously infected cysts when the infection has all resolved. The cyst periphery will be more difficult to identify because it is often attached by scar tissue to the surrounding tissues. It is often only possible to take the whole cyst out with an ellipse of skin, as long as it is not too big (Figure 20.12). In effect, this is an excision of an area of scar tissue. The walls of the cyst may be very friable. The cyst can usually be lifted out with the skin excision; any remaining cyst wall will need to be removed with blunt dissection with or without curettage. The excision tends to be larger than expected and to bleed more than usual.

Remember to send the excised material for histological examination; it is possible for some lesions (acantholytic squamous cell carcinomas, for example) to mimic a post-infected cyst.

Acne cysts

Acne vulgaris is commonly associated with troublesome cysts that can be deep, inflamed, and chronically infected. It is important not to excise these lesions until the acne is under control. In the acute phase, incision and drainage may be helpful, and sometimes injection with triamcinolone (see below) is indicated. Once the acne has settled down, residual lesions can be considered for excision. Acne that is associated with cyst formation requires more aggressive treatment (such as isotretinoin).

Non-surgical treatment of cysts

The use of intralesional steroids has been documented to reduce inflammation by using small quantities of triamcinolone injected directly into the cyst. It is not usually recommended for quiet, non-inflamed lesions. When used in carefully selected cases, this technique can sometimes result in complete resolution. It is particularly helpful for cysts that have previously ruptured and those which have become inflamed and swollen in the past but have never developed into an abscess with release of pus (by rupture or surgical drainage).

A total of 10–20 mg of triamcinolone 10 mg/ml is injected into the cyst contents. Care should be taken with very tense cysts as the volume of steroid can cause rupture. It is also important to avoid extravasation of the steroid outside the cyst as this has the potential to cause fat atrophy and pigmentary change.

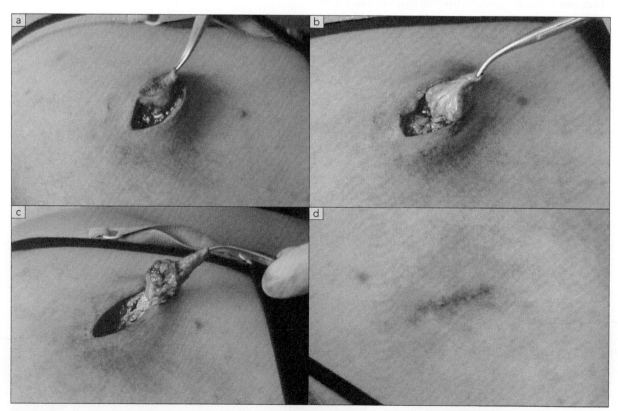

Figure 20.12 Excision of a previously infected cyst by ellipse excision.

MANAGEMENT OF MYXOID/MUCIN CYSTS

Myxoid cysts are increasingly considered to be ganglions of the distal interphalangeal (DIP) joint. More information about these relatively common lesions can be found in Chapter 9. Historically, a range of different treatments have been used for these lesions, but many of these are associated with a high recurrence rate. Spontaneous regression in asymptomatic cysts appears to be common, with several series suggesting that the likelihood of spontaneous regression may approximate 50%.

This section considers a range of management options. There is debate in the literature regarding the optimal treatment approaches, and different approaches to treatment may be necessary depending upon how symptomatic the condition is. If there is any doubt about management, the advice of an expert nail or hand surgeon should be sought.

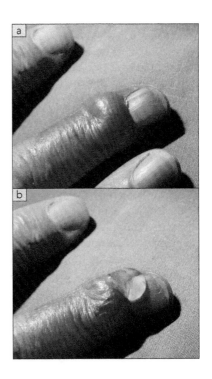

Figure 20.13
Digital mucous cyst (a) before and (b) after needle incision with the expressed, clear contents visible in (b).

/// Needle aspiration/injection

The cyst is usually easily punctured with a wide-bore needle, and the clear, glutinous contents are easily expressed (Figure 20.13); however, the cyst is highly likely to recur. Alternatively, the cyst can be traumatised at multiple sites with a wide-bore needle until resolution is achieved. The needle results in dispersal of the cyst contents, and hopefully scarring will then lead to destruction of the cyst wall.

Another technique is cyst aspiration with a large-bore needle, followed by instillation of corticosteroids (triamcinolone or hydrocortisone with or without lidocaine). Injecting corticosteroids or proteolytic agents, such as hyaluronidase or sclerotherapy agents, is not recommended because if the cyst communicates with the joint, leakage of any of these agents may cause problems.

/// Cryosurgery

This has been used with some success to treat small digital mucous cysts. The technique involves destroying the cyst by the use of liquid nitrogen cryotherapy, and creating an inflammatory response and scarring to try to prevent the lesion from recurring. Short freeze/thaw cycles should predominate when cryotherapy is applied to avoid possible scarring of the nail matrix. Cryosurgery of the cyst has reported cure rates of between 56% and 86%.

/// Curettage and cautery

Some clinicians, particularly dermatologists, favour curettage of the cyst, which may or may not be combined with electrodesiccation/cautery. Caution should be exercised to reduce the risk of scarring. The patient should be warned of possible nail deformity after this procedure.

///// Surgical excision

Formal surgical excision of the cyst is reported as having better success rates. A range of surgical procedures have been recommended, from simple excision of the cyst to wide, radical excision with possible graft or flap reconstruction using rotation or rhomboid flaps depending upon the location of the lesion. Another approach is marsupialisation, or excision of the whole proximal nail fold, with subsequent healing by secondary intention.

Excision and debridement of joint osteophytes has been recommended by some authors as a necessary adjunct, to reduce the risk of recurrence. Indeed, some hand surgeons believe that excision and debridement of the marginal osteophyte without removal of the cyst itself may be the best intervention. This may result in less postoperative impairment of joint motion and fewer nail deformities, as it is dissection around the germinal matrix that may injure the underlying nail matrix and cause scarring. In general, it is reported that although more aggressive dissection leads to lower recurrence rates, more nail deformity is likely to occur.

Surgical interventions, albeit possibly slightly more effective in preventing recurrence, are associated with complications including restriction of joint mobility and nail dystrophy. The patient must be warned of this. Radial or ulnar deviation of the DIP joint with resulting impairment of joint motion can occur. Although some nail deformities may be corrected by surgery, residual nail deformities may persist or be caused by the surgery. Other complications include tendon injury, superficial infection, DIP septic arthritis, increased arthritic symptoms in the joint, and persistent swelling, pain, numbness, and stiffness.

Identification and repair of the leak of joint fluid

An exciting new treatment by nail surgeons, with good results, is to treat recurrent or refractory cysts by repairing the causative leak of synovial fluid in such lesions (De Berker and Lawrence, 2001). This involves injecting methylene blue into the DIP joint space to identify the link between the joint and the cyst. A flap of skin is then raised over the cyst to identify the communication, which is closed by suturing. The flap of skin is then replaced.

Suggested management plan

Conservative treatments are likely to be associated with the least morbidity. Consequently, a reasonable treatment plan for symptomatic cysts overlying joints may entail initial needling or aspiration and injection. If this approach fails, patients may be referred to a hand or nail surgeon for surgical intervention, and the benefits and risks of any surgical procedure discussed so that the patient can make an informed decision about how to proceed. Cysts closer to the nail fold can also be treated by simple incision, curettage, and cautery.

MANAGEMENT OF MEIBOMIAN CYSTS

A meibomian cyst is a cystic swelling occurring within the upper or lower tarsal plates of the eyelids (Figure 20.14). It represents a retention cyst of the meibomian glands and is generally precipitated by lid margin disease in the form of blepharitis and meibomianitis.

Meibomian cysts should initially be treated conservatively with hot compresses and antibiotic ointment. If secondary infection has occurred, a course of systemic antibiotics may be necessary.

In its chronic form, a meibomian cyst appears as a well-localised nodule. The overlying conjunctiva may be engorged, but at the centre of the cyst the pressure of its contents often causes a central pallid patch on the tarsoconjunctival surface. It is essential to examine the tarsoconjunctival surface before proceeding with incision and curettage; with atypical or recurring meibomian cysts, it is particularly important to consider the rare diagnosis of meibomian gland carcinoma.

//// Surgical treatment

Incision and curettage of a meibomian cyst is generally best performed through the tarsoconjunctival surface, although if the lesion has discharged through the skin, incision and curettage should be performed through the skin using an incision parallel to the skin margin.

Anaesthesia

Local anaesthesia is generally achieved with a solution of 1% lidocaine containing adrenaline (epinephrine) 1:200,000 accompanied by topical anaesthesia using one or two drops of topical anaesthesia into the eye (Figure 20.15a). A 2 ml volume of 1% lidocaine with adrenaline is infiltrated into the lid skin around the meibomian cyst using a 25 G needle (Figure 20.15b). To reduce the discomfort from the local anaesthesia, the solution should be warmed to body temperature and if necessary a preinjection using a dilute solution of 1% lidocaine with normal saline (1:10) can be employed. After infiltration, gentle pressure on the eyelid helps to disperse the local anaesthetic agent.

Technique

A chalazion clamp (Figure 20.16a) is applied over the cyst with its open surface on the tarsoconjunctiva. The lid is then everted and the cyst incised vertically through the tarsoconjunctiva perpendicular to the lid margin,

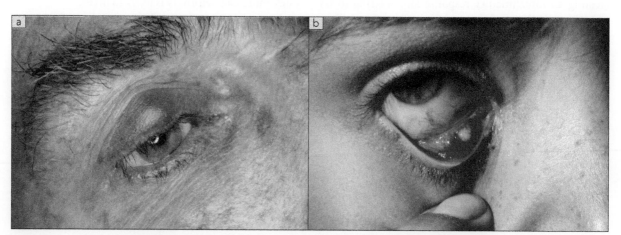

Figure 20.14 Appearance of a meibomian cyst (a) externally on the upper lid and (b) over the tarsal surface of the lower lid.

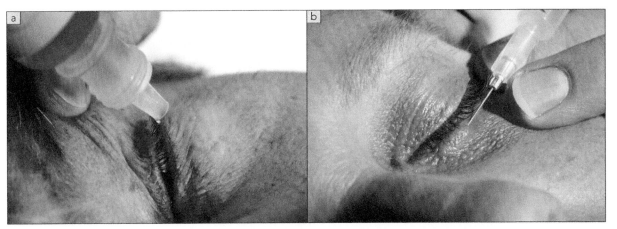

Figure 20.15 Excising a meibomian cyst: (a) topical and (b) infiltrational anaesthesia.

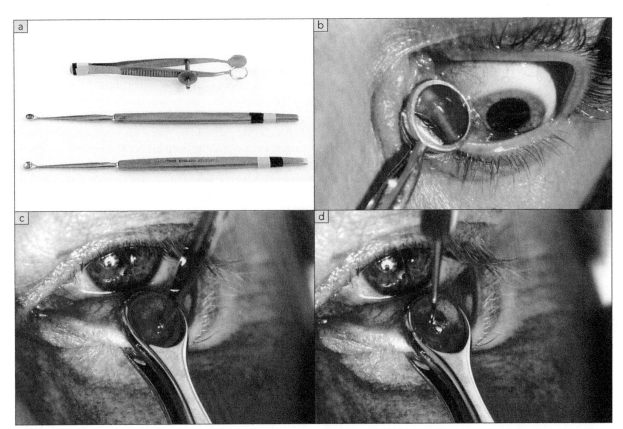

Figure 20.16 (a) Chalazion or Meibomian clamp and curettes. (b) Meibomian clamp in place with cyst in the centre. (c) The cyst is incised using a No. 11 blade. (d) Using a Chalazion curette, the contents are removed and the cyst wall curetted.

taking care not to involve the lid margin in the incision (Figure 20.16b). Once the cyst has been opened, the contents are evacuated and the walls of the cyst are scraped using a sharp chalazion curette (Figure 20.16c). Any abnormal tissue should be sent for histology to exclude malignancy.

Postoperative care

Antibiotic ointment is then inserted and a pressure dressing using two eye pads put in place for 15 minutes. The eye is then re-dressed with a lighter pad and antibiotic ointment, generally ophthalmic chloramphenicol, is inserted into the eye and continued twice a day for 3 days.

SURGICAL EXCISION OF LIPOMAS

Indications

The clinical presentation and diagnosis of lipomas are considered in Chapter 9. Surgical removal is indicated in the following clinical situations:

- Symptomatic relief (particularly important in the rare Dercum's disease, which is associated with multiple painful lipomas).
- Large lipomas, greater than 5 cm in diameter, that are enlarging (as there is a rare possibility of malignant change).
- Biopsy of large lipomas or those tethered to fascia to rule out a liposarcoma.
- Cosmetic nuisance.

⫻ – ⫻⫻ Surgical technique

Standard removal of a lipoma involves the following procedure.

Identification and marking

As with surgical removal of cysts, it is important to identify the extent of the lipoma before you begin by palpating the outer edge of the lipoma (Figure 20.17a). You should then mark the outermost edge of the palpable lipoma (Figure 20.17b). The lipoma is going to be squeezed out through a linear excision, so you should next mark your planned incision along the line of relaxed skin tension.

Local anaesthesia

Inject the local anaesthetic around the peripheral border of the lesion and the planned incision (Video Clip 20.4 [http://goo.gl/k0TWU; http://goo.gl/tpcjL]). Large lipomas may require deeper anaesthesia, which can be achieved painlessly after the intradermal injections have been completed.

Making the incision

Incise the skin across the diameter of the lipoma (Video Clip 20.5 [http://goo.gl/VAdSn; http://goo.gl/jh6DN]). It is a mistake to make this incision too small, especially if the lipoma is situated deeply. If the lipoma is encapsulated (and they are often lobulated), it will be identified immediately below the dermis and will often bulge out through the incision. Avoid cutting too deep initially. If the lipoma is not immediately identifiable, the subcutaneous fat will need to be carefully explored.

Mobilisation

Once the lipoma has been identified, blunt, curved-ended strabismus scissors can be used to gradually ease around the lipoma (Figure 20.18a, and Video Clip 20.6). Particular care should be taken when undertaking blunt dissection around the deep aspect of a lipoma as significant structures (arteries, nerves, and lymphatics) must be avoided. For this reason, it is safer to express the lipomas out through the wound if possible (Figure 20.19 and Video Clip 20.7).

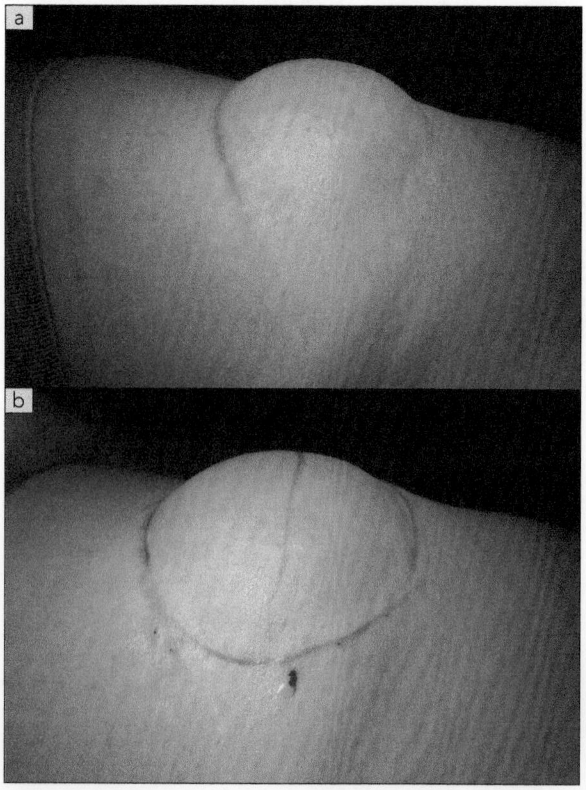

Figure 20.17 Lipoma (a) before and (b) after skin marking circumferentially and along the relaxed skin tension line.

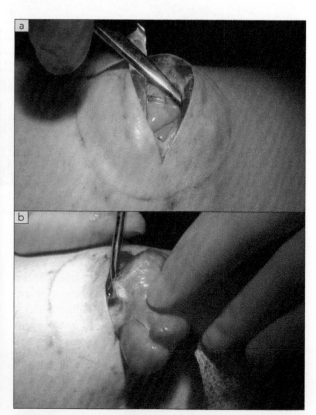

Figure 20.18 Mobilising the lipoma. See Video Clip 20.6: http://goo.gl/Zw17I; http://goo.gl/XL8Zp; http://goo.gl/CgIVk; http://goo.gl/Smzza; http://goo.gl/UITMy.

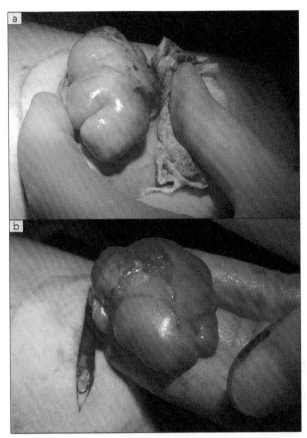

Figure 20.19 Expressing a lipoma, (a) using gauze to help hold the lipoma; (b) after removal. See Video Clip 20.7: http://goo.gl/sWBaH.

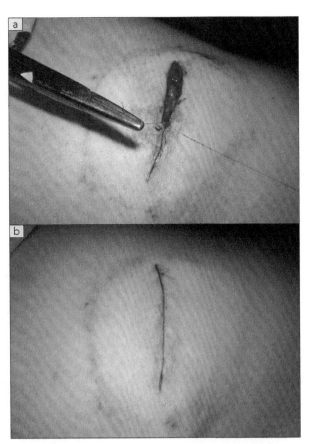

Figure 20.20 Closure of the lipoma wound, (a) using deep, absorbable sutures; (b) after closure.

Pedunculated or protuberant lipomas are best removed as ellipse excisions, taking the underlying lipoma out with the skin defect.

Closure

Care needs to be taken to ensure that wound cavities are closed, by using deep sutures, closing in layers, or using mattress sutures. Figure 20.20 shows the lipoma wound being closed with buried monofilament absorbable sutures.

Figure 20.21 shows a large lipoma being removed from the neck. After removal, the redundant skin is estimated (Figure 20.21h) and removed. The cavity is then closed with buried monofilament absorbable sutures and a final layer of skin sutures.

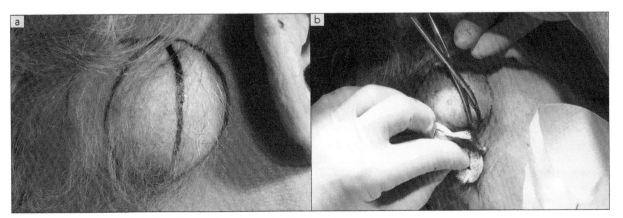

Figure 20.21 (a–j) Removal of a large lipoma from the neck. *(Continued on next page.)*

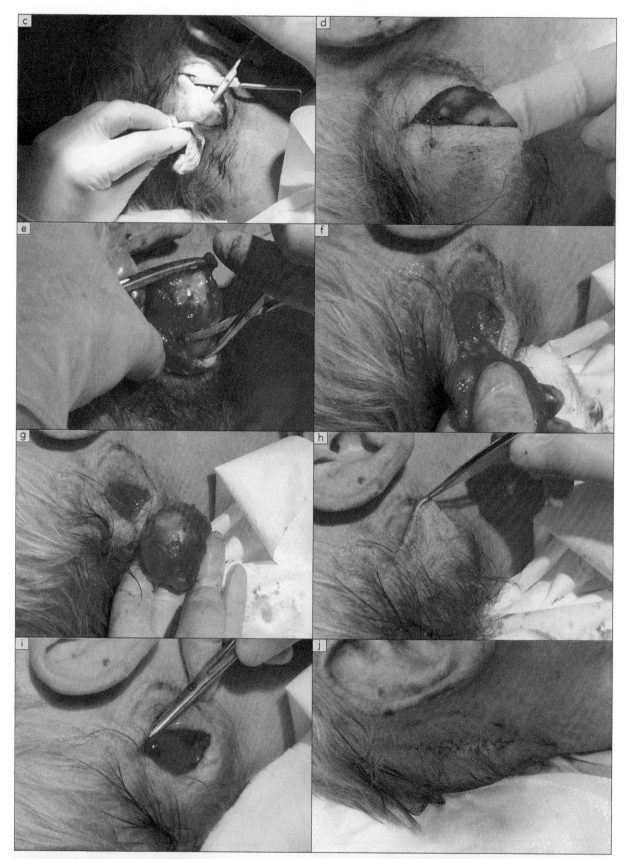

Figure 20.21 Removal of a large lipoma from the neck (continued). c) Bluntly mobilising skin with curved strabismus scissors. (d) Sterile gloved finger mobilising deep aspect. (e) Artery forceps to hold the lipoma for further blunt dissection. (f) Lipoma almost removed, deep attachments exposed. (g) Lipoma removed. (h) Skin edge drawn across to assess redundant skin. (i) Closure with deep sutures to obliterate cavity, and (j) skin sutures.

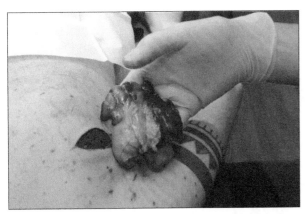

Figure 20.22 Large lipoma.

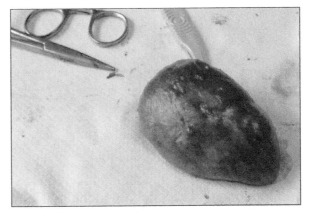

Figure 20.23 Encapsulated lipoma.

///// Large and/or encapsulated lipomas

- Large lipomas (Figure 20.22) may not fit into standard formalin-containing specimen pots. If the appearance is entirely in keeping with the diagnosis, it is acceptable to send a representative section to histology.
- Some lipomas are very clearly encapsulated (Figure 20.23), whereas others are more lobulated (Figure 20.24). Some can be extremely adherent and difficult to mobilise. In the author's experience, excision of lipomas situated over the forehead (Figure 20.25) should be avoided as they tend to be deep-seated and adherent to the aponeurosis.

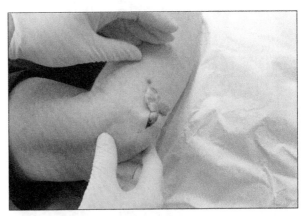

Figure 20.24 Lobulated lipoma.

Liposuction

Liposuction can be used for the treatment of medium (i.e., 4–10 cm) and large (i.e., bigger than 10 cm) lipomas in order to reduce the need for a large incision. For small lipomas, no advantage has been reported because these tumours can be extracted through small incisions. The exception is small facial lipomas, where favourable aesthetic results can be obtained using carefully placed incisions.

Laser lipolysis

Lipomas can be dispersed via a ND:YAG laser treatment. A narrow laser wand is inserted into the lipoma via a small skin incision, the laser wand is passed through the lipoma, disrupting the cells, liquifying the fat which will be absorbed by the body in the following months or via liposuction at the time of the laser treatment.

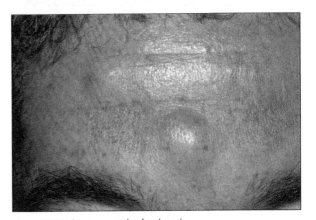

Figure 20.25 Lipoma on the forehead.

Outcomes

The outcome and prognosis are excellent because lipomas are benign. Recurrence is uncommon at the same location.

REFERENCES

De Berker D, Lawrence C (2001) Ganglion of the distal interphalangeal joint (myxoid cyst) therapy by identification and repair of the leak of joint fluid. *Archives of Dermatology* 137: 607–10.

LINKS TO VIDEO CLIPS

VC 20.1 VC 20.2 VC 20.3a VC 20.3b
VC 20.3c VC 20.3d VC 20.4a VC 20.4b
VC 20.5a VC 20.5b VC 20.6a VC 20.6b
VC 20.6c VC 20.6d VC 20.6e VC 20.7

VC 20.1: Marking a cyst
http://goo.gl/iRBGb

VC 20.2: Epidermoid cyst excision
http://goo.gl/qn8OM

VC 20.3a,b,c,d: Pilar cyst incision and dissection
http://goo.gl/U6Kel
http://goo.gl/NhgY2
http://goo.gl/o4axP
http://goo.gl/DDLCk

VC 20.4a,b: Lipoma anaesthesia
http://goo.gl/k0TWU
http://goo.gl/tpcjL

VC 20.5a,b: Lipoma incision
http://goo.gl/VAdSn
http://goo.gl/jh6DN

VC 20.6a,b,c,d,e: Lipoma mobilisation, dissection, and ligation of pedicle
http://goo.gl/Zw17I
http://goo.gl/XL8Zp
http://goo.gl/CglVk
http://goo.gl/Smzza
http://goo.gl/UlTMy

VC 20.7: Lipoma expression
http://goo.gl/sWBaH

Minor casualties

INTRODUCTION

Minor casualty attendances should be anticipated, and the scenarios described in this chapter will be familiar to most GPs and practice-based nurses. The skills described will enable any of those staff to know how to manage urgent, unplanned minor casualties in a logical and safe manner.

Levels of difficulty are indicated by scalpel ratings. The more scalpel blades, the more difficult the procedure and the more practical experience will be required to become competent at the technique.

INFECTIONS

Abscess

Large necrotic abscesses, so familiar in the nineteenth century, are now fortunately rare. Common sites for abscesses include the perineum and fingers—dealt with separately as paronychia—and a reasonable proportion of abscesses seen in primary care will be the result of infected surgical wounds (Figure 21.1).

Although antibiotics have revolutionised the treatment of most soft-tissue infections, there remains the challenge of resistant organisms such as meticillin-resistant *Staphylococcus aureus* (MRSA) and catastrophic infections such as necrotising fasciitis. If either of these situations is suspected, emergency hospital advice should be obtained.

Spreading cellulitis and induration with lymphangitis is best treated with antibiotics, but once pus has collected it should be released, usually by incision.

/// Technique to treat an abscess
Anaesthesia
Unlike almost every other surgical skin procedure, incising an abscess rarely involves the injection of local anaesthesia. Indeed, the presence of infection produces an acidic soft tissue, which results in local anaesthetic such as lidocaine not being effective. Most local anaesthetics are administered as water-soluble hydrochlorides, from which the active amine base is released, unionised, to diffuse through the nerve sheaths in healthy, alkaline tissue fluids. In acidic tissue fluids surrounding an infection, the anaesthetic remains ionised and unable to cross the nerve sheath.

If the overlying skin is already tense and thinned by the underlying collection of pus, anaesthesia may not be necessary. If this is not the case, cryoanaesthesia can be considered (Chapter 15). For deeper abscesses associated with systemic symptoms, general anaesthesia may be necessary. If a general anaesthetic is considered inappropriate, careful local or regional anaesthesia, cryoanaesthesia, or inhalational anaesthesia (nitrous oxide) may sometimes suffice.

Incision and drainage
If the abscess is superficial, distending the overlying skin, which has become thinned, incision using a pointed No. 11 scalpel blade (either on a size 3 handle or as a disposable scalpel) is all that is necessary. Once the abscess has been incised, the pus should be expelled by gentle pressure applied by a gloved hand, and a bacterial swab should be taken for culture.

Once it has been drained, management of the abscess cavity will depend on its size. A suitable drain and/or a sterile pack will sometimes need to be inserted to prevent premature closure of the wound and allow any remaining infected material to drain. For smaller abscesses, some authorities recommend incising the abscess, curetting the lining, and instilling an antibiotic gel such as fusidic acid. In this situation, a drain is unnecessary, a dry dressing is applied, and healing often occurs rapidly.

Aspiration
Aspiration using a wide-bore needle can sometimes be a useful technique. This is particularly the case with Bartholin's abscesses and may avoid the need for more radical surgery.

Abscess complicating an epidermoid cyst

If the abscess has complicated an epidermoid cyst (Figure 21.1b), the contents may be partly fluid and partly solid. Every attempt should be made to clear all the contents, and for this to succeed a reasonable width of incision is required. On occasions, it may even be possible to carefully lift out the cyst wall with fine forceps, thereby minimising the chance of recurrence. Be sure that the history is consistent with a previous cyst, now infected, as malignant tissue can sometimes have the appearance of an abscess (especially over the breast).

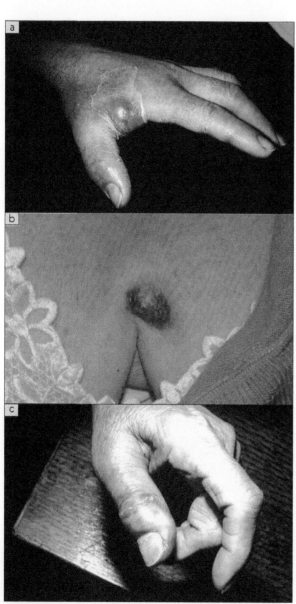

Figure 21.1 (a) Hand abscess suitable for simple incision and drainage. (b) Infected epidermoid cyst on the chest, suitable for incision, drainage, and if possible removal of the cyst wall. (c) A large thumb paronychia with pus collection, suitable for incision and drainage.

Paronychial abscess

Paronychia is a soft-tissue infection that develops around the proximal nail fold, with infective organisms entering a damaged nail fold (Figure 21.1c). Acute paronychia is usually the result of bacterial infection, and this may manifest as cellulitis (characterised by redness, swelling, and pain but no pus) or, particularly with staphylococcal infections, a classical paronychial abscess. Here the skin also tends to be hot, swollen, and painful, but the swelling is usually localised, it may be fluctuant, and if particularly superficial will have a green/grey/brown discoloration.

Management of a paronychial abscess

The surgeon should gently cut through the thinnest area of discoloured skin with the sharp, bevelled edge of a wide-bore (21 G or 19 G) hypodermic needle. Successful incision will result in the pus (which has given the distended skin its grey/green colour) being released, and with it relief of the throbbing pain. A swab of the pus should be taken for bacteriological culture.

Once all the pus has been expressed, a simple, non-absorbable dressing, held on by a tubular finger gauze, should be provided. The patient should be given a short course of antibiotic effective against staphylococci, such as flucloxacillin.

Pilonidal sinus

Pilonidal sinuses may vary from a small, ingrowing hair in the natal cleft to tortuous, multibranched long sinus tracts. The modern understanding of the aetiological factors leading to pilonidal sinus formation links the presence of hair growth along the midline to the warm, moist, bacteria-laden skin and the physical effect of sitting and standing creating a pit around the hair follicle. Subsequent localised pressure changes between sitting and standing allow material within the pit to be forced into the soft, subcutaneous tissues where sinuses can form virtually asymptomatically. Infection within the sinus tract produces pain, pus, and the need for treatment.

Management of a pilonidal sinus

Surgical management traditionally involved incision along the length of the tract, excising the sinus tract, and leaving the open wound to heal through secondary intention—a very slow process. The incisions were aimed away from the midline (where healing tends to be very problematic), and surgery was based on the presumption that the diseased deep tissues needed to be excised. Understanding that the shape of the natal cleft and the hair-bearing skin rather than the deeper tissues cause the condition has led to modified surgery, aimed at mobilising the skin of the natal cleft away from the midline by excising the main sinus (if not all the sinus tracts) via an ellipse of skin from the medial edge of the buttock on the most affected side. The ellipse is closed by mobilising and bringing the natal cleft skin across to close the ellipse, thereby moving non-hair-bearing buttock skin to cover the now less deeply valleyed natal cleft. Details of this technique are outside the remit of this text. The original articles by Karydakis, who described the surgical repair based on extensive personal experience, Bascom, who pioneered modifications, and Kitchen, who further developed them, should be studied for further details (Karydakis, 1973, 1992; Bascom, 1983; Kitchen, 1996).

Smaller pilonidal sinuses presenting for the first time may be suitable for day-case surgery.

SIMPLE ACUTE WOUNDS

This section deals with patients presenting with a minor injury, rather than the management of accident or serious injury victims. The patient should be carefully assessed according to the following three important points:

- Are there any *serious injuries* that require urgent management in a more acute or specialist setting?
- Are you going to be able to achieve *haemostasis* in the setting in which you are offering care?
- Is there any *damage* to deep structures that requires more specialist care?

The following patients should always be referred to an acute facility:

- Those in whom haemostasis cannot be achieved or the bleeding point cannot be identified. The patient will require the wound to be explored in a theatre equipped for general anaesthesia and fluid replacement.
- If there is any chance of a penetrating foreign body remaining in the wound. In this case, exploration of the injury will be required, often with radiographic (fluoroscopy) imaging.
- If a deep, penetrating injury has occurred, even without the presence of external bleeding. A small external wound may mask a deep wound, resulting in life-threatening bleeding or infection.
- If the injury is deep and nerve or tendon injury is suspected. A full assessment should be made of motor and sensory functions.
- If there is extensive tissue necrosis and devitalised tissue. In these situations, it is better to undertake surgical exploration and debridement in hospital.

✎–✐✐✐✐ Repairing lacerations

Provided the factors listed above are taken into account, there will be a range of small lacerations that can be safely repaired in a minor surgery setting. Techniques for debridement/cleaning of the wound and skin closure are described below.

Anaesthesia

The area will need anaesthetising before exploration. Although this can in theory be undertaken virtually painlessly by injecting through the raw edges of the wound, this temptation should be resisted as the needle will carry any infected material within the wound deep into subcutaneous tissues. The local anaesthesia should be injected around the wound following the principles described in other parts of this text and should only be undertaken after assessing for any nerve damage, both sensory and motor.

Wound cleaning

This requires a suitable sterile solution and sterile gauze. Strong cleaning solutions should be avoided as these may damage delicate tissues. Irrigation with sterile normal saline can help to clean a wound, and research has suggested that this is as effective as using antimicrobial solutions. If the wound is contaminated, it should first be irrigated with sterile saline to remove loose items before the wound edges are manually cleaned (Figure 21.2). If the wound edge is jagged or there is dead or devitalised tissue, a small amount of debridement may be required before repair.

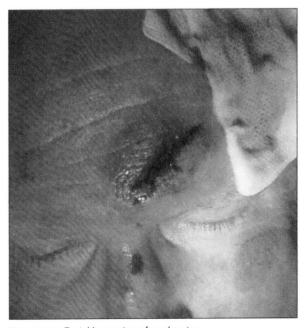

Figure 21.2 Facial laceration after cleaning.

Identifying and removing foreign bodies

Foreign bodies may be present in the wound, especially if the laceration has been caused by a fragile or brittle material such as glass. Patients can often feel the presence of a foreign body within their wound. If the presence of radio-opaque matter is suspected, a plain radiograph should be taken prior to wound closure. Wood and plastic are not likely to show on a radiograph, and if there is uncertainty, the patient should be treated in hospital.

The removal of small pieces of glass or metal can be extremely difficult if the operating field is covered with blood. Attempts to locate or remove such objects usually provoke further bleeding. Creating a bloodless operating area on a limb or digit by the use of a rubber tourniquet can facilitate the location and removal of any fragments. Further details related to different types of foreign body are included below.

Skin closure

The method of skin closure should be chosen according to the likelihood of wound infection and take account of any tension that might be created in closing the wound.

Wound glue

Simple clean, non-bleeding lacerations can be closed using wound glue, applied in layers to build up the strength of the bond.

Adhesive strips

Adhesive strips (e.g., Steri-Strip™, Leukostrip™) applied across a laceration can be the simplest and most effective method of closure, particularly where the skin is thin and friable (e.g., the pretibial area; Figure 21.3). They will not work on hair-bearing skin, and their adhesiveness can be improved by pre-treating the surrounding skin. Tincture of Benzoin or OpSite® spray, applied around the wound and allowed to dry, will improve adhesion.

Sutures

If sutures are required, they should be chosen to minimise the amount of foreign material within the wound. It is therefore best to use monofilament non-absorbable, interrupted skin sutures. Interrupted sutures allow any fluids to escape (unlike continuous subcuticular sutures), and non-absorbable sutures ensure that the material is removed. Particular care should be taken during the postoperative period to detect any early signs of wound infection.

Timing of skin closure

This will depend upon the state of the skin and the cleanliness of the wound. If the wound cannot be closed immediately, it should be kept packed and covered. Without packing, the wound will start to repair naturally within 24 hours. A clean laceration suitably covered with a sterile dressing can be closed up to about 48 hours after injury.

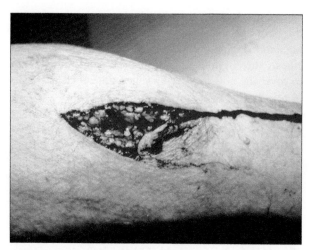

Figure 21.3 Pretibial laceration suitable for Steri-Strip™ closure.

Postoperative care

Patients should be told what to look out for postoperatively in terms of wound infection (pain, swelling, redness). Rapid commencement of oral antibiotics may prevent abscess formation and breakdown of the wound, the latter leading eventually to the wound closing slowly by secondary intention.

HAEMATOMAS

Soft-tissue haematomas are very variable in size, commonly occur after a relatively superficial injury, and can cause significant swelling (Figure 21.4). A careful assessment should be made before any treatment is undertaken. If they are left alone, and as long as the overlying skin remains intact, haematomas will eventually be reabsorbed, but this process may take several months. If the clinical assessment suggests that there is a significant chance of the skin breaking down or being damaged by the underlying swelling, drainage of the haematoma should be considered. If the patient presents acutely, it may be possible to drain the blood via a large-bore needle and large syringe before it clots, but more commonly the patient presents with the haematoma after it has begun to clot. In these circumstances, it is important to be sure that no further bleeding is taking place.

//–//// Incising and draining a haematoma

The skin should be cleaned and anaesthetised, with a large number of gauze swabs being made available. A small (about 1 cm) incision should be made where the overlying skin is at its thinnest, and pressure should be gradually applied from the edge toward the centre (Figure 21.5). The blood clot is then evacuated using firm pressure through the incision. This usually requires pressure being applied by two hands, one each side of the swelling, pushing down and toward the incision.

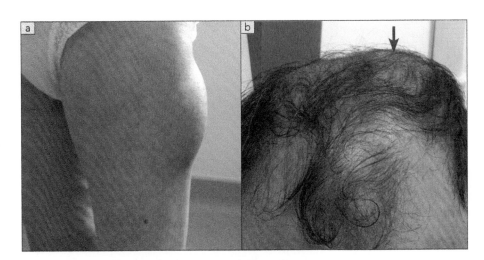

Figure 21.4 Large haematomas of (a) the thigh and (b) the scalp.

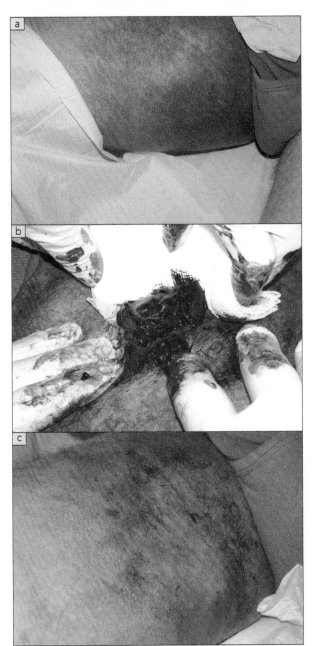

The surgeon should then cover the incision with gauze as the clot may be ejected with some velocity, along with bloody, serous fluid. The clot tends to come out as small bits of jelly-like material. The haematoma cavity should be systematically 'massaged' empty, taking care not to cause the patient undue pain through excess pressure. If possible, the whole haematoma should be completely evacuated. It is better to overestimate the number of absorbent gauze swabs required.

After the haematoma has been fully expressed, the incision should be covered with a sterile dressing and a pressure dressing applied. This will ensure that any residual haematoma can drain while minimising the risk of wound infection.

Complications

The two main complications of haematoma drainage are:

- *Postoperative infection*. This can be significant and deep and may require intravenous antibiotics.
- *Seroma*. This is a very difficult complication to resolve as it may cause a permanent fistula draining clear serous fluid; resolution may involve extensive surgery (Figure 21.6).

Figure 21.5 Large haematoma (a) with a high chance of breakdown being incised and drained (b); (c) post-drainage.

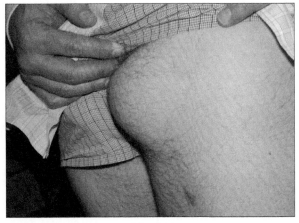

Figure 21.6 Large seroma of the thigh.

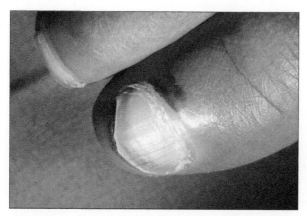

Figure 21.7 Subungual haematoma.

Subungual haematoma

A subungual haematoma (Figure 21.7) usually occurs as a result of direct injury to the affected digit (usually a finger) and can be extremely painful due the pressure caused by the haemorrhage under the nail. As with other haematomas, a decision should be taken on the possibility of draining the blood, but with a subungual haematoma this decision needs to be taken within hours of the injury as the pain tends to subside and the blood becomes organised and less amenable to evacuation.

A small hole is made in the nail over the haematoma; local anaesthetic is not usually required. There are two commonly used methods of evacuating the haematoma, trephining and cautery, described below.

Evacuating a subungual haematoma
Trephining

The simplest method involves using a large-bore (19 G or 21 G) hypodermic needle. When pressed gently against the nail and rotated back and forth, the bevelled end of the needle will gently cut a hole. Care should be taken to avoid pushing the needle through the hole as the underlying nail bed is exquisitely sensitive. The needle can be rotated around the hole to ensure that the hole formed is large enough to allow the clot to escape. A small bleb of blood will often escape as the nail is penetrated, giving the patient immediate relief.

Cautery

This simple 'first aid' technique involves an unbent paper clip and a flame source. The tip of one end of the paper clip is heated to a red-hot temperature and then quickly and gently applied to the nail. This is best done several times, each time using the minimum of pressure so that a very small hole is burnt with minimal heating of the nail and nail bed.

Within the clinical setting, an electrocautery unit allows a much more controlled method of burning a small hole (Figures 21.8). Again, this is best undertaken with very brief applications of a cautery tip to avoid undue painful heating of surrounding tissues.

Once a hole has been created by trephining or cautery, the pressure under the nail will cause evacuation of any blood or serous fluid. There should be no need to force the blood out. The small hole that remains can either be left or sealed with a drop or two of cyanoacrylic skin glue.

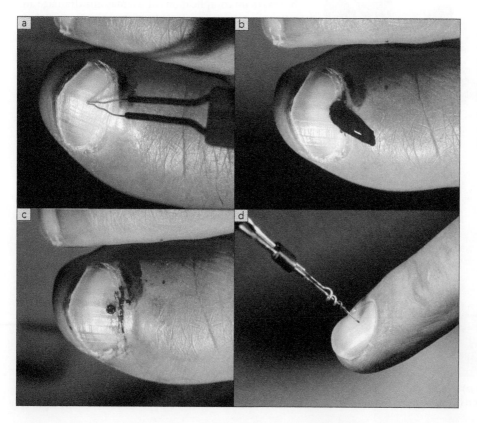

Figure 21.8 Electrocautery. (a) Fine wire electrocautery tip rested against the nail. (b) Blood released from the haematoma. (c) The residual hole is allowed to grow out. This can be sealed with nail varnish or tissue glue. (d) A cold-tip cautery point can also be used.

Perianal haematoma

Perianal haematomas have also been known as external thrombosed haemorrhoids. These are small haematomas close to the external anal margin (Figure 21.9). They are usually caused by the bursting of a blood vessel while straining at stool. They are only worth treating if the patient presents acutely (within a day or two) and is in pain. In appearance, the perianal haematoma is a purplish-grey, tender swelling close to the anus, which can make both sitting and evacuating the bowel painful. The pain from these lesions can be relieved by releasing the small blood clot.

Some haematomas form in pre-existing anal skin tags, in which case the treatment should consist of removing the skin tag with the blood clot within it.

❶–⓫ Draining a thrombosed external haemorrhoid or perianal haematoma

If a decision is made to incise the haematoma, assistance will be required to ensure that the buttocks are sufficiently parted to allow access. The area should be cleaned and routine anaesthesia injected gently around the haematoma.

Using a No. 11 or 15 scalpel blade, the haematoma can be incised, the incision following the skin creases radiating out from the anus (Figure 21.9c). The haematoma is often very simply evacuated through the incision as a small blood clot. Alternatively, the clot may exist in a number of thin-walled superficial dilated veins. These can usually be incised and drained or removed by gentle traction with a small pair of artery forceps.

Bleeding tends to be minimal and can if necessary be stopped with a few rapidly absorbable sutures (used to close the incision as well as to stop bleeding). Despite the number of bacteria found in this location, these wounds tend to heal rapidly and without infection. The patient should be advised to keep their bowel actions soft while the area heals and to use infant 'wet wipes' to clean the skin gently after bowel evacuation.

Haematoma within a skin tag

Where the haematoma is located within an existing skin tag, it will project out from the skin as a swollen, painful, dark-coloured tag as opposed to a bulge in the skin.

The base of the skin tag should be infiltrated with anaesthetic as described above. Once anaesthetised, the tag should be grabbed with a pair of mosquito forceps and pulled gently away from the anal margin. The scalpel should be used to cut the edge closest to the anus. Applying gentle traction with the forceps, the first suture can be inserted close to the initial incision. After this, the incision is continued a little further and another suture is placed, and so on until the haematoma within the skin tag has finally been cut free.

By using this 'cut a little, then suture' approach, closing of the wound is made simple. If the skin tag is cut off first, the cut base tends to retract back close to the anal margin, and suturing the defect can prove difficult.

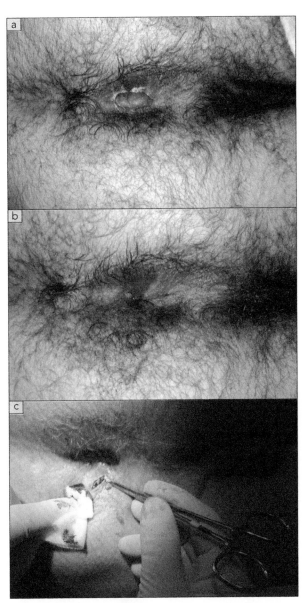

Figure 21.9 Perianal haematoma (a) before and (b) after incising. (c) The perianal haematoma has been incised and drained, and the redundant skin removed prior to suturing.

Haematomas

SPLIT EARLOBE

Two common traumatic complications can occur with pierced ears. In the first, an earring can be torn through the lobe, which, if left untreated, leads to an unsightly V-shaped defect in the earlobe because the edges of the V heal by secondary intention, causing a permanent defect. In the second, a partial tear, often occurring as a result of wearing heavy earrings, causes a enlarged, elongated piercing. Both conditions can be treated, but only by bringing together freshly cut surfaces.

/// Fully split earlobe

The anterior and posterior edges of the split should be marked with a fine skin marker. Local anaesthetic (lidocaine with adrenaline [epinephrine] can be used here) is infiltrated around both sides of the split. The resultant swelling of the tissues makes clear the need for careful skin marking.

A V-shaped of skin lining the split needs to be cleanly cut away (Figure 21.10). This should extend up to and include the original piercing. The raw edges of the lobe can then be sutured together as a line, from the anterior point of the original piercing, out along the anterior aspect of the ear to the tip of the lobe and then back around along the posterior aspect. A small-sized 6-0 monofilament non-absorbable suture will be suitable for closing the defect with a series of interrupted sutures. The sutures should remain in place for 5–7 days before removal. No attempt should be made to re-pierce the ear for some weeks after repair.

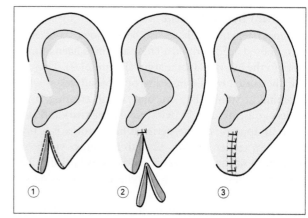

Figure 21.10 Repair of a split earlobe.

/// Enlarged ear piercing

Where the earlobe has not fully split, repair involves cutting out the skin lining the defect (Figure 21.11).

A skin marker is used to draw around both front and back edges edge of the hole. The size of the hole is then measured and a similar-sized biopsy punch prepared. Local anaesthetic is injected around the defect, and the volume of liquid infiltrated will usually close the hole. The punch biopsy is then used to cut out a small, central core including the enlarged hole. The edges should then be sutured together, first anteriorly and then posteriorly, using a fine monofilament suture, the sutures being left *in situ* for 5–7 days. Once again, any attempt at re-piercing should be delayed, and for both split lobes and enlarged piercings should be at a site just distant from the original defect, because the scar tissue will be weak.

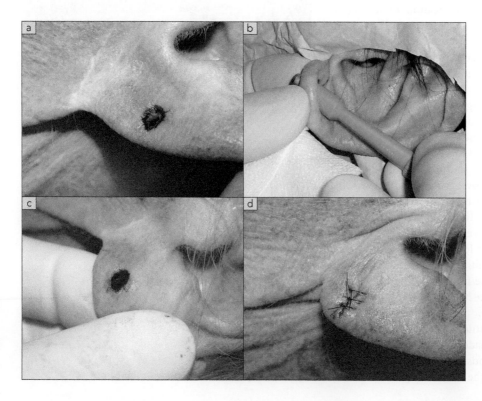

Figure 21.11 Repair of an enlarged ear piercing. (a) Hole anaesthetised and marked out. (b) Biopsy punch in use.(c) Defect punched out. (d) Anterior suturing.

REMOVING OBVIOUS FOREIGN BODIES

Unless a foreign body can be easily located, removal will prove to be difficult. The best form of locating is by direct vision, and the second best by palpation. Remember that after local anaesthetic has been injected (prior to surgical removal of the foreign body), the patient will no longer be able to indicate pain when the foreign body is identified, so careful skin marking prior to anaesthesia is essential.

∕–∕∕∕ Techniques to remove foreign bodies

Wood

Splinters of wood should be removed as soon as possible as delay will result in the wood slowly being broken down and eventually absorbed. Every attempt should be made to remove a splinter via its entry point and at the same angle as the entry.

A hypodermic needle can be used to both snag and then withdraw the splinter. Failing this, the needle tip may be used to gently enlarge the entry point (utilising the sharp bevelled point of the needle), allowing either another attempt with the needle or the use of very fine-tipped forceps to grasp the splinter. Pressure applied to the skin overlying the deep aspect of the splinter may also help push it to the surface, but care must be taken to avoid the splinter breaking.

If the splinter is located under a nail, it is usually possible to use a hypodermic needle to reach and tease out the splinter. Failing this, it may be necessary to cut a wedge from the overlying nail in order to facilitate grasping the splinter.

If the splinter has been in the skin for more than a few hours, it will tend to become surrounded by exudate or pus. In this scenario, exploration will result in pus-like fluid being released. Pressure around the opened entry site may result in the splinter being pushed up and out of the wound. If present for more than a week or two, it is likely to be reduced to a soft mass of partially lysed material.

Metal

Metal fragments, shards, and wire can all penetrate the skin through minor injury. If possible, these should be removed by teasing out with a small hypodermic needle through the original penetration site. Injecting local anaesthetic will not only swell and distort the skin, but also remove the sensation of pain, which tells the clinician he or she has reached the fragment.

Once a piece of metal has been present for some weeks, it will tend to become encapsulated by scar tissue, which will need to be surgically removed.

Glass

Glass fragments can be even more difficult to remove than metal ones as they can be very difficult to visualise and locate. Once again, exploration of the site can be awkward unless undertaken with a hypodermic needle and without the swelling that the injection of local anaesthesia causes. If the glass fragment is symptomless and difficult to locate, it should be left *in situ*.

Fish hooks

Most modern fish hooks have a sharp barb that stops the hook coming out once it has entered the skin. There are three main methods of extraction, all of which are facilitated by infiltrating the entry site with local anaesthesia.

Push-through method

Here the curvature of the hook is used to remove it (Figure 21.12). The hook is grasped firmly in an old pair of needle forceps. The tip of the hook is then rotated up and out through the skin. As soon as the barb has emerged, the tip of the hook, with the barb, can be cut off using a pair of wire cutters that have been cleaned with surgical spirit. The barbless hook remnant can now be rotated in reverse, out of the original entry point, with the needle forceps.

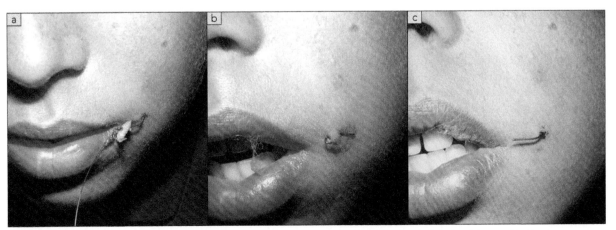

Figure 21.12 (a) Fish-hook—complete with maggot—embedded in the cheek. (b) One end of the hook is cut off with wire cutters. (c) The hook may now be pushed through and removed.

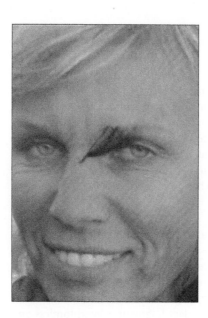

Figure 21.13
(a) Fish hook buried in the eyebrow, subsequently removed with the barb-cover method.

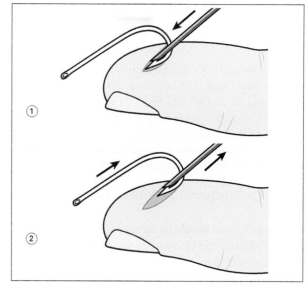

Figure 21.14 The barb-cover method.

Barb-cover method

In this method, a large-bore hypodermic needle (19 G or 21 G) is passed down the entry point of the hook along the concave surface until the bevelled tip reaches and covers the barb (the barb tip effectively sitting inside the hypodermic needle; Figures 21.13 and 21.14). The hook can then be rotated back out through the entry point with the hypodermic needle covering the barb. This has the benefit of leaving only one point of skin penetration, and the hook also remains undamaged!

String-yank technique

This technique is often performed in the field and is believed to be the least traumatic because it creates no new wounds and rarely requires anaesthesia. It may be used to remove any size of fish hook, but especially small and medium-sized ones. It works well for deeply embedded fish hooks but cannot be used on certain appendages of the body (e.g., the earlobe).

A string such as fishing line or strong silk suture is wrapped around the midpoint of the bend in the fish hook (Figure 21.15). The free end of the string is held tightly; a strong grip on the string can be achieved by wrapping the ends around a tongue depressor. The area of skin should be well stabilised, and the shank of the fish hook should be depressed against the skin. Continue to depress the eye and/or distal portion of the shank of the hook, taking care to keep the shank parallel to the underlying skin. A firm, quick jerk is then applied in line with the shank while continuing to exert pressure on the eye of the fish hook.

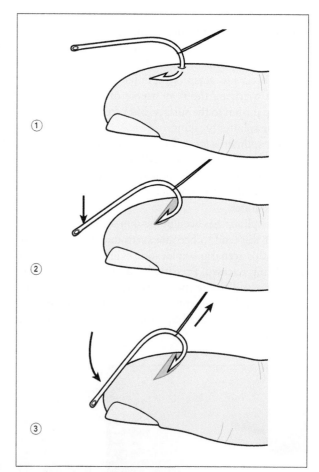

Figure 21.15 The string-yank method.

TETANUS AND ANTIBIOTICS

Wounds contaminated with soil or manure are at particular risk of containing *Clostridium tetani*, which can cause tetanus infection. Prevention of tetanus requires a full course of immunisation, which consists of a total of five doses of vaccine given at the appropriate intervals. This is considered to provide lifelong immunity. Tetanus immunisation programmes are well established around the world, and there may be variation in the immunisation schedule from country to country.

Tetanus vaccine is widely offered at the time of injury if there is risk of tetanus infection. However, it is unlikely that immunisation at the time of the injury will boost immunity rapidly enough to give additional protection within the incubation period of tetanus. In practice this means the following:

- If an individual has received a full five-dose course of tetanus vaccine and suffers a tetanus-prone wound, no further doses of vaccine are recommended.
- If the risk of tetanus is especially high, for example the wound is contaminated with manure, human tetanus immunoglobulin should be given to provide immediate additional protection.

The risk of tetanus is deemed higher in the following situations:

- Where there has been contact with soil or manure likely to harbour tetanus organisms, particularly if the wound was sustained more than 6 hours prior to surgical treatment.
- Any wound at any interval after injury showing one or more of the following characteristics:
  - A significant degree of devitalised tissue.
  - A puncture-type wound.
  - Clinical evidence of sepsis.

Prophylactic antibiotics

Unnecessary use of prophylactic antibiotics should be avoided. Wounds at particular risk are those whose primary closure has been delayed (beyond 3–6 hours).

If an antibiotic is used it should be chosen on the basis of likely pathogens, in particular staphylococci. For this reason, the use of ampicillin, flucloxacillin, or amoxicillin with clavulanic acid should be considered in penicillin-tolerant patients. In those who are penicillin-allergic, a cephalosporin or macrolide should be considered, bearing in mind that a small percentage of such patients may be allergic to a first- or second-generation cephalosporin. Within emergency rooms, this is often administered as a single parenteral injection followed by a short course of oral treatment.

REFERENCES

Bascom JU (1983) Pilonidal disease: Long term results from follicle removal. *Diseases of the Colon and Rectum* 26: 800–7.

Karydakis GE (1973) New approach to the problem of pilonidal sinus. *Lancet* ii: 1414–15.

Karydakis GE (1992) Easy and successful treatment of pilonidal sinus after explanation of its causative processes. *Australian and New Zealand Journal of Surgery* 62: 385–9.

Kitchen PRB (1996) Pilonidal sinus – Experience with the Karydakis flap. *British Journal of Surgery* 83: 1452–55.

Chapter 22

Carpal tunnel syndrome, Dupuytren's contracture, trigger finger, and ganglia: skills

Tim T. Wang and Simon Eccles

INTRODUCTION

In this chapter, we look at treatments for these common conditions. Each section is proceeded by instructions for non-surgical treatments (where these exist). The surgical procedures need to be learned with a mentor over many operating sessions. The trainee surgeon should keep a logbook of procedures observed and undertaken.

CARPAL TUNNEL TREATMENT

With all but the most severe cases of carpal tunnel syndrome (CTS), injection should be considered before surgery. Severity includes muscle wasting and permanent numbness in the median nerve distribution. Wasting of the thenar muscles tends to be permanent, even after decompression (Figure 22.1). In cases such as these, the priority is urgent referral for surgical carpal tunnel decompression (CTD).

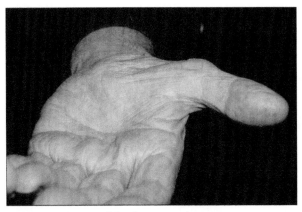

Figure 22.1 Wasting of the thenar muscles.

If injection has been tried, and has failed or is successful but the symptoms keep recurring after injection, surgical decompression should be recommended to avoid the possibility of permanent nerve damage.

The technique for injection is simple, but remember that steroid injection is less likely to be effective in those with severe symptoms, elderly patients, diabetic patients, and those whose symptoms have lasted for over 1 year.

Corticosteroid injection

A small volume of potent steroid (e.g., 20 mg triamcinolone 40 mg/ml) is drawn up into a 1 ml syringe. To this is attached a narrow-bore hypodermic needle (23–27 G) 30 mm in length.

The patient places their hand palm up and in slight extension. First the palmaris longus tendon should be identified (but note that some individuals do not possess this tendon, or only possess it unilaterally). It can be identified by opposing the thumb and little finger, and then flexing the wrist.

The needle should be inserted just to the radial side of the tendon, at the distal wrist crease. If inserted at 45° toward the metacarpophalangeal joint of the middle finger, there should be no resistance and no sharp median nerve pain. If there is sharp pain, gently withdraw the needle a bit. The steroid is injected as a bolus. If no palmaris longus is present, the mid position of the wrist should be estimated (it is reliably located by the main skin crease created by bringing the tips of the thumb and little finger together).

After injection, the wrist and hand should be rested. Two weeks should be allowed for the steroid to act before re-examining the patient. If the treatment is successful, the injection can be repeated as required.

Direct injection into the median nerve itself is a risk but is minimised by observing the advice above. The patient should be fully informed of the risk, and consent obtained.

Symptoms will recur in about half of all cases, but this treatment can be useful for delaying surgery and is also useful diagnostically in difficult cases. Prognostically, those who respond well to injection but progress to surgery tend to have a more successful outcome.

Surgical decompression

There are both open (traditional) and closed (endoscopic) methods for dividing the carpal ligament (also known as the flexor retinaculum). The open procedure is less likely to cause inadvertent nerve damage; it requires less specialised surgical equipment and is described below.

Some patients following a hospital pathway of care will have had formal nerve conduction studies (electromyography) performed in the neurophysiology department. There is controversy over the value of such studies in those with a straightforward history and findings but, as stated in Chapter 11, such studies are of help where there is diagnostic uncertainty. This includes those with diabetes who have possible diabetic neuropathy, younger patients, and situations where the clinician fears there may be a heightened medicolegal risk.

Basic requirements

Staffing requirements

It is recommended that a nurse assist at operations; they may also be trained to perform nerve conduction studies (see below) if these are required.

Operating facilities

It is not a prerequisite for existing facilities to have dedicated ventilation systems (as long as a suitable risk assessment has been carried out) as CTD is usually classified as minor surgery rather than a day-case procedure. However, when designing new facilities, it may be prudent to incorporate ventilation systems providing a minimum of 10 air changes per hour.

Prepacked CTD kits with single-use instruments are readily available. Alternatively, reusable instruments will need cleaning and sterilisation, usually via a local Central Sterilisation Service Department (CSSD).

Carpal tunnel patient pathway

Initial assessment

A waiting time to first appointment of less than 4 weeks should be deliverable. At the first appointment, the history should include:

- The patient's handedness.
- Occupation.
- Duration of symptoms.
- Distribution of tingling.
- Numbness, pain, and weakness (ideally there will be ulnar sparing).
- Timing of symptoms—disturbance of sleep being typical—and any provoking and relieving factors.
- In addition, it should be noted where there is any co-pathology that might complicate management, for example osteoarthritis, old fracture, diabetes, other neuropathy, neck/elbow problem, hypothyroidism, or Raynaud's syndrome.

Examination looks for deformity, muscle wasting (particularly of the thenar eminence), weakness of thumb and finger abduction, and weakness of grip. Sensation to light touch is compared between parts of the hand innervated by the median and ulnar nerves: in moderate to severe carpal tunnel, it is frequently diminished in the median territory. Tinel's and Phalen's tests should also be performed (see Chapter 11).

Carpal tunnel operative management

Several points should be noted here:

- Explain to the patient what will happen and gain their informed consent. Make sure you are operating on the correct side.
- Remove any jewellery from that hand.
- Consider asking the patient to clean their hand and wrist with alcohol rub.
- Arrange the patient on the couch with their arm resting on the operating trolley or an attachable arm support.
- Some surgeons use a tourniquet, but this is a personal choice.

Instruments

- No. 15 blade.
- Size 3 blade handle.
- Derf needle holder 12.5 cm.
- McDonald dissector 19 cm.
- Adson dissecting forceps 12 cm.
- Wullstein retractor, blunt.
- Monofilament 3-0 nylon suture (blue) with 19 mm three-eighths circle cutting needle (and/or alternative non-absorbable suture).
- Plus drapes, towel clips, gauze, gallipots, and sponge sticks.

Anaesthesia

A volume of 10 ml 1% lidocaine with adrenaline (epinephrine) is injected by the surgeon using a 29 G needle, inserting 8 ml in the midline of the wrist, distally to the distal palmar crease and perfusing the tissues into the palm (Figure 22.2), and a further 2 ml proximally from the same point to anaesthetise the upper end of the carpal tunnel. This is often the tightest and most sensitive point for the patient later on during the decompression procedure.

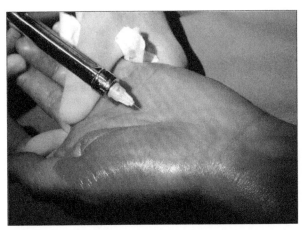

Figure 22.2 Infiltrating the line of the incision with local anaesthesia.

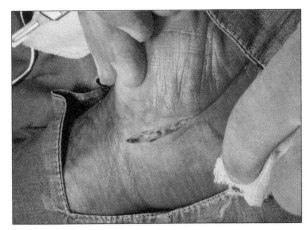

Figure 22.3 The incision is made in the proximal palmar crease as shown.

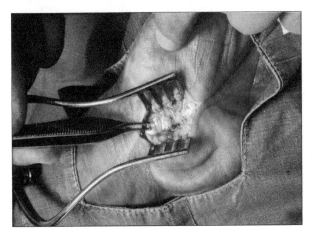

Figure 22.4 A self-retaining retractor allows visualisation.

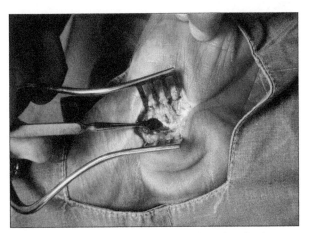

Figure 22.5 The McDonald's dissector is slipped under the ligament and above the nerve.

Procedure

First, the surgeon gowns up and prepares the instrument trolley. The patient's entire hand is then cleaned with chlorhexidine or Betadine and draped.

Using a marking pen, the distal wrist crease and Kaplan's cardinal line (KCL) are marked out. Kaplan's cardinal line is an extension of the ulnar border with the thumb in full extension. The superficial palmar arch is marked by the junction of the KCL and the radial border of the ring finger. The intersection of the KCL with the radial border of the middle finger is the landmark for the recurrent branch of the median nerve. The skin incision is marked 2–5 mm ulnar to the thenar flexor crease extending from the distal wrist crease to the KCL.

An incision is made from the distal wrist crease, in the midline of the wrist, in line with third and fourth interdigital clefts, for not more than 3 cm distally into the palm (Figure 22.3). The incision is deepened in the vertical plane, staying *perpendicular* to the plane of the hand. *Beware the hand's tendency to pronate,* which causes the scalpel to drift out of the perpendicular and cut towards the ulnar border of the hand instead.

Bleeding must be controlled by siting and resiting the retractor as needed. (Bipolar diathermy must be on stand-by; do not use unipolar diathermy close to the nerve.)

GOLDEN RULE ✳

Watch out for the occasional aberrant thenar branch of the median nerve at the proximal end of the incision. It must not be divided, as thenar muscle atrophy and weakness of the thumb will result.

The incision will expose the carpal ligament, the palmaris longus tendon (if present), and the underlying deep fascia. Self-retaining or individual hand-held retractors are placed in the wound and opened to expose the underlying fatty tissues and dense fibrous transverse fascia (Figure 22.4).

Carpal tunnel treatment

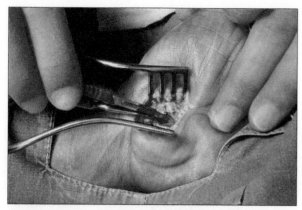

Figure 22.6 With the McDonald's dissector protecting the nerve, the ligament is divided with a small scalpel blade.

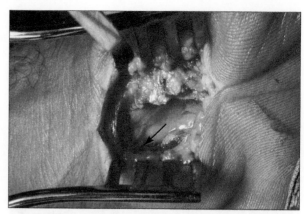

Figure 22.7 The size of the nerve can be appreciated after division.

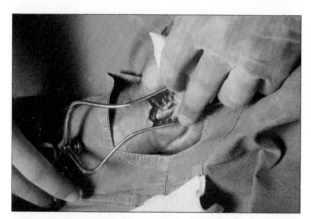

Figure 22.8 The retractor is now removed.

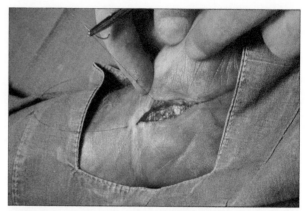

Figure 22.9 Skin closure with a single layer monofilament suture, here subcuticular.

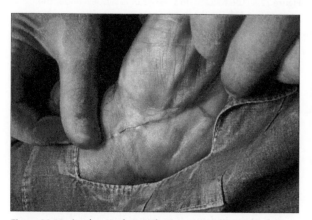

Figure 22.10 A subcuticular stitch gives a neat scar.

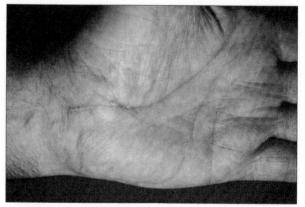

Figure 22.11 Appearance of the scar at 6 weeks.

This fascia is opened just proximal to its junction with the carpal ligament by carefully nicking it with the scalpel to create an opening through which the flat McDonald dissector can be slid (Figure 22.5) so that it lies beneath the ligament and above the median nerve, thereby giving it complete protection. This occasionally hurts and extra local anaesthetic should be administered. The carpal ligament is then divided (Figure 22.6). The nerve will be seen lying embedded in connective tissue, which need not be disturbed (Figure 22.7).

The wound is closed with a single layer of mono-filament 3-0 or alternative non-absorbable sutures as mattress sutures or subcuticular sutures (Figure 22.8 to Figure 22.10). A light dressing is then applied.

Full aftercare instructions and exercises should be given verbally and in writing, with spare dressings, a contact number, and an appointment for the removal of stitches on day 8. Be prepared to provide an off-work certificate if needed. Initial elevation can help to reduce pain and swelling, so consider the use of a high-arm sling support.

Aftercare

Non-absorbable sutures should be removed at 8 days and the wound only covered again if there is a clinical need to do so. The patient's progress since the operation should be assessed and any complications dealt with. Encourage an early mobilisation and return to work.

Patient should be given a postoperative questionnaire (as all CTS surgery should be followed by an outcome analysis). Figure 22.11 shows the appearance of the scar at 6 weeks.

Early complications

- *Postoperative bleeding.* A slight ooze is common, but heavy bleeding requiring re-exploration and bipolar diathermy is very rare. Pressure and re-dressing should suffice.
- *Wound infection.* Superficial infection may occur in around 5% of patients and should be swabbed and treated with oral antibiotics. Deep infection and abscess formation are very rare and need hospital admission for intravenous antibiotics.
- *Pain from the wound or the decompressed nerve.* This should be treated with analgesics and reassurance after reviewing and ruling out infection.
- *Numbness or shock-like pains.* These are not uncommon early on and should resolve. The patient should be reassured.
- Rarely, *motor branches of the median nerve* may sustain damage during surgery.

Late complications

- Scar tenderness and 'pillar pain' (tenderness and pain adjacent to the actual ligament release site) are quite common and are best treated by desensitising the scar, for example by rubbing it with a toothbrush.
- Residual patches of numbness should eventually resolve.
- Weakening of the grip and general stiffness of the hand should gradually recover, although in some patients this may persist.
- Autonomic neuropathy, now known as complex regional pain syndrome, is a rare problem in which the whole or part of the hand feels a neuropathic type of pain with disturbance of temperature and sweating control. It is difficult to treat. The patient should be referred to a hand therapist and should be started on gabapentin, pregabalin, or a similar drug. The surgeon should try to follow up the patient until the symptoms have resolved.
- The original symptoms may fail to improve or show only partial relief. This may be due to the diagnosis being wrong or the carpal ligament not being fully divided at operation. Such cases should be reviewed with the mentor.
- Patients report partial relief in approximately 30% of cases, and recurrence of CTS occurs in approximately 1 in 250 cases.

DUPUYTREN'S CONTRACTURE SURGERY

Although scalpel-free treatments are available (needle fasciotomy and collagenase therapy) (see Chapter 11 for more information), their long-term place in treatment is still uncertain, so we shall deal with surgical treatment in this section.

Operative management

Surgery for Dupuytren's contracture (Figure 22.12) is complex, and various techniques have been described. Prior to the procedure, the surgeon must formulate a clear surgical plan detailing the management of the skin, management of the fascia, and finally management of the affected joints. For this reason, the majority of procedures for Dupuytren's disease are performed in a specialist hand unit with an allied hand therapy unit in order to obtain the best postoperative results.

There is no single perfect approach for Dupuytren's contracture, and given long enough follow-up all cases will eventually recur. Achieving total clearance of diseased tissue is not possible. Therefore, the aim of surgery is primarily to release joint contractures, improve hand function, and significantly delay recurrence of the disease.

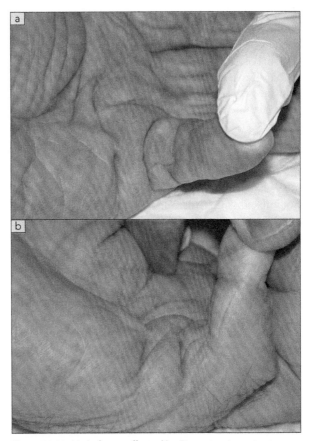

Figure 22.12 Little finger affected by Dupuytren's contracture, viewed (a) anteriorly and (b) laterally.

Of the various procedures, a regional fasciectomy is the most commonly performed. Severe and recurrent disease may require dermofasciectomy with full-thickness skin grafting. For the purposes of this chapter, we will describe a standard procedure of a regional fasciectomy affecting the palmar fascia of a single digital ray.

Instruments

- Aqueous chlorhexidine or Betadine solution.
- Local anaesthetic (50:50 of 1% lidocaine and 0.25% bupivacaine without adrenaline).
- Pneumatic tourniquet.
- Esmarch® bandage.
- Scalpel blade No. 15 and scalpel handle.
- One pair of tenotomy scissors.
- One pair of curved artery forceps.
- Two skin hooks.
- Two Kilner double-ended retractors (cat's paw retractors).
- Bipolar diathermy.
- One pair of needle holders.
- One pair of suture scissors.
- One pair of Adson forceps.
- Surgical suture: 4-0 non-absorbable monofilament suture.
- Saline, gauze, Velband® dressing, and crêpe bandages.

Anaesthesia

A patient will only tolerate the tourniquet for 20 minutes if he or she is not anaesthetised. Therefore, extended Dupuytren's excisions and surgery for recurrent disease should be performed under general anaesthesia or regional blocks.

The procedure is explained to the patient, and informed consent is obtained. The surgical site and incisions are then marked. Designing an incision is very complex and varies with each case. Common incision patterns include a zig-zag incision or a longitudinal incision broken up by 'Z'-plasties to reduce postoperative linear wound contractures.

Next, a padded tourniquet is applied to the arm but not inflated. The sterile field is prepared, and the affected hand is painted with aqueous chlorhexidine solution. Local anaesthetic is injected on both sides and along the entire incision. The limb is elevated and exsanguinated through tight and overlapping application of the Esmarch® bandage from distal to proximal. The tourniquet is inflated to 250 mmHg and the Esmarch® bandage removed.

If the doctor requires a bloodless field and anaesthesia in a limb, the area should be infiltrated with local anaesthesia, and then an orthopaedic tourniquet and Esmarch® bandage applied. This is particularly effective for decompression of the carpal tunnel, release of trigger finger, and exploration for foreign bodies.

Procedure

Anaesthesia is confirmed with the tip of the scalpel. A zig-zag incision is made in the palm and along the finger (Figure 22.13 and 22.18). Skin flaps are dissected in the plane between the fat and the fascia to preserve vascularity, and are subsequently reflected sideways.

The longitudinal pretendinous cord is dissected out using both sharp and blunt dissection from proximal to distal. The affected cord is subsequently elevated (Figure 22.14). The transverse fibres of the palmar aponeurosis are left intact as they are rarely contracted. Neurovascular bundles lie just deep to these transverse fibres, and the authors prefer to identify and expose the bundles at intervals in order to protect them. The extent of dissection along the longitudinal palmar cord varies greatly.

A pair of curved arterial forceps is placed underneath the longitudinal cord and spread maximally. Using the tip of the scalpel, the cord is divided under tension at its superior and inferior ends over the teeth of the forceps (to protect the underlying structures).

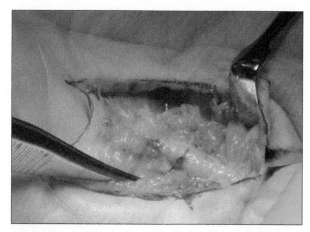

Figure 22.13 Dupuytren's contracture: a zig-zag incision is made in the palm.

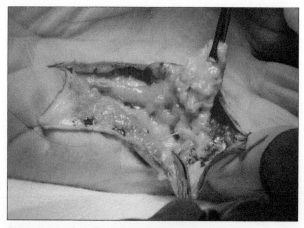

Figure 22.14 The affected cord is seen being elevated.

Dissection continues distally to the proximal phalanx (Figures 22.15 and 22.16). Great care must be taken during this level of dissection to carefully follow the neurovascular bundles through affected tissue as they are often displaced medially by a second lateral or spiral cord. The authors advocate the extent of dissection as the point at which the joint contracture is satisfactorily released.

The affected finger will never be completely straight (Figure 22.17 shows the finger now fully extended, prior to wound closure). If the release of the joint contracture is unsatisfactory, look for additional cords in the area.

Once excision has been completed, the tourniquet is deflated. Careful haemostasis is then achieved using the bipolar diathermy, and the wound is washed out with saline.

Skin closure is achieved with intermittent non-absorbable monofilament sutures (Figure 22.18). Many surgeons will leave the transverse palmar part of the wound open (the 'open-palm' or McCash technique) to assist postoperative mobilisation and allow any haematoma to drain. A wound dressing is applied with a non-adherent material, for example Jelonet®, gauze, Velband, or crêpe bandage.

The patient is sent home with a high-arm sling for elevation and simple analgesics. The sutures are removed in 10 days, after which the patient is encouraged to use the hand normally. Hand therapists play a crucial role in the rehabilitation of these patients.

Specific complications

- The recurrence rate is possibly 100%. Given long enough, it is possible (but not proven) all cases of Dupuytren's contracture will recur.
- Neurovascular injury.
- Haematoma formation.
- Stiffness.
- Complex regional pain syndrome, especially for open-palm fasciectomy.

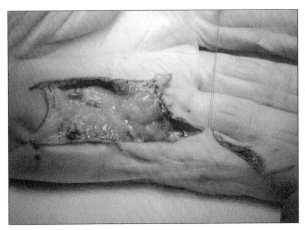

Figure 22.15 Incision extended along the proximal phalanx; suture used to expose tendon.

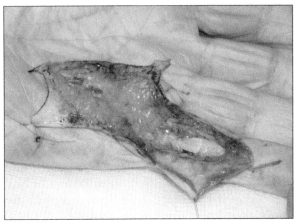

Figure 22.16 The tendon sheath with exposed tendon can be seen over the proximal phalanx, cleared of affected Dupuytren's tissue.

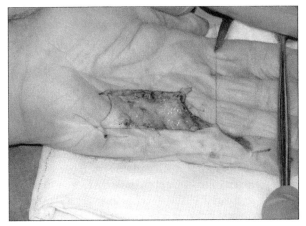

Figure 22.17 Wound, prior to closure, showing finger fully extended.

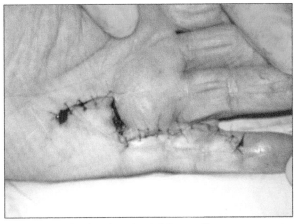

Figure 22.18 The skin closed with 5-0 monofilament sutures, the zig-zag approach limiting scar contracture.

TREATMENT OF TRIGGER FINGER

With early triggering of a finger or thumb, non-surgical therapy in the form of corticosteroid injections should always be given an opportunity to work. When this approach fails, surgery should be considered.

Corticosteroid injection

The patient rests the hand palm up. The clinician identifies the location of the triggering tendon—a small nodule will often be palpable as it passes through the pulley, over the metacarpal head.

A narrow-bore needle and syringe is used to draw up steroid (10 mg triamcinolone) and up to 1 ml of 2% lidocaine. The combined 1 ml, 29 G diabetic needle and syringe are ideal for this. The needle is inserted through the A1 pulley. It can be inserted and directed either distally or proximally.

Once the clinician is confident that the needle is within the pulley, the patient can be asked to gently extend and flex the digit. If the needle is in the correct plane, the tendon will pass easily in the direction of the needle (the clinician can feel the tendon scraping along the tip of the needle), but catch the tip of the needle in the opposite direction (take care as this can be painful for the patient). This simple manoeuvre ensures that the steroid is not injected into the body of the tendon. The syringe content is injected as a bolus; excess pressure required for the injection suggests the needle is incorrectly placed.

Immediately afterwards, the patient may report an improvement in the pain and movement thanks to the expanding effect of the volume of fluid injected and the anaesthetic. The effect of the steroid may take several weeks to be fully realised. Failure to improve or very short-term improvements are indications to refer for formal surgical treatment.

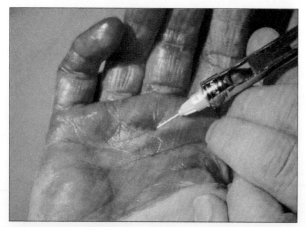

Figure 22.19 The line of the distal palmar crease is infiltrated with local anaesthetic (without adrenaline) using a dental syringe and 30 G needle.

Surgical release

Some clinicians advocate using a needle bevel under local anaesthetic to try to release the proximal edge of the A1 pulley (percutaneous release). There is, however, a potential risk of damage to the neurovascular bundle, so the majority of surgeons prefer to rely upon an open procedure to open up the pulley, as described below.

Instruments

- Aqueous chlorhexidine or Betadine solution.
- Local anaesthetic (50:50 of 1% lidocaine and 0.25% bupivacaine without adrenaline).
- Pneumatic tourniquet.
- Esmarch® bandage.
- Scalpel blade No. 15 and scalpel handle.
- One pair of tenotomy scissors.
- West or Weitlaner self-retaining retractor.
- Two Kilner double-ended retractors (cat's paw retractors).
- Bipolar diathermy.
- One pair of needle holders.
- One pair of suture scissors.
- One pair of Adson forceps.
- Surgical suture: 4-0 nylon or Prolene™.
- Saline, gauze, Velband dressing, and crêpe bandages.

Anaesthesia

The procedure, including the risk of recurrence, is explained to the patient. Informed consent is obtained, the surgical site is marked, and a short transverse 10–15 mm incision is drawn. Trigger finger release may be performed under either a wrist block or local infiltration of anaesthetic—the authors prefer the latter technique. The exact technique of performing a wrist block is outside the remit of this chapter.

A padded tourniquet is then applied to the arm but not inflated. A sterile field is prepared, and the affected hand is painted with aqueous Betadine solution. Local anaesthetic is injected in the line of the distal palmar crease (Figure 22.19). The limb is elevated and exsanguinated through a tight and overlapping application of the Esmarch® bandage from distal to proximal. The tourniquet is inflated to 250 mmHg, the Esmarch® bandage is removed, and the clock time is noted.

Procedure

The proximal edge of the A1 pulley for the ring and little fingers lies at the distal palmar crease; for the index finger, it lies at the proximal palmar crease; and in the middle finger, it lies between the two creases.

Anaesthesia is confirmed with the tip of the scalpel. A small transverse incision approximately 15 mm in length is made just distal to the distal palmar crease, or along the palmar crease (to produce the most cosmetic scar; Figure 22.20). Note that a longitudinal incision may be used instead.

Using the tenotomy scissors, the entire length of the incision is bluntly dissected through the subcutaneous tissues and palmar fascia to reveal the flexor sheath (Figure 22.21). Care is taken to avoid and protect the neurovascular bundles running parallel to the flexor sheath on either side. Using retractors to hold the tissues and neurovascular bundles to the sides, the A1 pulley is revealed—use a self-retaining West retractor if you are operating alone or the blunt end of cat's paw retractors if you have an assistant.

The entire length of the A1 pulley overlying the flexor tendon is released using either the tip of the scalpel, or scissors, under direct vision. The pulley is approximately 10 mm in length, and the surgeon will know the entire pulley has been released when the tissues become noticeably thinner and the border of the oblique cruciate pulley, marking the start of the A2 pulley, can be identified. Note that the A1 and A2 pulleys are continuous in approximately 50% of individuals. Avoid dividing the A2 pulley as this will lead to bowstringing of the digit.

Under direct vision, ask the patient to actively flex and extend the digit through its entire range of motion. The flexor tendons should now glide smoothly with no visible nodules or areas of thickening seen on them. There are usually two flexor tendons to each digit: flexor digitorum superficialis which flexes the proximal interphalangeal joint, and flexor digitorum profundus which flexes the whole digit.

After confirming free movement of the digit, the tourniquet is deflated. Careful haemostasis is achieved using bipolar diathermy if necessary, and the wound is washed out with saline. Skin closure is achieved with intermittent 4-0 non-absorbable monofilament sutures, as either individual sutures or horizontal mattress sutures (Figure 22.22).

A wound dressing is applied with a non-adherent material, for example Jelonet®, gauze, Velband, and crêpe bandage. Make sure the dressing leaves the digits free to move. Immediate hand motion is advised.

The patient is sent home with a high-arm sling for elevation and simple analgesics. The sutures are removed in 10 days, after which the patient is encouraged to use the hand normally.

Specific complications

- Bowstringing of the affected digit (more likely if the A2 pulley has been divided during surgery).
- Loss of sensation/digital nerve injury (recovery of sensation may be slow); radial digital nerve injury in the thumb.
- Recurrence.
- Scar tenderness and erythema.
- Although major complications are rare, minor complications including pain and loss of movement are not uncommon.

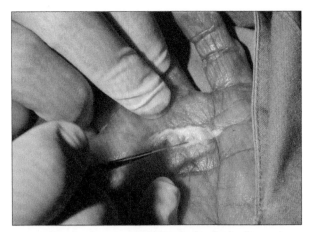

Figure 22.20 Small transverse incision in the distal palmar crease.

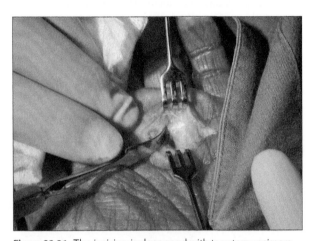

Figure 22.21 The incision is deepened with tenotomy scissors.

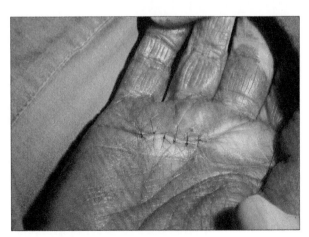

Figure 22.22 Wound closed with interrupted sutures.

TREATMENT OF GANGLIA

Untreated, many ganglia disappear spontaneously; many others appear not to trouble the patient and may be left alone. Treatment is indicated if the patient is complaining of unacceptable symptoms, usually pain or limitation of function.

Non-surgical treatments

Rupture

Rupture of a ganglion by striking it with the holy Bible is no longer recommended! If located over the dorsal aspect of the wrist, rupture of the ganglion may be possible by holding the wrist in flexion, thereby tensing the skin over the ganglion. The doctor then places both hands around the wrist with the thumbs placed one on top of the other and on the distal side of the ganglion. The doctor then pushes down and away with their thumbs, thereby rapidly compressing and hopefully rupturing the ganglion. Failure to succeed the first time will usually necessitate abandoning this approach—it is painful for the patient and he or she is unlikely to welcome a second attempt.

Aspiration

The edge of the ganglion is cleaned with a surgical wipe, and a small volume of lidocaine is injected by a diabetic needle and syringe to raise a bleb (Figure 22.23). A white (19 G) hypodermic needle (attached to a 5 ml or 10 ml syringe) is inserted through the bleb and into the middle of the ganglion. With a reasonable aspiration vacuum, clear gel-like material can be aspirated. After the ganglion has collapsed and the needle has been withdrawn, the area should be covered with a small dressing and pressure bandage for a day or two. It is likely that the risk of recurrence decreases with each subsequent aspiration (if required).

If sclerosant (sodium tetradecyl sulphate) is to be injected, a syringe with a small quantity should be attached to the white needle before it is withdrawn. The sclerosant is injected and then the needle withdrawn and a pressure dressing attached.

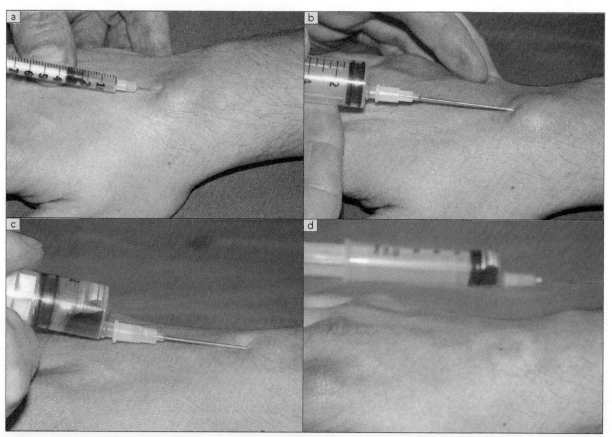

Figure 22.23 A recurrent ganglion being aspirated. (a) The bleb of anaesthetic. This is the same ganglion as seen in Figure 11.14, but many months after the first aspiration (it is smaller and the clear gel contents are now minimally bloodstained compared with the first aspiration). (b) The 19 G needle about to penetrate the ganglion via the anaesthetised bleb. (c) The lightly bloodstained gel-like contents. (d) The post-aspiration appearance.

Surgical treatment

Many treatments have been advocated, but all carry a risk of recurrence, so many surgeons recommend excision as offering the best chance of cure.

It is essential to have a bloodless operating field, secured by a pneumatic tourniquet, as the dissection can be quite difficult and the ganglion may extend more deeply than anticipated. Thus, a general anaesthetic or tourniquet and local infiltration are required, the latter being the method chosen by the average GP.

Many patients will assume that excision of a ganglion will be no different from that of a small sebaceous cyst. It is therefore important to let them know that it is quite a complicated procedure, that they should not drive a car immediately following the operation and that, despite a meticulous dissection, recurrence is still possible.

Instruments

- Aqueous chlorhexidine or Betadine.
- Dental syringe and 30 G needle.
- Cartridge of local anaesthetic (without added adrenaline).
- Orthopaedic tourniquet.
- Esmarch® bandage.
- Sterile pads, bandages, and gauze.
- Scalpel handle size 3.
- Scalpel blade No. 15.
- Self-retaining retractor (West, Weitlaner, or similar).
- *Or* two Kilner double-ended retractors (cat's paw retractors).
- Two pairs of Halstead mosquito artery forceps, curved, 5 inch (12.7 cm).
- One pair of stitch scissors.
- One Kilner needle holder, 5¼ inch (13.3 cm).
- One pair of fine-toothed Adson dissecting forceps, 4¾ inch (12 cm).
- One surgical suture 4-0 monofilament nylon or Prolene™ on a curved cutting needle.

Technique for producing a bloodless anaesthetic field

Any rings are removed from the fingers of the patient's affected hand, and the procedure is explained in detail to the patient.

An intravenous premedication injection of fentanyl 100 μg and midazolam 2–4 mg is given slowly over 1–2 minutes into a vein in the opposite arm. If an intravenous cannula is inserted at this stage and taped in position, the doctor then has access to the circulation for the remainder of the operation. This is valuable should the action of the midazolam need to be reversed.

The skin overlying the ganglion is painted with chlorhexidine or Betadine and infiltrated with local anaesthetic (without added adrenaline) using a dental syringe and 30 G needle. The skin is painted a second time with povidone-iodine in spirit and covered with a sterile pad.

The orthopaedic tourniquet is applied over a layer of cotton wool over the upper arm and bandaged in position. The arm is raised, keeping the sterile pad in position, and the Esmarch® bandage is applied tightly from the fingertips to the lower edge of the orthopaedic tourniquet. The tourniquet is then pumped up to above arterial pressure (approximately 300 mmHg). The Esmarch® bandage is unwound, the sterile pad removed, and the clock time noted.

Procedure

The overlying skin is liberally painted with chlorhexidine or Betadine, a sterile drape is applied over the area, and full aseptic precautions are observed. A surgical gown, mask, and gloves should be worn by the surgeon.

The incision should follow a skin crease, normally transverse (Figure 22.24), about 4 cm long, and any underlying nerves are dissected free. The extensor retinaculum overlying the ganglion is incised and a self-retaining retractor inserted (Figure 22.25, next page). The bulk of the ganglion is seen superficial to the tendons, but when these are retracted, the deeper part of the ganglion may be seen extending to the wrist joint or intercarpal joint. Gradually, the main part of the ganglion is dissected free using a scalpel, applying traction with toothed dissecting forceps.

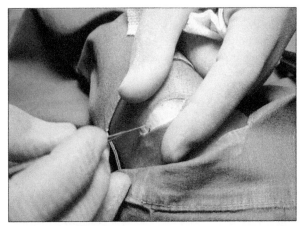

Figure 22.24 A transverse incision is made over the ganglion in the line of a skin crease.

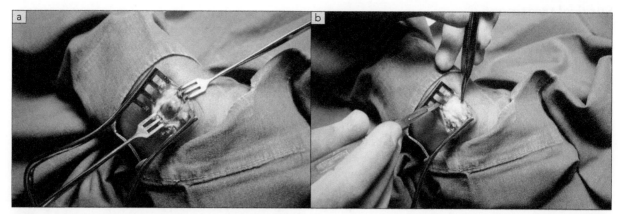

Figure 22.25 (a) A self-retaining retractor is inserted. (b) If necessary, two 'cat's paw' retractors may be used as well to aid access.

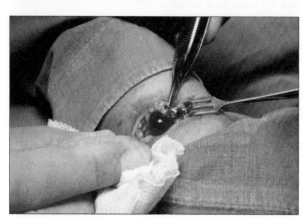

Figure 22.26 The ganglion has been opened and bloodstained jelly is seen, indicating previous trauma.

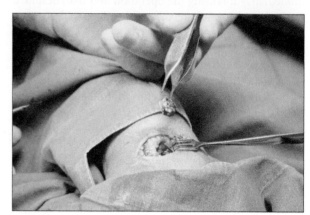

Figure 22.27 The ganglion detached.

At this stage, the capsule is usually incised, liberating the typical clear jelly (Figure 22.26). This is often an advantage and makes the remaining dissection easier. The ganglion is now detached (Figure 22.27), excising part of the joint capsule as well. It is quite in order to leave adjacent tendons without a synovial covering.

Closure is by one subcuticular Prolene™ or monofilament polyamide suture, strengthened by skin-closure strips (Figure 22.28). A sterile dry gauze dressing is applied, covered with cotton wool and an elastocrêpe bandage. The assistant now applies direct pressure over the site of the incision, and the doctor releases both tourniquets.

If all is well, the dressings are left undisturbed until the 10th postoperative day, when the suture is removed, leaving the Steri-Strips™ in position. A light sterile dressing is reapplied over these for 4 more days and then removed.

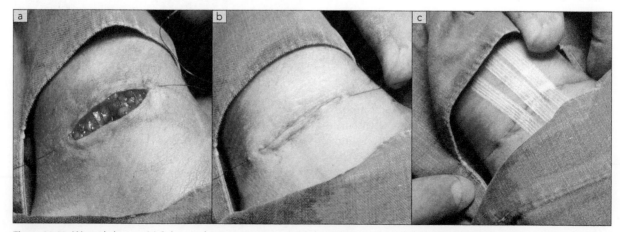

Figure 22.28 Wound closure. (a) Subcuticular suture prepared; (b) skin edges approximated; (c) additional support may be given by skin-closure strips.

Chapter 23

Vasectomy: skills

Laurel Spooner and Tony Feltbower

INTRODUCTION

Chapter 12 considered the definition, indications, anatomy, and risks of vasectomy surgery, as well as patient counselling. This chapter details the surgical procedure.

Levels of difficulty are indicated by scalpel ratings. The more scalpel blades, the more difficult the procedure and the more practical experience will be required to become competent at the technique.

BEFORE THE PROCEDURE

Following on from pre-vasectomy counselling, the patient should be booked for a dedicated vasectomy appointment. Informed written consent should be obtained (see Appendix 1 of this chapter).

It is essential, prior to operating, that the genital area is examined (preferably before the surgeon has scrubbed up and put on sterile gloves, or even at the preoperative counselling appointment) to ensure that:
- The surgeon is familiar with the anatomy.
- There are not likely to be any 'surprises' from abnormal anatomy.
- The vas deferens can easily be identified and palpated on each side.
- The patient is provided with information on how the surgeon is likely to be handling and manipulating the scrotum.

CONVENTIONAL VERSUS 'NO-SCALPEL' VASECTOMY

The two most common surgical techniques for accessing the vas during vasectomy are the *traditional incisional method* and the *'no-scalpel vasectomy'* (NSV) technique. The conventional incisional technique involves the use of a scalpel to make one or two incisions, whereas the NSV technique uses a sharp, forceps-like instrument to puncture the skin.

A Cochrane Review (of two randomised controlled trials; Cook *et al.*, 2007) indicates that NSV is associated with a significantly lower risk of early postoperative complications (postoperative haematoma, pain during surgery, postoperative scrotal pain, and wound infection) than the standard incision technique. Based on the same review, NSV is a faster procedure than the conventional surgery. However, there was no significant difference in the effectiveness (azoospermia or absence of motile sperm) of the two procedures.

The World Health Organization Reproductive Health Library (WHO RHL) concludes that, compared with the traditional incisional method, NSV results in less bleeding, haematoma formation, and pain during or after the procedure (Xiaozhang, 2009). The operative time is shorter, and these vasectomised men are able to resume sexual activity more quickly.

NO-SCALPEL VASECTOMY: EQUIPMENT

Where appropriate, single-use instruments are preferable unless adequate sterilisation facilities are available to allow the use of reusable instruments.

Essential equipment
- Heat pad (optional; to place over the genital area while the surgical trolley is being prepared, in order to keep the testicles well descended into the scrotum).
- Dressing pack to include cotton wool balls and gauze swabs.
- Warm aqueous antiseptic solution such as povidone–iodine, chlorhexidine, or Savlon.
- 10 ml syringe.
- Green and orange needles.
- Warm lidocaine, 5–10 ml of 1% or 2% solution.

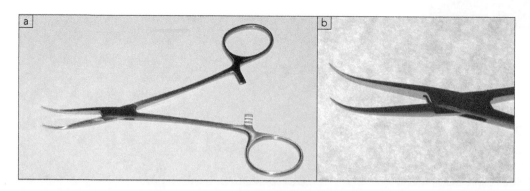

Figure 23.1 Sharp dissecting forceps (also known as NSV sharp haemostat) to puncture and spread the scrotal skin and deliver the vas deferens.

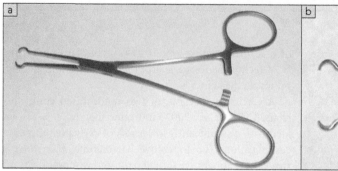
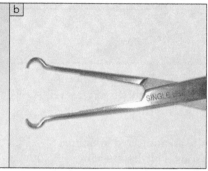

Figure 23.2 Extracutaneous ring forceps (ring clamp): the ringed tip (b) encircles and grasps the vas deferens.

- NSV sharp haemostat to puncture and spread the scrotal skin and deliver the vas deferens (Figure 23.1).
- NSV ring forceps 4 mm, the ringed tip being used to encircle and grasp the vas (Figure 23.2).
- Unipolar diathermy device with needle tip (Figure 23.3).
- Sterile polo towel (also called a fenestrated drape).
- Adequate ventilation/extraction facilities.

Figure 23.3 Unipolar diathermy unit, with smoke extraction unit below.

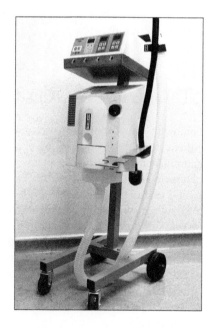

Additional equipment

The following should also be available in case they are required, but they need not necessarily be put out on the trolley with the above instruments:

- Mosquito artery forceps.
- Needle holder.
- Surgical suture material: monofilament absorbable. (e.g., Monocryl™ 4-0).
- Pair of suture scissors.

Electrosurgery: cutting and coagulation

A reminder is necessary that different waveforms are required for cutting and coagulation (see Chapter 1). An online eLearning module on this is available on the internet (Medicines and Healthcare products Regulatory Agency, undated).

Not all electrosurgical machines can deliver both the continuous sine wave required for cutting and the intermittent sine wave for coagulation. A machine that cannot produce a cutting or blended coagulation/cutting wave will produce excessive amounts of tissue charring and adhesion of tissue to the cutting electrode, resulting in drag as the electrode is passed through the tissue. With a cutting waveform, a small amount of steam is generated that separates the electrode from the tissue.

Unipolar diathermy is popular with vasectomy surgeons and designed for desiccation, fulguration, and coagulation but not cutting (see Figure 1.14, Chapter 1). The surgeon may sometimes use the electrode tip to press against the vas wall to enter the lumen. A machine that can deliver a cutting waveform will theoretically cause less tissue charring and therefore less postoperative discomfort, but studies have yet to be carried out to investigate whether the results warrant the increased cost of the more expensive machine.

NO-SCALPEL VASECTOMY: TECHNIQUE ⁄⁄⁄⁄⁄

A definitive technical guide to NSV is available on the internet (EngenderHealth, 2003). This chapter will explore the numerous issues surrounding NSV rather than reproduce this 'NSV Guide' in detail.

All instruments should either be sterile single-use or sterilised by autoclave according to recommended sterilising procedures. In addition, an absolutely aseptic technique should be employed throughout as the most common postoperative complication is a haematoma complicated by infection, which can have disastrous consequences.

It is recommended that the scrotal area is not shaved, but, if the surgeon wishes hair to be removed, should only be clipped just prior to operating, as it has been shown that shaving skin prior to an operation can increase the risk of postoperative infection.

While the surgeon is scrubbing up, it can be helpful to place a heat pad over the scrotal area to ensure the area remains warm, otherwise anxiety and cold can cause the testicles to retract, causing difficulty for both surgeon and patient. The heat pad can also be used to warm local anaesthetic ampoules and aseptic sachets prior to use.

A right-handed surgeon would normally stand to the right of the patient as this allows the non-dominant left hand to manipulate the vas deferens and scrotum while operating with the dominant right hand.

It can be helpful if the penis is gently taped onto the abdomen to prevent it entering into the operating area. If this is done, it is important that the scrotal skin is not stretched as this can make it difficult to isolate the vas between the fingers and manipulate it into position. In addition, tape should not be placed over the glans.

The genital area is swabbed with the aqueous antiseptic solution and the polo towel placed over the patient, with the scrotum easily 'available' through the hole in the towel (Figure 23.4a).

Using the three-finger technique described by Li Shunqiang, the left vas deferens is identified and held in position in the midline (Figure 23.4b). Lidocaine is first injected as a bleb just under the skin (Figure 23.4c). The needle is then gently inserted more deeply alongside the vas deferens, and more lidocaine is injected. Alternatively, local anaesthetic can be injected using Hypospray equipment or a Dermojet® unit (Figure 23.5).

Time is required to allow the anaesthetic to adequately numb the area. Because of the localised surgery, this effect should occur within seconds of the injection being completed.

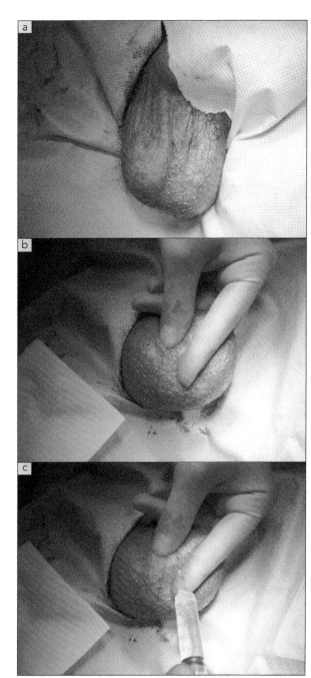

Figure 23.4 (a) Surgical drapes in place. (b) Vas deferens identified and held in position. (c) Vas deferens injected.

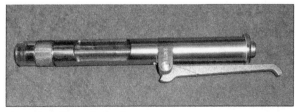

Figure 23.5 Dermojet® unit.

No-scalpel vasectomy: technique

///// Approach for 'no-scalpel vasectomy'

Incision

Both the Cochrane Review and the WHO RHL refer to comparison with the traditional *incisional* method. In addition, the NSV Guide states explicitly that NSV is a *surgical approach for isolating and delivering the vas* that uses conventional methods of vas occlusion. Therefore, 'NSV' is independent of the method of occlusion of the vas.

With regard to the incision to access the vasa, there are two factors to consider.

Site of incision

The NSV Guide specifies that the vasa should be isolated using the three-finger technique under the midline raphe for the local anaesthetic vasal block, and therefore this is the site of the scrotal skin incision through which each vas is grasped with the ring clamp (Figure 23.6). Surgical wisdom states that midline raphe incisions of any length for a variety of scrotal operations bleed less and heal with a good postoperative scar.

Variation

It is recognised that anatomical variation can result in difficulty in bringing the vas deferens anteriorly to lie just below the midline raphe. The options then lie in either bilateral incisions, as the vas can be brought into a subcutaneous position much more easily in the lateral position, or in making a midline raphe incision and reaching for the vas through a short distance with the ring clamp. The former approach results in two wounds that are not in the ideal site of the midline raphe for healing, but the latter is associated with a higher risk of haematoma formation through trauma from instrumentation, especially if the vas has proved difficult to encircle.

Method of skin incision

The NSV Guide describes puncturing the skin with one blade of a sharpened curved artery forceps (see Figure 23.1) and advancing this blade through the midline of each vas into its lumen. This depth of the puncture is important in order to avoid common pitfalls described in detail in the NSV Guide. Both tips of the forceps are then inserted into the puncture wound to the depth of the vasal lumen, and the tissues are spread gently until the opening in the skin and vasal sheath is twice the diameter of the vas.

Variation

The variations of this technique include a stab incision with a scalpel blade and spreading with artery forceps, or making the incision through the skin with a unipolar electrocautery device (Figure 23.7).

The scalpel stab and spread technique should be no different from that described in the Guide. There may be bleeding from the skin edges or the dartos muscle, this being controlled by pressure or a horizontal mattress suture at the end of the operation.

Although it is dogma in skin surgery to avoid the diathermy of bleeding vessels in the skin edge for haemostasis as dead, burnt skin does not heal as well, some practitioners find that incision through the skin with unipolar electrocautery minimises this source of bleeding, albeit at the price of a wound that is slower to heal.

At this point, it serves to be reminded of the tissue layers between the skin and the vas that need to be divided to expose and deliver the bare vas for division. From superficial to deep, the layers are the skin, dartos muscle, external spermatic fascia, cremasteric fascia, cremaster muscle, internal spermatic fascia, and finally vas deferens. Any of these layers can bleed, and fastidious haemostasis is required to minimise haematoma formation.

Delivery of the vas deferens through the incision

In the NSV Guide, the vas deferens is elevated out of the incision by skewering it with one blade of the sharpened artery forceps and rotating the handle of the forceps through 180° through supination until the tips face upwards (Figure 23.8). This movement, combined with a simultaneous release of the ring clamp, delivers a loop of vas through the incision site. This coordinated sequence requires practice to perfect it.

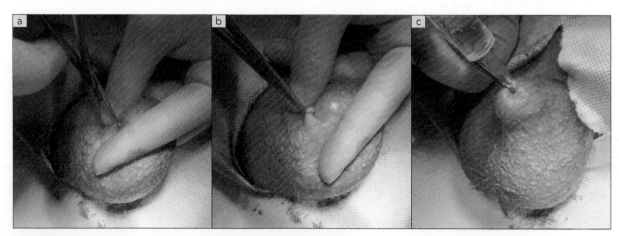

Figure 23.6 (a,b) Ring forceps applied in the midline. (c) Further anaesthetic injected.

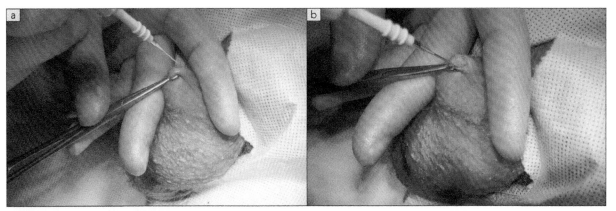

Figure 23.7 Radiosurgical incision through the scrotal layers to the vas deferens, which is exposed in a bloodless field.

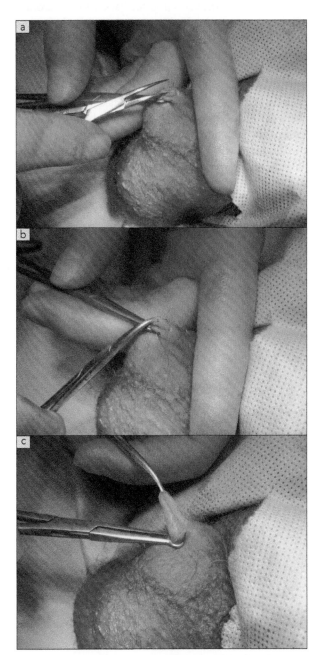

Figure 23.8 Vas deferens initially (a) 'skewered' by fine dissecting forceps, then (b) lifted, and finally (c) fully lifted and exposed.

Variation

Grasping the exposed vas with toothed forceps or another ring clamp will also allow delivery through the skin incision. The hazard here is inadvertent trauma to the vascular internal spermatic fascia, or mesentery as it is also known.

The vas must be free of its sheath, and any significant blood vessels need to be identified and gently pushed away or down from the vas (using a piece of gauze or blunt dissection) to avoid damaging them when cauterising the vas as these are the main cause of bleeding. However, the process of stripping needs to be carried out gently as this in many cases causes the bleeding.

Once free, the vas should be gently pulled to confirm that the testicle on the expected side moves. This is to ensure that the same vas is not operated on twice by mistake, as can sometimes happen if the vasa lie very posteriorly toward the midline.

Occlusion

Division of the vas deferens

Regardless of the method of occlusion used, the vasa have to be divided. This can be carried out by electrosurgery or with a scalpel.

Excision of a segment of vas deferens

The NSV Guide recommends that up to 1 cm of vas deferens is excised. However, the published literature reveals a range of opinion between the following:

- No association between the length of the vas segment excised and the risk of recanalisation (Labrecque *et al.*, 2003).
- At least 15 mm of vas needing excision in order to maximise success. Excised segments of vas less than 15 mm in length were associated with an up to 25-fold greater incidence of failure (Kaplan and Huether, 1975).

No-scalpel vasectomy: technique

Methods of occlusion

There are three main methods of occlusion of the vas: ligation, fascial interposition, and intraluminal cautery. The NSV Guide describes all three, but the published literature concludes that fascial interposition—the use of the fascial sheath to create a natural barrier between the cut vasal ends—and intraluminal cautery have similar effectiveness, with a combination of the two representing the gold standard with the lowest failure rate (Labrecque *et al.*, 2004).

Ligation

No studies have been shown to assess the best suture material for ligation of the vasal stumps. However, the risk of the ligature being too loose and falling off, or too tight causing ischaemic necrosis and falling off, explains the higher failure rate associated with this technique.

Fascial interposition

It is not necessary to bury either end of the vas under fascia, although some surgeons prefer to bury the lower end and stitch a layer of fascia over it such that the two ends of the vas are in different fascial planes.

There are several techniques for fascial interposition. The one illustrated in the NSV Guide has the advantage of not requiring suture needles but being carried out in conjunction with ligation. The use of a suture needle increases the risk of trauma to the small vessels in the fascial sheath, causing bleeding and haematoma formation.

Intraluminal cautery

This is done by inserting a needle electrode or cautery device into the vasal lumen and desiccating the luminal mucosa of the vas as it is withdrawn to create a firm scar that will occlude the vas (Figure 23.9). Damage to the muscle of the vas must be avoided as this can lead to necrosis, with subsequent sperm leakage, granuloma, and recanalisation.

Open-ended technique

Leaving the testicular vasal end open has been shown to reduce the incidence of epididymal congestion (Figure 23.10). The risk of both early and late recanalisation is not affected by this technique provided that intraluminal cautery and fascial interposition have been used on the prostatic vasal end.

Irrigation of the vas deferens

Irrigating the vas during vasectomy may decrease the postoperative sperm count but does not reduce failure rates or time to clearance.

Haemostasis

Once cauterised, the vas is inserted back into the scrotum (Figure 23.11) and withdrawn again to check for any bleeding, as sometimes a tourniquet effect at the base of the loop of vas deferens can mask small bleeding vessels, which only become evident when the vas is inserted back into the scrotum and then gently withdrawn.

As much care as possible must be taken to ensure that there is no evidence of active bleeding before the ring forceps is released from the vas. Any bleeding vessels can be cauterised with diathermy or tied with an appropriate absorbable monofilament suture. It is preferable, if any bleeding vessel is to be tied, that it is grasped with mosquito artery forceps and the suture is tied around the vessel without using a needle to avoid damaging deeper structures.

Using the same three-finger technique described above, the right vas deferens is now identified and manipulated to lie under the same midline scrotal opening. Lidocaine is then injected along and into the outer sheath.

Once anaesthetised, the vas is drawn out and cauterised as for the left side, before being placed back into the scrotal sac once haemostasis has been ensured.

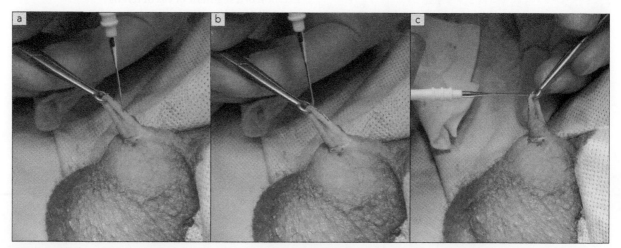

Figure 23.9 (a) Vas deferens incised by radiosurgery while being held by the repositioned ring forceps. (b,c) The vasal lumen is cauterised down both sides from the ring clamp.

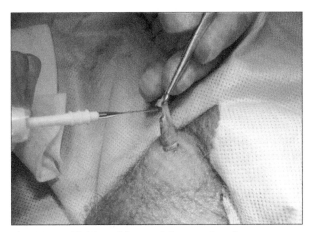

Figure 23.10 Division of the vas deferens using electrosurgery.

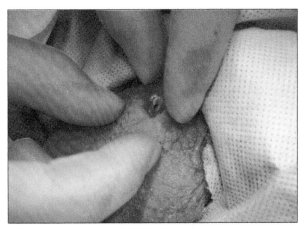

Figure 23.11 Vas deferens returned to the scrotum.

Closure

The incision (single midline) or incisions (bilateral lateral) are small but can sometimes continue to bleed and cause a small haematoma (Figure 23.12). This can be minimised by choosing a site with no visible vascular markings before making the incision, but bleeding can still occur as a result of stretching the tissues.

It is not necessary to stitch the skin edges as they do not usually bleed, the opening is usually small, and the patient can be assured that the edges will heal naturally within a few days, although there may be slight blood-staining at first. Despite this, some surgeons prefer either to stitch the edges (using a horizontal mattress suture), to use cyanoacrylic tissue adhesive (Figure 23.13), or to cauterise the edges if there is significant oozing.

Histology

Routine histology on vasectomy specimens represents an unacceptable burden on both laboratory staff and time and is also expensive. Therefore in the United Kingdom the Royal College of Obstetricians and Gynaecologists' guidance (2004) recommends that 'excised portions of vas should only be sent for histological examination if there is any doubt about their identity.'

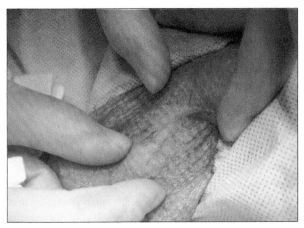

Figure 23.12 Checking the wound for any bleeding.

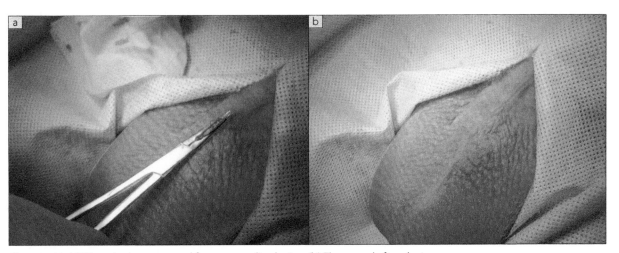

Figure 23.13 (a) Wound edges prepared for cyanoacrylic glueing. (b) The wound after glueing.

No-scalpel vasectomy: technique

POSTOPERATIVE CARE

After the procedure a pad is provided which the patient will keep inside close-fitting underpants (or a scrotal support). The patient is then allowed to slowly get up, dress, and move to the recovery room. Here he should rest for about half an hour following the vasectomy and only be discharged after his vital signs have been checked and found to be normal. This rest period may be a good time for him to complete a postoperative questionnaire for audit purposes.

In addition, the patient should receive and understand the instructions for postoperative care (see Appendix 2) and the need for seminal fluid analysis to confirm sperm clearance. He also needs to be given instructions on what to expect (a little pain and bruising) and when to seek medical advice (if there is fever, a bloody or purulent discharge from the wound, or excessive pain or swelling).

It can be beneficial for the patient to apply cold packs (crushed ice, frozen peas, or gel packs wrapped in a cloth to avoid direct contact between the ice pack and the skin) pressed against the scrotal area for 15–20 minutes per hour between the time of the operation and going to bed on the night after the vasectomy. In addition, use of a cold pack in the recovery room has the benefit of minimising swelling and bruising without delay, and showing the patient where to position the pack.

Physical exertion should be limited in the period immediately after a vasectomy. This reduces the risk of haematoma formation and is most beneficial in the immediate postoperative period, with a graded return to activity over the following few days. The clinician should suggest minimal exertion on the day of the surgery, avoidance of running and heavy lifting the following day, and avoidance of anything that still causes discomfort for the third day. Although sexual intercourse and competitive sports and vigorous exercise are advised against for a full week, it is not unknown for patients to resume these activities much earlier without any adverse effect, and everyone heals at different rates.

The surgeon should make an appropriate record of the operation, including any difficulties encountered and any complications or additional procedures that might have been required (e.g., tying a bleeding vessel), as well as any abnormal findings on initial examination that might have a bearing on the operation itself.

Seminal fluid analysis

Men should be advised to use effective contraception until azoospermia has been confirmed.

Seminal fluid analysis is intended to quickly identify men who have persistent motile sperm as a result of technical failure or early recanalisation. In the past, two consecutive clear samples have been recommended as a requirement, but recent evidence confirms that a single azoospermic sample at 3–4 months is sufficient to confirm infertility. Compliance with a second sample collection is poor, and therefore UK guidance advises the minimum number of tests. Reminders for patients who default on testing may increase uptake.

Postal samples have the advantage of higher return rates, but they rely on azoospermia to confirm sterility as the samples will never be analysed 'fresh'. This becomes a problem if sperm are still present at 7 months, and in these circumstances arrangements have to be made for a fresh sample to be analysed.

In situations where semen analysis is not available, the consensus view is that alternative methods of contraception can be stopped after 30 ejaculations following successful vasectomy.

Special clearance

A small percentage (2.0–2.5%) of men have persistent non-motile sperm in their seminal samples. Evidence now confirms that if a fresh semen sample (i.e., taken within the previous 2 hours) collected at least 7 months after vasectomy is inspected, and there are fewer than 10,000 immotile sperm/ml present, the risk of pregnancy is the same as if there were azoospermia (Royal College of Obstetricians and Gynaecologists, 2004). In this way, 'special clearance' can be given to the patient (the American Urology Association state fewer than 100,000 immotile sperm/ml for special clearance [AUA, May 2012]).

In one study, no pregnancies were reported for over 600 men followed up for 1–3 years when contraception was discontinued after fewer than 10,000 non-motile sperm/ml had been found in a fresh specimen examined at least 7 months after vasectomy. Medicolegally, it is prudent to present this evidence to the patient and allow him to choose whether to discontinue contraception or continue with testing until azoospermia is reached.

REFERENCES

Cook LAA, Van Vliet HHAAM, Lopez LM, Pun A, Gallo MF (2007) Vasectomy occlusion techniques for male sterilization. Cochrane Database of Systematic Reviews (2): CD003991. Available from: http://onlinelibrary.wiley.com/doi/10.1002/14651858.CD003991.pub3/abstract (accessed July 2012).

EngenderHealth (2003) No-scalpel vasectomy. An illustrated guide for surgeons, 3rd ed. Available from: www.engenderhealth.org/files/pubs/family-planning/no-scalpel.pdf (accessed July 2012).

Kaplan KA, Huether CA (1975) A clinical study of vasectomy failure and recanalization. *Journal of Urology* 113: 71–4.

Labrecque M, Hoang DQ, Turcot L (2003) Association between the length of the vas deferens excised during vasectomy and the risk of postvasectomy recanalization. *Fertility and Sterility* 79: 1003–7.

Labrecque M, Dufresne C, Barone MA, St-Hilaire K (2004) Vasectomy surgical techniques: A systematic review. *BMC Medicine* 2: 21.

Medicines and Healthcare Products Regulatory Agency (undated) Electrosurgery. Available from: http://mhra.gov.uk/learningcentre/ESUGenericModule/player.html (accessed July 2012).

Royal College of Obstetricians and Gynaecologists (2004) Male and female sterilisation. Evidence-Based Clinical Guideline No. 4. Available from www.rcog.org.uk/files/rcog-corp/uploaded-files/NEBSterilisationFull060607.pdf (accessed July 2012).

Xiaozhang L (2009) Scalpel versus no-scalpel incision for vasectomy: RHL commentary. Geneva: World Health Organization, WHO Reproductive Health Library. Available from: http://apps.who.int/rhl/fertility/contraception/lxhcom/en/index.html (accessed July 2012).

FURTHER READING

Male Contraception Information Project (2006) Frontiers in nonhormonal male contraception: The next step.

Naz RK, Rowan S (2009) Update on male contraception. *Current Opinion in Obstetrics and Gynecology* 21: 265–9.

Vasectomy Information (2001) Vasectomy and vaso-vasostomy (reversal surgery). Available from: www.vasectomy-information.com/pages/wellconn2001.pdf (accessed July 2012).

Within the United Kingdom, a national training standard for vasectomy was first published in 1999, since when training modules have been developed, along with a syllabus and log book. The minimum number of supervised operating sessions is 10, or 40 vasectomy procedures for doctors with no prior special surgical experience (with a minimum of eight supervised sessions for those with prior vasectomy experience).

APPENDIX 1: CONSENT TO TREAT

Date of procedure: ....

Name and address of patient: ....

PATIENT'S DECLARATION

Being an adult, I ....
hereby consent to undergo the operation of
VASECTOMY under local anaesthetic, the nature
and effect of which has been explained to me by

Dr ....

- I have been counselled regarding alternative forms of long-term *reversible* contraception, e.g., coils/implants, and have read and understood the information leaflet.

- I also consent to such further alternative measures as may be found necessary or advisable during the course of the operation, and to the administration of a local anaesthetic for any of these purposes.

- I have been told that the object of the operation is to render me sterile and incapable of further parenthood, and I understand that the effect of the operation may be irreversible.

- Furthermore, I confirm that I acknowledge there is a rare but accepted failure rate associated with non-scalpel vasectomy reported to be in the order of 0.05% (1 in 2000) and therefore a small risk of pregnancy in the future even after being given the 'all clear'.

- No assurance has been given to me that the operation will be performed by a particular surgeon, and I understand that no guarantees can be given that the operation will be successful or that it will be free from side effects.

- I acknowledge that there is a small risk of significant complications such as severe infection and excessive bleeding/bruising (common to any surgical procedure—for non-scalpel vasectomy, less than 1%), a small risk of developing chronic testicular pain, and extremely rarely testicular atrophy.

- Any complication may require further medical treatment, hospitalisation, or further surgery.

- I understand that I should not abandon other methods of contraception prior to receipt of notification that at least one sperm count at least 4 months after my vasectomy has proved negative, or special clearance has been given to me after 7 months.

- I understand that I can change my mind at any time and decide not to proceed with the vasectomy.

MEDICAL HISTORY

Allergies: ....

....

Current medication: ....

....

Contraception currently used: ....

Alternatives to vasectomy discussed: Yes / No

Children: ....

- ☐ Procedure*
- ☐ Risks*
- ☐ Failure rate*
- ☐ Irreversibility*

* All explained as above

DOCTOR'S CONFIRMATION

I confirm that I have explained to the patient/and partner the nature and effect of vasectomy as detailed above. Furthermore, I confirm that the patient has read (or had read to him) the above form, and I am satisfied that he understands what is proposed, has no further questions, and is happy to proceed with a vasectomy.

Signature of doctor: ....

Date:...

PATIENT'S CONFIRMATION

I confirm that I have read (or had read to me) and understand the above form and I am satisfied with the conditions stated therein.

Signature of patient: ....

Date: ....

Any additional signature (e.g., interpreter):

....

Date: ....

Name: ....

Role: ....

APPENDIX 2: PATIENT INFORMATION GUIDE—POSTOPERATIVE CARE

Name of clinic: ....

Address of clinic: ....

....

Tel: .... E-mail: ....

After your operation

- Following a local anaesthetic, you can leave the surgery after a short rest. You should not drive home but ideally arrange for someone to collect you and be with you for the rest of the day.

- You are likely to experience some pain or discomfort during the first few days, and occasionally some swelling develops. It is sensible to plan to relax at home for a few days before returning to work. We advise that you avoid strenuous exercise, heavy lifting, or driving long distances for 1–2 weeks.

- To minimise swelling and discomfort, it is advisable to wear tight-fitting underpants, swimming trunks, or a jock strap (brought with you on the day of your operation). You should continue to wear these day and night for about 1 week. If you have a heavy manual job, you may need to take more time off work if 'light duties' are not available.

- About 1–2 hours after the operation, when the local anaesthetic wears off, you will normally have some discomfort or pain. It is OK for you to take your usual painkillers, e.g., paracetamol, ibuprofen, or co-codamol, in the normal dosages (these are all available from the chemist without needing a prescription). Use of an ice pack on the scrotum for 10–20 minutes every 1–2 hours for the first day can help to reduce swelling and discomfort. Remember to place a tea towel (or something similar) between the ice pack and the skin.

- Some swelling (up to the size of a testicle) and bruising of the scrotum and testicles is normal, but if it is severe during the first few hours after the operation you should contact the surgeon. If you are unable to contact him or her, please contact a doctor through your own surgery.

- Where the tubes have been cauterised and cut, some scar tissue will form. This may be felt as a slightly lumpy, sometimes tender, area just above the testicle. This is quite normal, but if you do become concerned about any unusual lumps, see your GP.

- There are no stitches to remove, and there is only a small cut that will heal itself, although it may gape open a little and cause a slight bloodstained discharge. You only need to seek medical advice if this is persistent, excessively smelly, or inflamed. You may also notice slight bloodstaining the first few times you ejaculate.

- Sperm can live for up to 70 days or longer and will still be released for a variable length of time after the operation when you ejaculate. In order to empty the 'reservoir' of live sperm within this period of time, it is recommended that you have intercourse/ejaculate on average three times a week.

- Sometimes it is found that, even with this frequency of intercourse, some men take longer to clear their 'reservoir' of live sperm, and you should not worry if you are asked for further specimens. Evidence shows that one fresh sample at 4 months that is completely clear of all sperm is sufficient. If small numbers of dead sperm persist, you may be given the 'all clear' after about 7 months. However, you must wait until this is confirmed by your own GP or by the surgeon.

- *Until you have received confirmation from your own GP or the surgeon, you should continue to take contraceptive precautions.*

- No assurance that you have become infertile can be given without these tests, and no responsibility will be accepted for failure of the operation if the required semen specimens are not submitted for analysis at the appropriate times.

The approximate date (not before) for your first semen specimen collection will be:

....

A letter will be sent to you in about 4 months' time to remind you. Full instructions regarding request forms and sample pots and where to take the samples will be included in the letter. Your own GP and the surgeon will have access to the results.

Phenol nail ablation

Chapter 24

Toenail surgery

Ian Reilly

INTRODUCTION

Chapter 13 outlined toenail pathologies that might benefit from surgery. Nail surgery can be separated into two distinct categories: first, destruction of the nail bed and matrix by physical methods such as the use of chemicals (phenol or sodium hydroxide), cryotherapy, and electrogalvanism, and second, excision of the pathological tissue using sharp instrumentation.

Levels of difficulty are indicated by scalpel ratings. The more scalpel blades, the more difficult the procedure and the more practical experience will be required to become competent at the technique.

OVERVIEW

The most common indication for nail surgery will be for chronic or recurrent ingrowing toenails (onychocryptosis). Although there are a range of other indications such as abnormal nail shape and structure, nail unit tumours, and nail plate deformity, this chapter will concentrate on the common techniques used to manage ingrowing toenails. The techniques described are for toenails and are not recommended for fingernails.

The most common nail treatment in the United Kingdom is non-invasive and involves nail avulsion and the use of phenol/alcohol. Eekhof *et al.* (2012) concluded in their systematic review that the evidence suggested that simple nail avulsion combined with the use of phenol, compared with surgical excisional techniques without the use of phenol, was more effective at preventing symptomatic recurrence of ingrowing toenails. This chemical ablation of the nail bed can be carried out in the presence of sepsis and is seen as a simpler procedure requiring less skill, with low morbidity and good patient acceptance. In the absence of frank pus, much of the inflammation of an ingrowing nail comes from a foreign body reaction (to the nail) rather than sepsis. There are, however, occasions when formal surgical incision technique may offer certain advantages over chemical treatment.

The ocurrence of nail regrowth following the segmental chemical ablation described and recommended here is low, with recurrence rates typically in the 2–5% range (Weaver *et al.*, 2004).

PHENOL NAIL ABLATION

Phenol

Phenol (C_6H_5OH) is an organic compound containing a hydroxyl group directly attached to a benzene ring. It is a colourless-to-white solid with a sweet acrid odour. It is thought that phenol may have been the first surgical antiseptic used by Joseph Lister in 1865 to sterilise his operating field. Phenol is toxic in concentrated solutions and causes burns to the skin and mucous membranes. It is this action that is exploited in the phenolisation of the nail matrix with or without the nail bed and also, in lower concentrations, in chemical peels. A chemical burn occurs when phenol is applied to the skin, with destruction of its chemical structure, absorption of water, and coagulation of proteins.

Phenol has been used since 1901 in the treatment of ingrown nails. There remains debate about the exact time for application of phenol when treating ingrowing toenails, with 30 seconds, 1 minute, 2 minutes, and up to 5 minutes all having been reported. Boberg *et al.* (2002) showed that with between 30 seconds and 1 minute there was a significant increase in the amount of tissue destruction, but little change from 1 to 2 minutes. They concluded that 1-minute applications are the optimum required for complete destruction of the germinal nail matrix.

Similarly, there is a lack of agreement on how the phenol is best applied: cotton-tipped applicators, syringe, or Blacks file. Furthermore, there is disagreement over whether the phenol should be applied and left to work or whether it needs to be rubbed over the area.

Principles of phenol nail ablation

Espensen *et al.* (2002) published a helpful review of the literature and suggested eight overarching principles:

1. Patient selection: along with patient's vascular and neurological status, the most important factor to establish is the ability of the patient to achieve wound healing.

2. The removal of the nail border (partial nail avulsion) or total nail plate should be carried out as aseptically as possible, a principle that holds true for all minor surgical procedures.

3. Following the removal of the nail and all hyperkeratotic tissue, curettage of the nail bed, nail fold, and groove should be carried out to remove as much of the nail matrix as possible. This will allow the phenol to come into contact with the remaining nail matrix.

4. Obtaining a dry, bloodless field using a tourniquet is standard clinical practice as it allows good visualisation of the area, and ensures that the chemical is not washed out by excessive bleeding and that bleeding does not carry the phenol out of the operative area, potentially leading to phenol burns around the nail unit.

5. It is worth considering use of a protective barrier for the surrounding skin. A petroleum jelly, bacitracin, silver sulfadiazine, or similar is suggested. Although good technique should prevent leakage to the surrounding tissue, it is argued that this is a simple and cheap method to avoid skin damage.

6. No definitive method for applying the phenol has been identified. Cotton-tipped applicators, wooden applicators, and even syringes with needles have been used, the important point being that the chemical must be carefully applied to the tissue. This will prevent unnecessary damage to the surrounding tissue. Wiping off excess chemical on pieces of gauze or cotton is also recommended.

7. The length of application of the chemical is considered. Curetting between applications is recommended to expose tissue that would not have been in contact with the chemical. Espensen *et al.* (2002) comment on the fact that there has to be a balance between applying the chemical for long enough to permanently destroy the nail matrix and prevent regrowth, against not causing too much tissue damage, which would result in a long period of wound healing. Application times can therefore vary from 30 seconds to 5 minutes.

8. The aftercare regime should include dry sterile dressings. Espensen *et al.* (2002) noted that moist wounds heal quicker than dry wounds. Therefore, the use of daily soaks is recommended. These soaks keep the wound moist, prevent the formation of dry crusts, and promote the drainage of fluid from the wound.

Partial nail avulsion
Equipment

The equipment required for this procedure is shown in Figure 24.1. In addition, the following are required:

- 80–100% phenol. Individually packed and sealed sterile containers of 90% liquid phenol with appropriately sized containers are available. These are safer to use than phenol in brown bottles
- Industrial methylated spirit (IMS).
- Tourniquet.
- Local anaesthetic (usually 1% lidocaine).
- Dressings.

/// Recommended technique

The area is prepared using a povidone-iodine solution, and a sterile field is applied.

Local anaesthetic is injected into the base of the toe using a digital nerve/ring block (Figure 24.2 and Video Clip 24.1). Lidocaine 1% is usually used, but *never with adrenaline (epinephrine)* (see Chapter 15). Some clinicians use a 50:50 mix of 0.5% plain bupivacaine and 1% or 2% lidocaine. Bupivacaine has a slow onset but is longer acting, whereas lidocaine is of quicker onset but is shorter acting. Combination of the two allows for immediate and postoperative anaesthesia.

After checking that anaesthesia has been achieved, an exsanguinating tourniquet (Esmarch® bandage) is applied for as short a period of time as possible, but certainly no more than 20 minutes (Figure 24.3 and Video Clip 24.2). Use of a sterile glove as a tourniquet is no longer considered appropriate.

The embedded margin of the nail (sulcus) is released using a Blacks file or spatula (Figure 24.4 and Video Clip 24.3). This allows the practitioner to ascertain the size of the nail plate—especially useful where hypergranulation tissue is abundant.

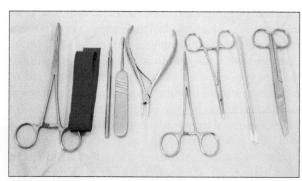

Figure 24.1 Equipment for partial nail avulsion with tourniquet phenolisation.

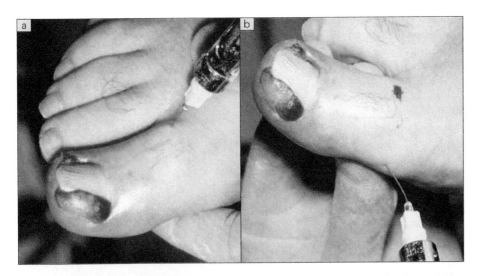

Figure 24.2 Digital block. See Video Clips 24.1a and 24.1b—http://goo.gl/jAdr5; http://goo.gl/6NvyR.

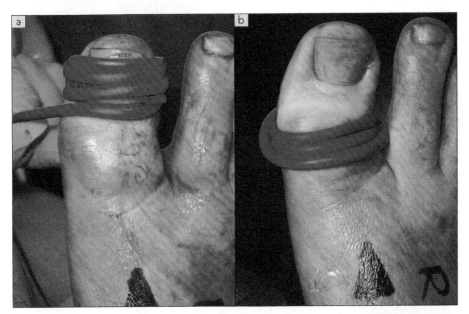

Figure 24.3 Applying a digital tourniquet. See Video Clip 24.2—http://goo.gl/8a7br.

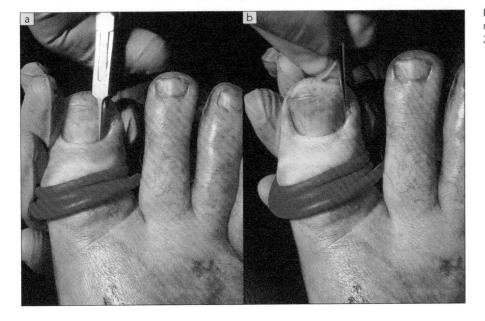

Figure 24.4 Freeing the nail margin. See Video Clip 24.3—http://goo.gl/d6JAX.

The nail plate is completely split longitudinally using Thwaites nippers (Figure 24.5 and Video Clip 24.4). The cut is continued proximally under the proximal nail fold with a chisel Beaver blade (fine) or a second cut from the nippers.

The section is clamped as proximally as possible with a pair of mosquito or Spencer Wells forceps and rotated toward the midline of the nail plate (Figure 24.6 and Video Clip 24.5). The section with a fragment of nail matrix attached will detach from the site—check that this is the case and that the entire proximal nail has been removed (Figure 24.7).

Any remaining particles are removed with a Blacks file or microcurette. Sharp resection of hypergranulation tissue is strongly recommended.

Phenol 80–100% is applied to the sulcus and exposed nail bed using a sterile cotton wool bud or orange stick to a dry field maintained by the tourniquet (Figure 24.8 and Video Clip 24.6). The phenol should be applied to any area of hypergranulation tissue resection in order to reduce postoperative bleeding. Consider protecting the proximal nail fold with vaseline. Three 1-minute applications are recommended, which is sufficient to blanch the area.

After irrigation with IMS, the area is dried and the tourniquet removed (Figure 24.9 and Video Clip 24.7) (remember to note the tourniquet time.) The phenol

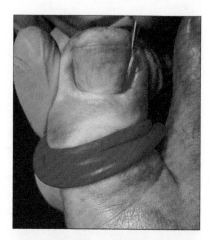

Figure 24.5 Splitting the nail longitudinally. See Video Clip 24.4—http://goo.gl/YlsJd.

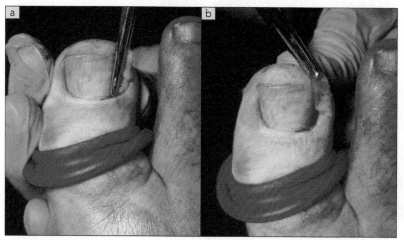
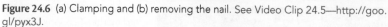

Figure 24.6 (a) Clamping and (b) removing the nail. See Video Clip 24.5—http://goo.gl/pyx3J.

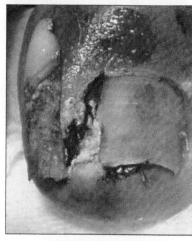

Figure 24.7 Length of the nail wedge.

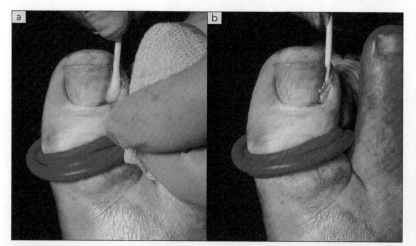

Figure 24.8 (a) Application of phenol with a cotton bud. (b) Cotton bud inserted. See Video Clip 24.6—http://goo.gl/Blq9c.

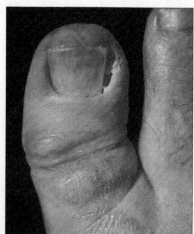

Figure 24.9 After removal of the tourniquet, the procedure is complete. See Video Clip 24.7—http://goo.gl/izkgF.

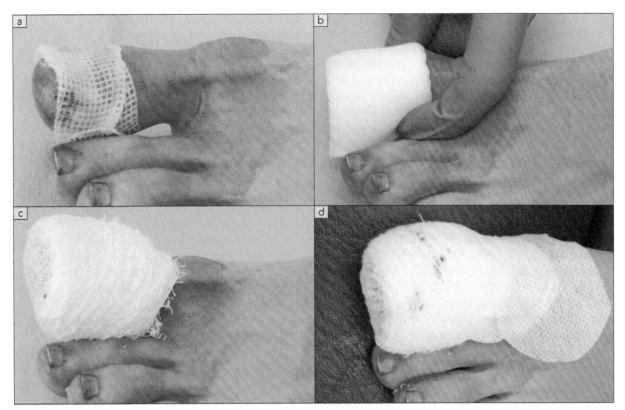

Figure 24.10 Applying the suggested dressing. See Video Clips 24.8a,b,c—http://goo.gl/3UzbR; http://goo.gl/c63Ay; http://goo.gl/qJ8bG.

itself is not neutralised as some authors believe, but should be removed with swabbing, and then diluted with 5 ml IMS. In the United States, the technique is known as the phenol–alcohol procedure.

The wound is dressed with a non-adherent primary dressing, gauze, and (light) pressure bandage (Figure 24.10 and Video Clip 24.8). Many authors have looked at dressing regimes, but the differences in healing times between one technique and another appear minimal.

Total nail avulsion with phenolisation

The technique is the same as for partial avulsion, save for the whole nail plate being removed using an elevator (Figure 24.11).

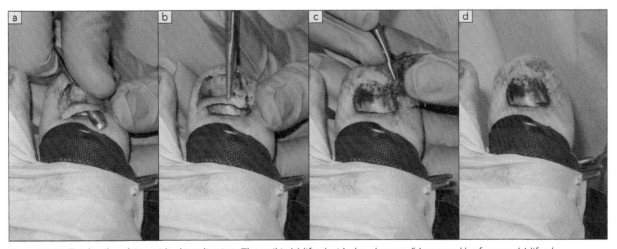

Figure 24.11 Total nail avulsion with phenolisation. The nail is (a) lifted with the elevator, (b) grasped by forceps, (c) lifted, and (d) removed.

Complications

The most common complication is delayed healing, which may be related to the phenolisation process. There is a need to balance the amount of destruction caused by phenolisation and the increased healing time against the risk of recurrence. Minimal destruction and a speedy healing time, using a small amount of phenol for a short period, may lead to recurrence. It is better to cause some destruction with a longer healing time than to run the risk of regrowth and further symptoms of an ingrowing toenail.

Diabetic patients suffering with ingrowing toenails are thought to be at risk from the procedure itself and from postoperative complications. It has been suggested that individuals with diabetes cannot tolerate the chemical burn caused by the procedure. Postoperative healing is thought to be reduced in these patients, leading to an increased risk of infection. The clinician will need to weigh carefully the risks and benefits of the procedure in diabetic patients after careful assessment of the peripheral circulation to the toe. Some clinicians suggest avoiding the use of phenol with diabetic patients. If there is any concern about possible poor healing, the surgeon should discuss the planned procedure with others involved in the care of the diabetic patient.

SODIUM HYDROXIDE AND ALTERNATIVE TREATMENTS

In the United States, sodium hydroxide is commonly used instead of phenol. The procedure is similar in that it is carried out under local anaesthesia, with the nail spicule/plate being removed, and 10% sodium hydroxide then being applied to the nail matrix for a period of between 3 seconds and 3 minutes, depending on which author one reads. Unlike phenol, sodium hydroxide can be neutralised. Acetic acid 5% is applied to neutralise the sodium hydroxide and prevent its further action. Some authors believe that this technique has a more predictable outcome and criticise the use of phenol for its unpredictability in terms of destruction, drainage, and healing times.

Other treatments such as electrodesiccation, negative galvanic current, and the carbon dioxide laser are reported but are beyond the scope of this chapter.

SURGICAL TECHNIQUES FOR NAIL ABLATION

There are numerous reported surgical techniques for invasive surgical ablation of the nail—either in part or in whole. The main advantage of incisional techniques is that they lead to quicker healing (by primary intention) compared with phenolisation. This is useful in patient groups prone to infection who thus need to heal as quickly as possible. Incisional techniques may therefore be indicated for some individuals with diabetes, steroid users, immunocompromised patients, and those with a sensitivity to chemical cautery.

Invasive techniques are also indicated when a piece of periungual tissue needs to be removed in conjunction with removal of the nail. They also allow access to a subungual exostosis and are more commonly used by orthopaedic and general surgeons, although there has been a move towards phenolisation by many within the medical and surgical communities (Dockery, 2001).

The main disadvantages are the higher recurrence rate compared with phenolisation, the greater pain, and an increased likelihood of bleeding. In the United Kingdom, the Winograd and Zadik procedures, for partial and total nail ablation respectively, are the techniques most commonly used by podiatric surgeons. The terminal Syme approach—removal of the nail unit and part or all of the distal phalanx—is especially useful for fifth toe deformity. Readers are advised to refer to more specialist podiatric surgery texts for further details of these procedures.

USE OF ANTIBIOTICS

Although appropriate antibiotics may be all that is required for a paronychia, their repeated use for true ingrown toenail is all too common and usually ineffective. Interestingly, the results of Reyzelman et al.'s study (2000) suggest that oral antibiotics do not reduce postoperative infection rates in the treatment of ingrown toenails, adding weight to the argument that the ingrowing nail acts primarily to cause a foreign body reaction. Furthermore, antibiotic prophylaxis against infective endocarditis is no longer indicated when performing procedures for ingrown toenail (National Institute for Health and Clinical Excellence, 2008).

REFERENCES

Boberg JS, Fredericksen MS, Harton FM (2002) Scientific analysis of phenol nail surgery. *Journal of the American Podiatric Medical Association* 92: 575–9.

Dockery GL (2001) Nails. In: Banks AS, Downey MS, Martin DE, Miller SJ, McGlamry ED, eds. *McGlamry's Comprehensive Textbook of Foot and Ankle Surgery*, 3rd ed. Philadelphia: Lippincott Williams & Wilkins, pp. 203–30.

Eekhof JAH, Van Wijk B, Knuistingh Neven A, van der Wouden JC (2012) Interventions for ingrowing toenails. *Cochrane Database of Systematic Reviews* (4): CD001541.

Espensen EH, Nixon BP, Armstrong DG (2002) Chemical matrixectomy for ingrown toenails: Is there an evidence basis to guide therapy? *Journal of the American Podiatric Medical Association* 92: 287–95.

National Institute for Health and Clinical Excellence (2008) Prophylaxis against infective endocarditis: Antimicrobial prophylaxis against infective endocarditis in adults and children undergoing interventional procedures. Available from: www.nice.org.uk/nicemedia/pdf/CG64NICEguidance.pdf (accessed July 2012).

Reyzelman AM, Trombello KA, Vayser DJ, Armstrong DG, Harkless LB (2000) Are antibiotics necessary in the treatment of locally infected ingrown toenails? *Archives of Family Medicine* 9: 930–2.

Weaver TD, Vy Ton M, Pham TV (2004) Ingrowing toenails: Management practices and research outcomes. *International Journal of Lower Extremity Wounds* 3: 22–34.

FURTHER READING

Park DH, Singh D (2012) The management of ingrowing toenails. *BMJ* 344: e2089.

LINKS TO VIDEO CLIPS

VC 24.1a,b: Digital block
http://goo.gl/jAdr5
http://goo.gl/6NvyR

VC 24.5: Clamping and removing the nail
http://goo.gl/pyx3J

VC 24.2: Applying a digital tourniquet
http://goo.gl/8a7br

VC 24.6: Application of phenol
http://goo.gl/Blq9c

VC 24.3: Freeing the nail margin
http://goo.gl/d6JAX

VC 24.7: Removal of tourniquet
http://goo.gl/izkgF

VC 24.4: Splitting the nail longitudinally
http://goo.gl/YlsJd

VC 24.8a,b,c: Applying the dressing
http://goo.gl/3UzbR
http://goo.gl/c63Ay
http://goo.gl/qJ8bG

Chapter 25

Advanced surgical procedures

INTRODUCTION

In this chapter, we look at more complex methods to close skin. In naming these procedures 'advanced,' we do not imply that they are in any way better than traditional elliptical closures. They are techniques that can be employed where simple elliptical excisions would not give a good result, either from distortion to surrounding structures or because a defect is too large to allow simple closure.

In developing these skills, the assistance of a surgical mentor is essential, and practice on pork belly or synthetic skin is highly desirable. When learning these skills, a surgeon will naturally look for opportunities to practise. With increased experience, the same surgeon will tend to look at similar opportunities in terms of the most simple and straightforward closure.

Levels of difficulty are indicated by scalpel ratings. The more scalpel blades, the more difficult the procedure and the more practical experience will be required to become competent at the technique.

ADVANCED EXCISION TECHNIQUES

When an elliptical excision is closed, the two edges of the excision are advanced to meet each other in order to close the defect. However, in certain body locations and for the excision of larger lesions, more complex closures may be necessary, involving more movement of the skin to effect closure. This chapter considers some more advanced surgical techniques, including crescentic excisions, M-plasty, and some simple flaps.

Careful thought, preparation, and marking of the skin are essential to achieve the best results. Experienced carpenters understand this principle—mark twice, but only cut once.

Crescentic excisions

It is not always appropriate to produce a linear scar—over the face in particular a curved scar may look more natural. By observing the natural skin creases, the surgeon can decide whether a curved scar should be created by the use of a crescentic excision. Locations where such curves are commonly found include the forehead, cheeks, nose, chin, and breast, the female breast posing a particular challenge.

Crescentic excisions and the female breast

Excisions under the breast, while easily hidden, need to be carefully planned to follow the curve of the breast, although excisions close to the nipple need to follow the circular curve of the areola or to form a segmental ellipse across it. Surgery over the upper breast is particularly difficult. Not only is this an area likely to develop hypertrophic or keloid scarring, but it is also subject to different skin tensions according to the patient's posture and clothing. In order to best assess the most natural incision line, it is essential to examine the breast while the patient is upright and not wearing a bra. The reason for such an examination should be carefully explained to the patient and every effort made to preserve her modesty while, at the same time, fully assessing the relaxed skin tension lines (see Chapter 6 for more details).

Demonstrating the relaxed skin tension lines over the upper medial aspect of the breast is facilitated by the patient bringing her shoulders forward and pushing the breasts together with her upper arms. The resultant skin creases tend to run almost vertically down in arcs. An excision made to follow these curved lines, supported by buried sutures, will usually produce the most subtle of scars. The wound can be supported by a combination of adhesive tape and silicone dressings to minimize scarring.

> ### GOLDEN RULES ✳
> - Only use these advanced procedures where you can be sure of complete and adequate excision.
> - Plan carefully.
> - Mark twice, cut once.
> - Anaesthetise widely, undermine widely,

//// Performing and suturing a crescentic excision

Carefully mark out the proposed excision (Figure 25.1a). The curved edge of the crescent will inevitably be longer than the straight edge. The more curved the crescent, the greater the disparity in length and the more difficult it is to match up both sides of the scar, and hence the more skin tension will be present. The rule of three times length to width should still be observed to allow closure with minimal tension.

After creating the incision in the skin, the lesion is excised in the usual way, except when undermining the wound edges prior to skin closure (25.1b,c). With a crescentic excision, most undermining takes place adjacent to the shorter, straighter edge to enable it to be advanced to meet the curved edge. For this reason, local anaesthetic should be infiltrated over a wide area adjacent to the shorter edge. To effect closure, the sutures will need to be fanned out along the length of the crescent and will be more closely grouped along the shorter edge (25.1d–f).

Every suture that is inserted to close a crescent could, in theory, produce a so-called 'dog ear' defect, so it is essential that the surgeon judges just how large a difference in wound edge length can be accommodated without forming a dog ear. With increased practice, it is possible to vary the distance between sutures in order to change the radius of the curve between each end of the scar.

A crescentic wound can be closed with buried sutures, but this requires meticulous care when placing the sutures, being careful to ensure that the sutures are in exactly the same plane on both sides of the incision and have equally sized 'bites' of dermis. A carefully performed crescentic dermal closure is particularly suitable for breast excisions, where a line of suture marks might be disfiguring.

On the face, where sutures are removed earlier, dermal closure is less important as interrupted sutures are less likely to cause unsatisfactory scarring. However, a few buried monofilament absorbable sutures will support the wound while it gains strength after the skin sutures have been removed after 5 days (Figure 25.2). Alternatively, the wound can be supported with adhesive tape after suture removal.

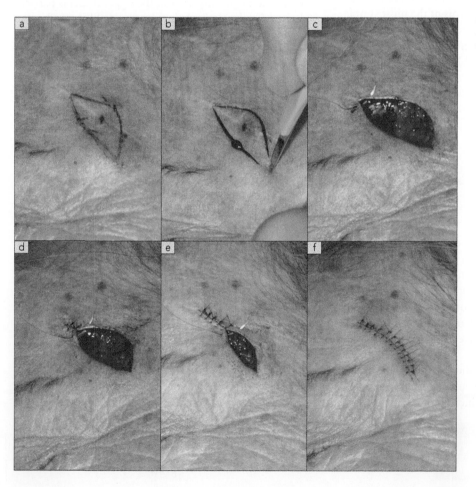

Figure 25.1 Crescentic excision on the lateral forehead.

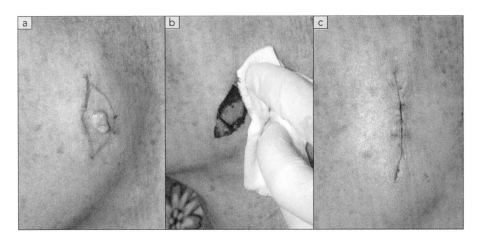

Figure 25.2 Crescentic excision on the cheek, closed with deep Monocryl™ sutures.

M-plasty

To successfully complete an ellipse excision, there needs to be enough space for both apices of the ellipse, but in some anatomical locations this can be very difficult. The classical problem areas include the nasolabial fold, the corner of the mouth, and close to the lateral border of the eye. If an ellipse is attempted in these areas, one apex of the ellipse would involve the nose, the mouth, or the eye, respectively. Truncating the ellipse (i.e., ignoring the three times as long as wide rule) to deal with this problem is likely to result in an ugly scar under too much tension. It is in these situations that an M-plasty is useful. The principle behind the M-plasty is to invert the second apex by turning the apex back in on the ellipse. This inversion creates the M shape, hence the name the M-plasty. In marking the skin, approximately one-third of the ellipse length becomes the M-plasty, ensuring that the inverted apex tip (Figure 25.3) is a suitable distance from the lesion.

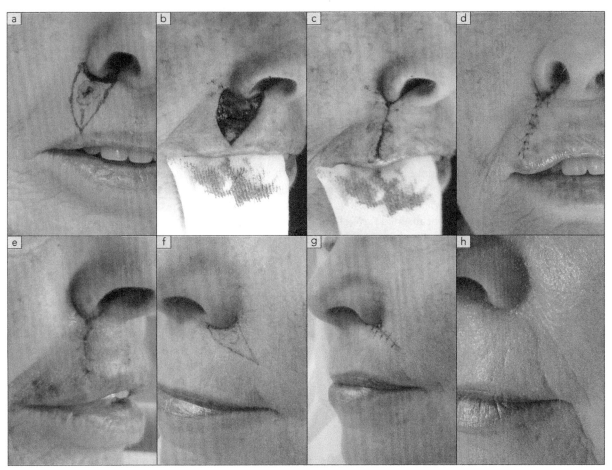

Figure 25.3 (a–d) M-plasty excision above the lip. (e) The site of the incision 1 week later. (f,g) M-plasty on the nasolabial fold. (h) The nasolabial fold 1 month after the procedure.

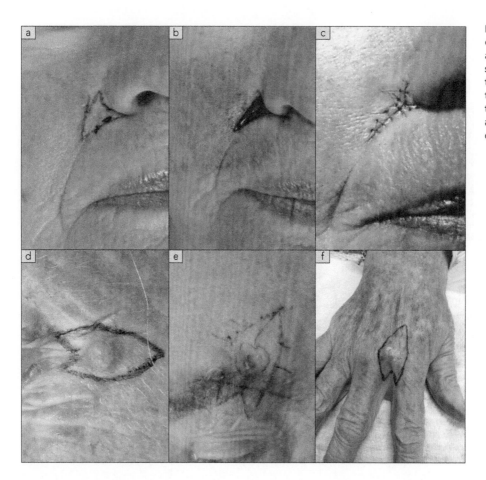

Figure 25.4 (a–c) M-plasty on the nasolabial fold (the arrow shows the three-point suture). (d) M-plasty lateral to the eye. (e) M-plasty within the eyebrow (with marking of the forehead creases prior to anaesthetising). (f) M-plasty on the hand.

/// Closure of an M-plasty

There are three steps to closure of the wound. The first is to close the original ellipse, and this is then followed by bringing together the two sides of the M. The resultant scar has a Y-shaped appearance (Figure 25.4). For all but one of the skin sutures, a standard suture and knot should be used, but a different suture should be used to suture the inverted apex. This suture is important to avoid rendering the tip of the apex non-viable by occluding the blood supply. The suture should be inserted through the dermal layer of the tip, avoiding the epidermis entirely.

The cosmetic result of the M-plasty tends to be very good. By turning the apex back in on itself, the M-plasty end of the wound has less skin tension, which in turn causes less distortion of the surrounding structures. In the nasolabial fold, the M disappears into the edge of the nose as it adjoins the cheek.

Simple flaps

There will be occasions when a simple ellipse, crescentic closure, or an M-plasty will be insufficient to achieve closure, either because of the size of the lesion being excised or because of its location. In these circumstances, it may be possible to achieve an excellent cosmetic result with minimum interference with function by moving a flap of skin around to cover the defect that has been created. This type of procedure should be observed and then practised on synthetic skin or pork belly before the surgeon ever uses the technique on a patient.

Performing a flap is more complex in terms of *planning*, but the actual surgery follows the same principles as ellipse closures. It is, however, essential that the surgeon has a clear understanding of the anatomy of the vascular supply and lines of skin tension before undertaking any surgical procedure involving the use of a flap. In addition, there needs to be full discussion with the patient about the planned surgery, the likely scarring, and any potential complications.

Simple flaps utilise the skin that lies adjacent to the lesion so that it is matched in terms of colour and texture. Four main types of flap are commonly used: transposition, advancement, rotation, and subcutaneous island pedicle flaps. The four types of flap have some common elements, and some procedures use a combination of techniques. Within this text, we describe a small number of techniques suitable for the experienced skin surgeon, but the advanced skin surgeon will use many more, and for these a specialist plastic surgery textbook should be studied. For all the techniques the use of a marker suture is important.

Marker suture

Because of the disruption to the anatomy caused by moving the skin to cover the defect, it is particularly important to ensure that the lesion is completely excised, especially if it is a skin malignancy. If a histology report shows incomplete excision or inadequate margins, it will be much more complicated to identify the location. This is also why all such excised specimens should be orientated using a marker suture (Figure 25.5). The specimen being removed should have a single suture inserted at a location that is clearly marked on both the clinical notes and the histology request form using suitably annotated diagrams.

///// Transposition flap

Skin adjacent to the defect is advanced by a combination of rotation and advancement. The simplest example is the finger flap (Figure 25.6), where a finger-shaped flap of skin is rotated and advanced to cover the defect (Figure 25.7). An alternative is the modified rhomboid flap, as described below.

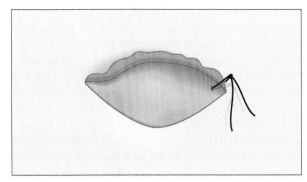

Figure 25.5 Marker suture.

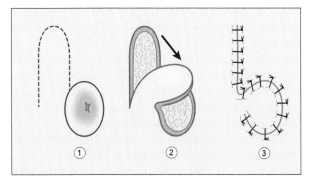

Figure 25.6 (1) Lesion excised. (2) Finger of skin mobilised and transposed across the defect. (3) Suturing.

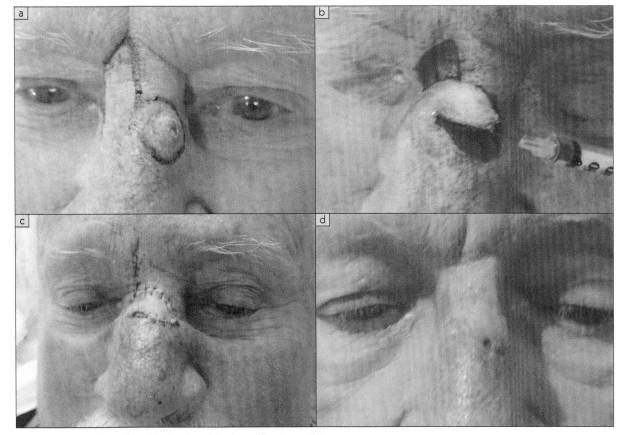

Figure 25.7 (a–c) Finger flap. (d) The site of the finger flap 1 month later.

The modified rhomboid flap (rotation/transposition)

The transposition flap aims to close defects by moving adjacent skin and subcutaneous tissue. Plastic surgeons originally attempted to construct these flaps based upon rigid mathematical and geometric principles, and the classical rhomboid flap is a good example of this (Limberg, 1946, 1966). The lesion is excised as a rhomboid shape (with the internal angles being $2 \times 60°$ and $2 \times 120°$ angles). Precise measurements are made in creating the flap, which will exactly mirror the rhomboid defect in both size and angle (Figure 25.8).

In 1987, Quaba and Sommerlad modified this classic design to create a much more adaptable flap. A circular defect is created by excising the lesion (along with a marker suture), and a smaller flap is raised. A flap can be taken at any point on the circle in any direction to permit the most favourable closure. The wound can then be closed with least disruption to the local anatomy. Quaba and Sommerlad's technique has been called putting a 'square peg into a round hole'. In this modified design, the flap is smaller than the defect, with the smaller, square-shaped flap causing less disfigurement.

The circular excision is also advantageous as it avoids unnecessary corners, which are less likely to heal well, and it produces a less angular and more natural final result. This flap is most useful around the head and neck, although there is no reason why the technique could not be used successfully elsewhere on the body. The main advantage over other techniques is its flexibility.

As mentioned previously, transposition flap construction requires planning and forethought. Accurate skin marking is essential, and although this will initially take time, it will

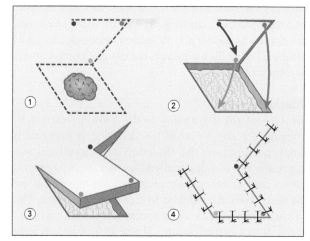

Figure 25.8 Classic rhomboid flap.

become easier to visualise the orientation of the incisions once the technique has been mastered. The surgical principles of incising correctly down to subcutaneous fat and undermining adequately are just the same as for ellipse excisions. The undermining tends to be greater, and this in turn means that the area anaesthetised needs to be generous.

Due to the excellent blood supply to the head and neck, it is difficult to render a flap ischaemic (although this can be caused by excessive skin tension or poorly located sutures). On the body, however, particularly for the limbs, the vascular supply may be less good, and this may create problems of ischaemia.

Figures 25.9–25.11 show the use of rhomboid flaps at various sites.

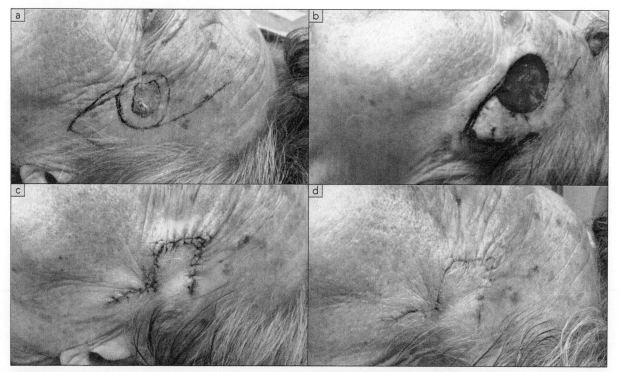

Figure 25.9 (a–c) Rhomboid flap over the temple. (a) Both a rhomboid flap and a Z-plasty have been considered and drawn out. (b) The lesion removed and the flap mobilised and (c) sutured. (d) The site of the flap after 1 week.

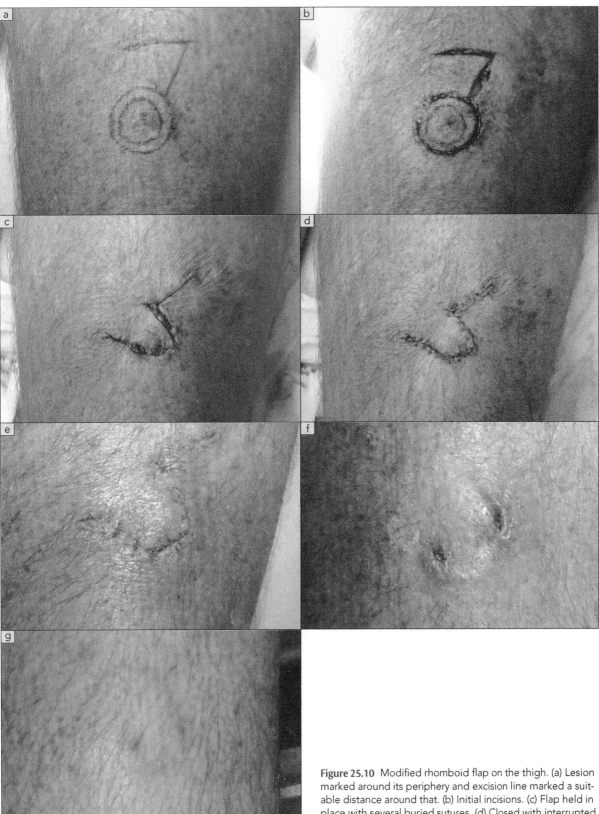

Figure 25.10 Modified rhomboid flap on the thigh. (a) Lesion marked around its periphery and excision line marked a suitable distance around that. (b) Initial incisions. (c) Flap held in place with several buried sutures. (d) Closed with interrupted skin sutures. The incision site at (e) 2 weeks, (f) 1 month, and (g) 4 months later.

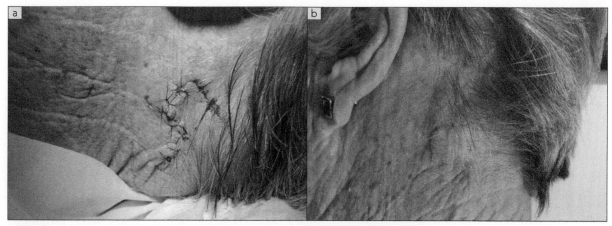

Figure 25.11 (a) Rhomboid excision on the neck. (b) Its appearance 1 week after the procedure, after the sutures had been removed.

///// Advancement flap

The principle of the advancement flap is that, after the specimen has been removed, the defect is closed by raising a flap from either one side (a single flap) or both sides (a double flap or H-plasty). In a single advancement flap, the movement of skin is entirely in one direction. The flap is advanced to cover the defect, with the ratio of width to length (of the defect) not usually exceeding 3:1 on the face or 2:1 on the trunk (some would say up to 1:1, but only where there is significant laxity). The forehead and cheek are both areas where an advancement flap may be utilized (Figures 25.12 and 25.13). There may be a tendency for dog ears to form from the base where the flap is advanced, but this risk can be minimised by cutting out small triangles of skin (Burow's triangles) at the base of the flap (25.12d–g).

It may be possible, with a double advancement flap, to avoid the need for Burow's triangles (Figure 25.12a–c), as the advancement distance for each flap is halved. The closure effectively consists of an end-to-end suture of the leading edges of the two flaps, followed by four

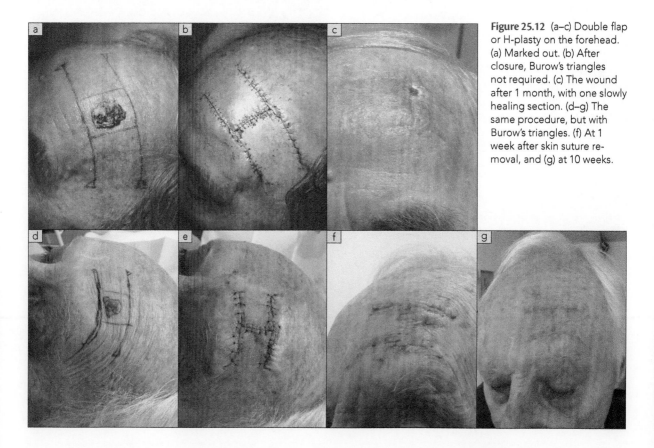

Figure 25.12 (a–c) Double flap or H-plasty on the forehead. (a) Marked out. (b) After closure, Burow's triangles not required. (c) The wound after 1 month, with one slowly healing section. (d–g) The same procedure, but with Burow's triangles. (f) At 1 week after skin suture removal, and (g) at 10 weeks.

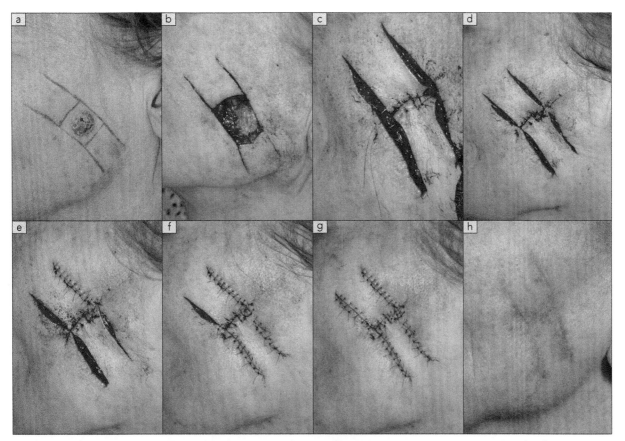

Figure 25.13 Excision using an H-plasty on the cheek. (a) Marked out. (b) Initial closure with stay sutures and the first four-point suture. (c) The two four-point sutures in place, leaving four 'crescentic' closures. (d–g) Each of these crescents is then sutured. (h) The wound at 1 month, with no distortion of the surrounding structures.

crescentic closures, one on each side of each flap. In order to achieve a successful advancement flap, there needs to be reasonable undermining of the skin around the sides of the wound. Undermining of the flap is possible as long as the surgeon is careful to avoid damaging the vascular supply, either by careless undermining or by too much stretch on the flap.

For single advancement flaps, a three-point suture will be required at each corner, and for double advancement flaps a four-point suture will be required at the two corners where the flaps meet (Figure 25.13).

//// Advancement: A to T plasty

Variations on the simple flap include A to T flaps (and O to T flaps). The A to T plasty is a double advancement flap in which only one side of each flap is cut and the excised lesion is removed as a triangular shape, not a square or a rectangle (Figure 25.14). This technique is useful when the excision is close to the edge of one of the facial units (e.g., above the eyebrow or close to the angle of the jaw; Figure 25.15) or where a T-shaped scar can be hidden more easily than an H-shaped one. The two flaps require less extensive undermining than with

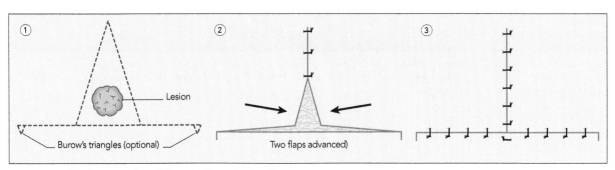

Figure 25.14 Employing an A to T flap with Burow's triangles.

an H-plasty (as they are mobilised on two, rather than three edges). Advancement is facilitated by cutting two small Burow's triangles. If the lesion is removed as a circular excision (the 'O' in O to T), it is advisable to excise further in order to create a triangular defect to avoid puckering on closure.

It may occasionally be sufficient, or desirable, to raise a single flap, especially if the skin is lax enough. This can produce a very cosmetically acceptable scar. Figure 25.16 shows such an excision, closed initially with buried absorbable sutures and then with supporting skin sutures.

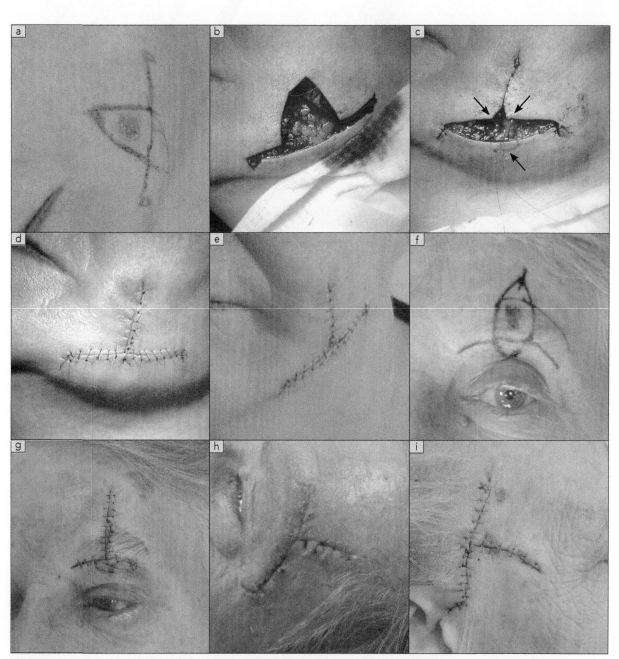

Figure 25.15 (a–e) A to T excision along the jaw line, showing the three-point suture inserted (c). (f,g) Use of an A to T flap through the eyebrow; skin creases have been drawn for alignment. (h) An A to T above the eyebrow at 1 week postoperatively. (i) Completed A to T flap over the temple.

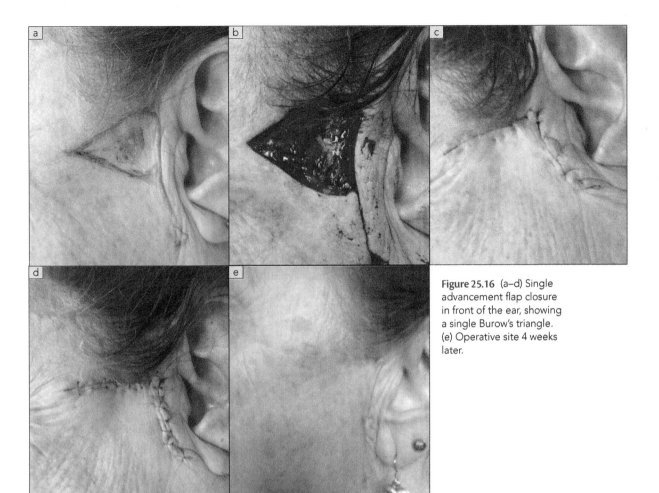

Figure 25.16 (a–d) Single advancement flap closure in front of the ear, showing a single Burow's triangle. (e) Operative site 4 weeks later.

Rotation flap

With the rotation flap, a circular excision is closed by rotating one or two curved flaps from the side of the excision.

///// Z-plasty rotation flap

The most frequent type of rotation flap is the Z-plasty. This can be particularly useful on the lateral forehead where the resultant Z-shaped scar may be hidden within the natural skin creases (Figure 25.17). The technique involves extensive undermining and careful planning of the two flaps to ensure that their length and width will be sufficient to allow closure of the defect. Like the modified rhomboid flap, the position of the flaps can be chosen to minimise skin tension. The tip of the flap(s) should not be too thin, otherwise it will be difficult to suture in place and create too large a difference in size between the flap and the defect.

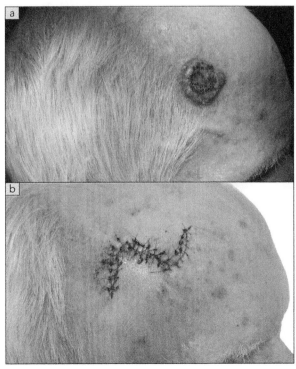

Figure 25.17 Z-plasty rotation flap used on the forehead.

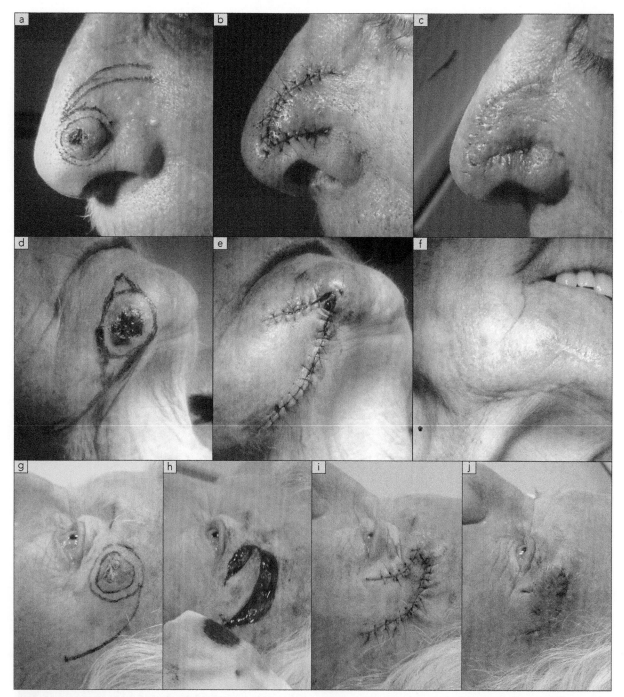

Figure 25.18 (a,b) Single rotation flap on the nose, and (c) on suture removal. (d–e) Single rotation flap on the chin, and (f) 1 month later. (g–i) Single rotation flap on the temple, and (j) after suture removal.

//// Single rotation flap

In some locations, it may be possible to close the defect by raising a single curved flap of sufficient area; the side of the nasal area suits this procedure. This is a single rotation flap (Figure 25.18). A temporary stay suture close to the apex of each flap helps position it. This leaves three wounds to close: two crescentic, and one elliptical. With the two crescentic closures, it is possible to place each suture (starting at the end furthest from the tips of the flaps) at an angle to help draw the flap forward, thereby reducing the tension for the final sutures. Two three-point tension-free sutures can now replace the temporary stay sutures.

///// Subcutaneous island pedicle flap

This can be a useful technique when one is faced with a large lesion that might otherwise need skin grafting, but only if a reasonable thickness of subcutaneous fat exists, without vital structures close to the surface, for example on the thigh. It is also possible to use a single triangular pedicle flap to close a circular defect on the face. The overall shape of this procedure is a diamond-shaped incision (Figure 25.19). The centre of the diamond consists of an hexagonal specimen that is completely excised. This leaves two small triangularly shaped pedicles of skin. These are the two flaps, and their viability is totally dependent upon the blood supply reaching them through the subcutaneous fat upon which they are situated. Undermining to allow closure therefore needs to take place around but not under the triangles.

After the initial incisions and the excision of the lesion, the surgeon tends to be left with a large defect and two diminutive triangles of skin. Do not despair. The two triangles should be sutured together with one or two suitably strong stay sutures. The two apices of the diamond can then be closed with conventional sutures. This will have the effect of not only reducing the size of the defect, but also pushing the triangles together, thereby helping to reduce tension on the stay sutures. Next, the corners of the triangles can be sutured using four-point sutures, thereby avoiding devitalizsing the tips. This results in four elliptical or crescentic wounds to be closed to complete the repair.

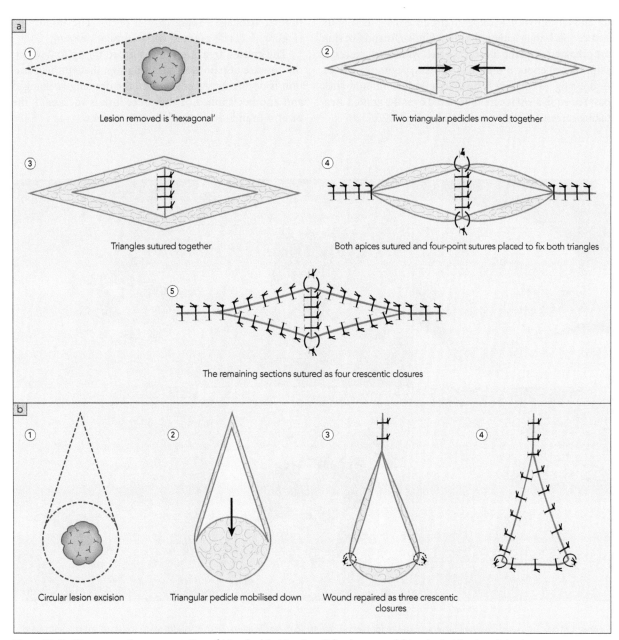

Figure 25.19 Diagrammatic representation of (a) a double island pedicle closure and (b) a single island pedicle closure.

PINCH-GRAFTING OF VENOUS ULCERS ////

Venous ulcers that stubbornly fail to heal are not uncommon (Figure 25.20). Occasionally, in suitable patients, pinch-grafts can promote and expedite healing and are well worth trying. Before attempting grafting, the base of the ulcer should be clean, granulating, free from infection as far as possible, and fairly shallow. This will provide the optimum conditions for applying the graft (Figure 25.21a).

The donor site is normally the upper outer thigh. An area is chosen and anaesthetised. This may be by infiltration, but a simple method of anaesthetising the skin is by using EMLA® cream under waterproof occlusion. This is applied 2 hours before the procedure.

Using a 21 G needle, a small piece of skin is picked up and cut off with a scalpel to produce the 'pinch-graft' tissue. This is then laid on the ulcer. Similar 'islands' of skin are prepared until the ulcer is covered with small pieces of skin, spaced about 5 mm apart or less (Figure 25.21b,c). A dressing of Inadine® (povidone-iodine in non-stick base) or equivalent is carefully placed over the grafted area, taking care not to dislodge the grafts (Figure 25.21d).

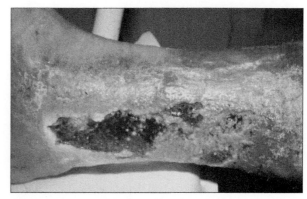

Figure 25.20 Non-healing venous leg ulcer.

A layer of sterile cotton wool or multiple layers of gauze are then applied, covered by an elastocrêpe bandage, which in turn is covered by an elasticated tubular bandage (Tubigrip™ E or F). The donor site (Figure 25.21e) is covered with a similar dressing.

The grafted area is left undisturbed for up to 2 weeks: the absence of pain is a promising sign that epithelialisation is occurring. After 2 weeks, the dressing is changed and another applied. If the procedure is successful, the ulcer is found to have healed after 6 weeks.

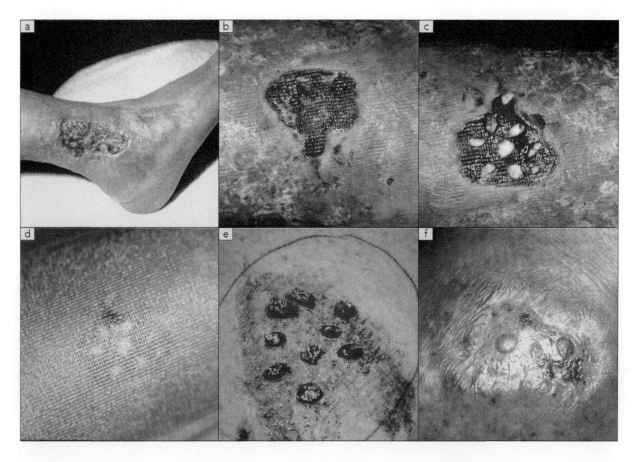

Figure 25.21 (a) Clean, shallow venous ulcer suitable for pinch-grafting. (b,c) Application of pinch-grafts to the ulcer. (d) Pinch-grafts held in place by Inadine® dressing. (e) Donor site wound. (f) Healed ulcer at 6 weeks after pinch-grafting.

TEMPORAL ARTERY BIOPSY

Polymyalgia rheumatica and temporal arteritis are relatively common in the elderly. Untreated, temporal arteritis may be followed by a sudden loss of vision, which is permanent and occurs without warning. Systemic steroids provide dramatic results and prevent the onset of blindness.

The diagnosis is usually made on clinical findings plus a markedly raised erythrocyte sedimentation rate and/or C-reactive protein level, but occasionally the diagnosis is not straightforward and it may be helpful to biopsy a branch of the superficial temporal artery. Biopsy of the artery should be taken preferably before, or within a few days of, starting oral steroids. It is desirable but not essential to biopsy the artery before starting steroids.

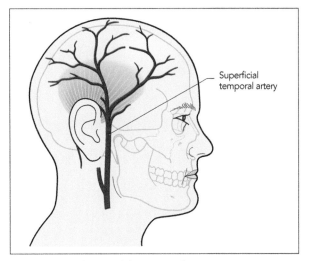

Figure 25.22 Anatomy of the temporal artery.

//// Technique of temporal artery biopsy

Identify the temporal artery by palpation. It lies above the deep fascia on the temporalis muscle (Figure 25.22) and is usually easily palpated along the frontal branch, although it may be non-pulsatile and tender if arteritis is present. Mark along the artery. Any overlying hair is clipped if necessary. The skin is prepared as usual and infiltrated with 1% or 2% lidocaine ± adrenaline.

An incision should then be made over the artery, ideally in a skin crease line. If possible, the edge of the wound should be retracted, either by an assistant or by using a small self-retaining retractor. The artery should then be freed by blunt dissection using a pair of curved Halstead mosquito forceps, and two ligatures of absorbable suture material should be applied spaced 1.5 cm apart (3-0 coated Vicryl™ or Monocryl; Figure 25.23). The isolated segment of artery can then be carefully excised and immediately placed in a histology pot with formalin. The wound is then closed with interrupted monofilament sutures. No other dressing is required.

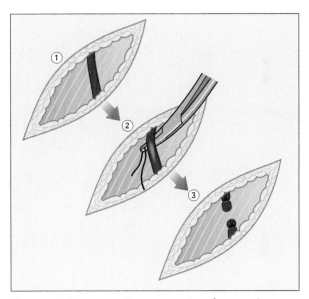

Figure 25.23 Diagrammatic representation of temporal artery biopsy.

REFERENCES

Limberg AA (1946) *Mathematical Principles of Local Plastic Procedures on the Surface of the Human Body.* Leningrad: Medgis.

Limberg AA (1966) Design of the local flaps. In: Gibson T, ed. *Modern Trends in Plastic Surgery.* London: Butterworth.

Quaba AA, Sommerlad BC (1987) 'A square peg into a round hole': A modified rhomboid flap and its clinical application. *British Journal of Plastic Surgery* 40: 163–70.

Chapter 26

Electrosurgery

INTRODUCTION

The term 'electrosurgery' covers a variety of processes used in minor surgery, ranging from the use of simple heated devices (electrocautery) through to uni- or bipolar radiosurgery (often referred to as diathermy).

In *electrocautery*, the electrode tip, rather than human tissue, serves as the source of electrical resistance. Current passes through two wires connected to the cautery tip, which has inbuilt resistance. The current produces heat as it passes through the resistance. The heated tip works by burning and contracting the tissues it touches. With *radiosurgery*, the tip remains relatively cool. Current passing through the tip meets resistance as it reaches the body surface, and it is here that heat is produced.

This chapter reminds the reader about the simpler forms of electrosurgery, but most of it describes the technique of radiosurgery using higher power equipment, which requires the development of new and different skills. It is important that the reader is aware of the need for additional training in this technique. Levels of difficulty are indicated by scalpel ratings. The more scalpel blades, the more difficult the procedure and the more practical experience will be required to become competent at the technique.

ELECTROCAUTERY

✦–✦✦✦ Technique

Electrocautery is the simplest form of electrosurgery and also the most limited in application. The unit consists of a high-power transformer that converts mains voltage to a low voltage (around 12–24 V) and a high current. The current passes through wires to a simple press-on switch in a handle. The equipment required for electrocautery is considered in Chapter 1, and the use of electrocautery following curettage and shave excision is considered in Chapter 19. A cutting tip is suitable for cutting through lesions (e.g., pedunculated lesions such as skin tags). A ball or flat spade tip can be used to achieve haemostasis following curettage (Figure 26.1), and the cold tip for localised cautery of spider naevi (Figure 26.2).

Electrocautery requires skill to adjust the power (via a simple rheostat) in order to produce sufficient heat to cut or coagulate. Too much heat and the burner tip will produce excessive local destruction; too little and it will 'stick' to the skin tissues. It is essential that the operator has sufficient support to be able to hold the burner tip very steady. It often helps to rest the operating hand against the other hand; this is especially true for cold-tip cautery. With this technique, a small coil of wire at the base heats up and conducts a focused point of heat to the pointed tip. The tip can be applied to the feeding vessel of a spider naevus for very localised cautery.

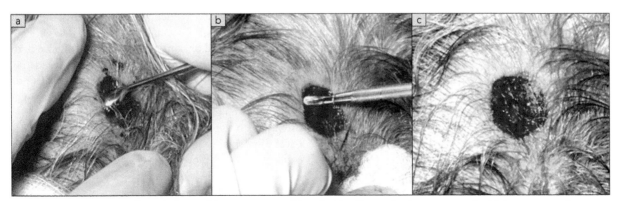

Figure 26.1 (a) Curettage of a scalp lesion. (b) Haemostasis achieved with a flat spade electrocautery tip. (c) Appearance after light cautery.

Drawbacks

The drawbacks of electrocautery include the following:

- It is difficult to sterilise electrocautery handles and battery-operated units.
- It is difficult to find sterile plastic sheaths to encase the handle.
- The burner tips should be autoclaved after use, but not all tips are autoclave-proof.
- The wires in simple loop tips are easily damaged.
- The point of the cold-tip burner is particularly prone to damage.
- The simple contact switch in the handle is prone to poor contact due to arcing as the circuit is made and broken.

Despite these problems, electrocautery can provide a very economical solution to cauterising the base of a curetted lesion or burning off a raised or pedunculated lesion. The mains-operated units have the advantage of not being reliant upon battery power but the disadvantage of being less transportable.

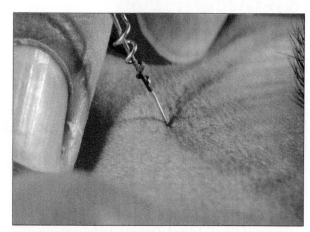

Figure 26.2 Cold-tip cautery of spider naevi.

RADIOSURGERY (INCLUDING DIATHERMY)

Overview

Modern radiofrequency electrosurgical devices transfer electrical energy to human tissue via a treatment electrode that remains relatively cool. In radiosurgery or diathermy, the patient is included in the circuit and current enters the patient's body.

Standard mains electrical current alternates at a frequency of 50 (United Kingdom) or 60 (United States) cycles per second (Hz). Electrosurgical systems could function at this frequency, but because current would be transmitted through body tissue at 50 or 60 cycles, excessive neuromuscular stimulation and perhaps electrocution would result. Because nerve and muscle stimulation cease at 100,000 cycles per second (100 kHz), electrosurgery can be performed safely at 'radio' frequencies above 100 kHz. An electrosurgical generator takes mains 50 or 60 cycle current and increases the frequency to over 200,000 cycles per second. At this frequency, electrosurgical energy can pass through the patient with minimal neuromuscular stimulation and no risk of electrocution.

In *unipolar diathermy*, the current passes from the instrument tip to the tissue, where resistance causes local effects. The current returns 'to earth' through the body either via a ground plate or through contact of the body with the operating table, etc. In *bipolar diathermy*, the two functions of the active electrode and the return electrode are performed at the site of the surgery by the two tines of the forceps. Only the tissue grasped is included in the electrical circuit. Because the return function is performed by one tine of the forceps, no patient-return electrode is needed. Bipolar forceps are favoured by many surgeons to produce a blood-free operating zone.

Power range

Low-power units

Small, relatively inexpensive unipolar diathermy devices include the Birtcher hyfrecator and Aaron Bovie diathermy unit. These units tend to work at lower frequencies (450 kHz) with power outputs of around 35 W. They are designed to work without ground plates, the return current leaking away over the contact area of the patient. If, however, patients touch a metal surface or even the surgeon (if the surgeon is less insulated from the ground) while the diathermy is being used, they may experience a small area of contact diathermy. This is likely to be no more than a tiny electric shock-like sensation and can be avoided by ensuring any contact is over a larger area or by the optional use of a ground plate.

High-power units

The technique now known as radiosurgery requires high power and higher frequency units. In 1978, Maness *et al.* showed that 3.8 million cycles per second (3.8 MHz) was the optimal frequency for cutting soft tissues (Figure 26.3). This frequency is still used in modern radiosurgery units.

These units will be considerably more expensive than the low-power units, but they are also far more versatile. The power output requires the use of a ground plate or dispersive electrode (Figure 26.4). This is usually a small plastic-covered plate or rubber mat that is placed in close proximity to the patient. It does not need to make electrical contact with the patient but acts like an antenna to concentrate the radiowaves.

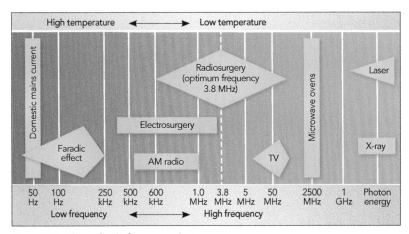

Figure 26.3 Chart of radiofrequency devices.

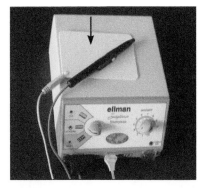

Figure 26.4 Radiosurgery device, showing the ground plate (arrowed).

	Waveform	Use	Oscilloscope configuration
1	Fully filtered and fully rectified	Cutting	
2	Fully rectified	Cutting and coagulation	
3	Partially rectified	Haemostasis	
4	Markedly damped (spark gap)	Fulguration and electrodesiccation	

Figure 26.5 Waveforms used in radiosurgery. A fully filtered and rectified pattern is favoured for pure cutting, mimicking the action of a scalpel blade. If fully rectified, both cutting and coagulation can be achieved simultaneously, aiding visualisation. A partially rectified waveform is only useful for coagulation.

Modern radiosurgical instruments are able to generate several different waveforms, each having different characteristic effects on the tissues, including incision, excision, and coagulation (Figure 26.5). High-power radiosurgery units can therefore provide an atraumatic method of cutting and coagulating soft tissues. No pressure is needed, and the cells are vaporised in the path of the radiowaves, causing them to split apart in much the same way as with a hot wire through polystyrene. Advocates of the technique suggest that this results in less trauma to the cells, less fibrous scarring, and less postoperative discomfort.

Radiosurgical waveforms

The four types of waveform commonly used in radiosurgery are as follows:

- A *pure filtered waveform* (pure microsmooth cutting; Figure 26.6a) is used for skin incisions and wire loop excisions where haemostasis is not expected to be a problem. This waveform gives the least lateral heat, and therefore produces the least tissue damage.
- A *fully rectified waveform* (blended cutting and coagulation; Figure 26.6b) is used for skin tags, papillomas, keloids, keratoses, and removal of naevi where slight bleeding might be expected. It cuts as well as coagulating small blood vessels and gives slight lateral heat to the tissues.

- A *partially rectified waveform* (hospital-type control of bleeding vessels; Figure 26.6c) is used primarily for haemostasis; it cannot be used for cutting, but is excellent for coagulation, telangectasia, and spider veins.
- A *fulgurating current* (spark-gap tissue destruction; Figure 26.6d) is very similar to unipolar diathermy (hyfrecator) and causes superficial tissue damage by holding the needle electrode close to the tissue and allowing a stream of sparks to burn the tissues. It is suitable for superficial haemostasis and the destruction of small basal cell carcinomas and cysts.

Bipolar coagulation

Very precise haemostasis may be obtained by using bipolar forceps (Figure 26.7). Each blade is connected to the radiosurgical unit so that the current passes between the points of the forceps. It is very useful for picking off individual bleeding vessels in microsurgery.

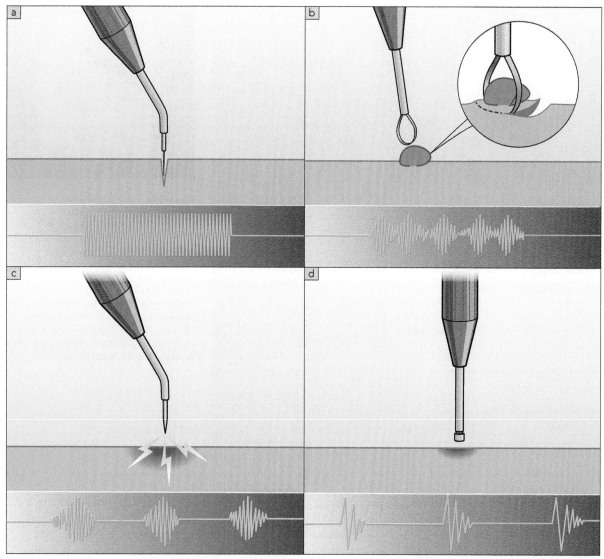

Figure 26.6 (a) Pure filtered waveform. (b) Fully rectified waveform. (c) Partially rectified waveform. (d) Fulguration waveform.

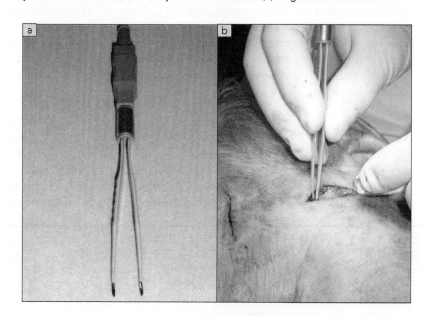

Figure 26.7 (a) Bipolar forceps. (b) Bipolar forceps in use on an elliptical excision.

Ancillary items

Ancillary equipment required is discussed in Chapter 1. When budgeting for electrosurgery, particularly radiosurgery, provision should be made for a smoke extraction unit. These vacuum devices remove smoke plumes and filter the air. They make the working environment safer and much more pleasant and are a prerequisite for performing radiosurgery.

Indications for radiosurgery

Some examples of specific uses are included at the end of this chapter. Advocates of the use of radiosurgery in minor surgery of the skin suggest the following two main uses:

- The first is the most simple—the shave removal of raised lesions from the surface of the skin instead of using a large scalpel blade or DermaBlade® (Figure 26.8). The radiosurgery unit allows the surgeon to achieve near-perfect shaving from the skin surface with minimal skin trauma. The cosmetic results can be excellent.
- Second, it is possible to excise lesions with a fine-wire electrode, using the wire instead of the usual No. 15 blade scalpel (Figure 26.9). This is particularly useful where the skin is very lax (e.g., on the face of an elderly person). Extreme care needs to be taken to avoid penetrating too deeply with the electrode (so it is advisable to have only a short-wire electrode).

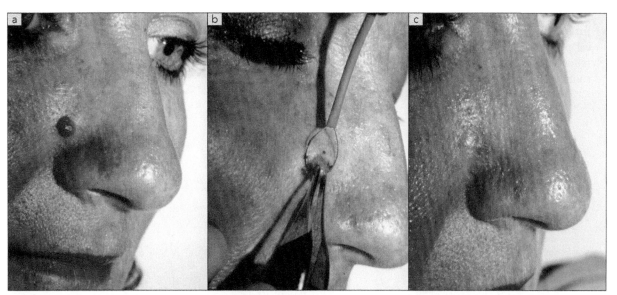

Figure 26.8 Intradermal naevus (a) before, (b) during, and (c) 3 months after radiosurgery.

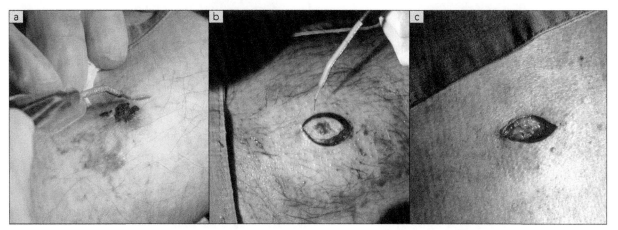

Figure 26.9 (a) Fine-wire tip cutting through skin. (b) Resultant ellipse with very clean lines. (c) Ellipse incision; note how both the sample and the surrounding skin retract.

Radiosurgery (including diathermy)

Learning the technique of radiosurgery

Radiosurgical instruments are powerful and require a totally different technique from that of conventional scalpel surgery; this has to be learned. Most poor results are entirely due to inexperience and faulty technique:

- The first major difference is that *no pressure must be used*. This is hard to learn for a surgeon who has been trained to press the scalpel firmly through the tissues. In radiosurgery, it is the radiowave that is doing the cutting.
- Second, there are no absolute power settings on the machine; these need to be learned by trial and error and experience. For example, a small moist lesion will require much less power to remove than a larger fibrous keratinised lesion.
- Third, if repeat incisions are to be made on the same lesion, time should be allowed to let the edges cool between cuts, usually up to 10 seconds.
- Fourth, rather than removing the whole lesion at the first attempt, better cosmetic results are obtained by first removing a representative sample for histological examination and then gradually 'planing' off the remainder of the lesion until it is flush with the surrounding skin.

One of the simplest teaching aids is a piece of raw steak placed on the passive base electrode (Figure 26.10). Starting with high power, different techniques of cutting and coagulation may be tried, and then, by reducing the power, the effects of too low or too high a current can be discovered.

A range of recorded material has now been produced demonstrating the technique of radiosurgery, and this can be highly recommended for teaching. Tuition by a colleague familiar with the technique of radiosurgery is well worth the time and effort, followed by treating several patients under supervision.

Warnings

First, no patient with a cardiac pacemaker should be treated with radiosurgery without prior consultation with their cardiologist. Fixed-rate pacemakers are least likely to experience problems, but demand-led pacemakers may well be affected and result in arrhythmias. It is, therefore, essential to ask every patient in advance whether they have a pacemaker.

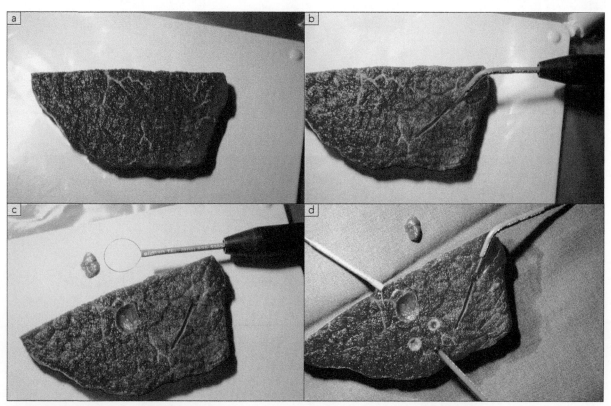

Figure 26.10 (a) Raw steak sitting on the ground plate. (b) Fine-wire cutting. (c) Loop excision. (d) All the above, plus the round tip for haemostasis.

No spirit-based or inflammable skin antiseptic should be used. In fact, it is probably unnecessary to use any form of skin preparation for simple shave excisions.

In addition, delayed bleeding can occur. This is usually light but can alarm the patient. It can be minimised by *not* using adrenaline (epinephrine) with the local anaesthetic (when the adrenaline wears off, the vasodilation can cause haemorrhage) and by applying a solution of aluminium chloride (Driclor®) on a cotton wool applicator at the end of the procedure. It is also helpful to advise the patient about applying finger pressure for 10 minutes should any oozing occur.

It must be remembered that explosion risks exist in the presence of bowel gases and/or oxygen, as they do with diathermy and electrocautery.

Electric shocks and burns can be minimised by not allowing any part of the patient to touch any metal, and by the operator wearing rubber gloves.

As with any new technique or procedure, it is essential that the operator has appropriate knowledge and experience of the procedure.

Avoidance of complications

As with all medical and surgical treatments, complications can occur, but the majority are avoidable, and careful preoperative assessment of both patient and equipment will prevent many mishaps. The following precautions should be taken:

- All wires should be checked, and any that are frayed or show a break in their insulation must be replaced.
- All electrodes must be checked. Broken wires will cause lacerations. Any worn tips should be discarded.
- Too deep an excision will result in unnecessary scarring.
- The doctor should watch the foot switch or finger switch. Both the operator and any assistants should be careful not to tread accidentally on the foot switch, as accidental burns can occur to the patient.
- The handpiece must be inserted in the correct socket.
- The doctor should check that the power control has not been increased at the end of a previous procedure (for example, to steam-clean the electrodes).
- Too much tissue destruction makes histology impossible. This may be due to an incorrect power or waveform setting, or a lesion that is too shallow. In this case, the top may be cut off with a conventional blade and then the base treated with the radiosurgical unit.
- The doctor must check that the patient does not have a cardiac pacemaker.
- The patient must not be taking aspirin or anticoagulants.
- Beware of lower limbs in diabetic patients (poor healing; see Chapters 5 and 6).

General guidelines for radiosurgery

- The correct waveform must be selected.
- Never try to cut with partially rectified (coagulation) waveform.
- The ground plate should be as near as possible to the operative site, but it does not need to have skin contact with the patient.
- Tissues should be moist. If a dry, keratotic lesion is being removed, the area should be kept moist with swabs dipped in saline.
- The unit must be activated before making contact with the tissues.
- The operator must never apply pressure but instead let the radiowave do the cutting.
- If there is resistance or 'drag', or tissue sticking to the electrode, the power setting is too low.
- If there is sparking, the power setting is too high.

Preparation of the patient

- It is essential to explain to the patient in advance the technique of radiosurgery and what to expect both during the procedure and the postoperative management.
- Where a vacuum extractor unit is being used, it is helpful to explain to the patient that most of the noise will be coming from that, and that the operative electrode and unit is silent (although most units produce a 'beep' when the foot or finger switch is depressed).
- Any rings and jewellery must be removed, particularly if situated near the operation site.
- The patient must be made comfortable and asked not to make any jerky or sudden movements if at all possible.
- The patient should be warned about the smell of burning and also to expect to see some smoke, even if the vacuum extractor is used.
- Preprinted preoperative and postoperative information sheets are invaluable and usually answer most of the patient's questions.

Anaesthesia

With few exceptions, local infiltration anaesthesia is required, exactly as with conventional surgery or electrocautery. To reduce the likelihood of postoperative bleeding, this should be with plain lidocaine rather than lidocaine with added adrenaline. The finest gauge needle should be used to administer the anaesthetic (30 G or finer). As described elsewhere in this book, the boundaries of the skin lesion should be marked with a skin marker pen before injecting the local anaesthetic.

Radiosurgery in conjunction with cryosurgery

Although excellent cosmetic results can be achieved with radiosurgery alone, even better results are said to be obtained if the area treated by radiosurgery is sprayed with liquid nitrogen immediately postoperatively. The rationale behind this is to blend the edges of the wound and make for a smoother junction between healthy and treated skin. In practice, the lesion is marked with a skin pen and removed or destroyed using the radiosurgical electrode; any bleeding vessels are coagulated using the ball-ended electrode, and the base is then frozen using liquid nitrogen cryospray, extending the freezing to 1 or 2 mm beyond the edge of the wound. Healing will then be a combination of the effects of radiosurgery and freezing.

Radiosurgery for specific indications

Intradermal naevi

Some of the most impressive results of radiosurgery are seen with the removal of intradermal naevi and other similar lesions. Because the amount of thermal damage is so slight, remarkable cosmetic results can be obtained (Figure 26.11).

A wire loop or diamond electrode is used, and this should be held at right angles to the skin. A smooth, light action is required with no pressure.

/// Treatment of intradermal naevi

1. The edges of the naevus are marked with a skin marker pen.
2. Lidocaine is infiltrated beneath and around the base of the naevus using a 30 G needle and dental syringe or a diabetic needle and syringe.
3. The ground plate electrode is positioned near the lesion. Skin contact is not necessary.
4. The assistant should have a histology pot available in which to preserve the specimen, and also have the vacuum extractor ready for use.
5. The naevus is moistened with a small gauze swab soaked in saline.
6. Holding the wire loop electrode at right angles to the lesion, the doctor makes one or two practice strokes to ensure accuracy and avoidance of shakes or unwanted movements.
7. The power is switched on using the foot switch or fingertip control.
8. The wire loop is passed smoothly through the lesion (Figure 26.12). If sticking occurs, the power may be increased; if sparking occurs, it should be reduced.
9. The specimen is placed in the histology pot and labelled.

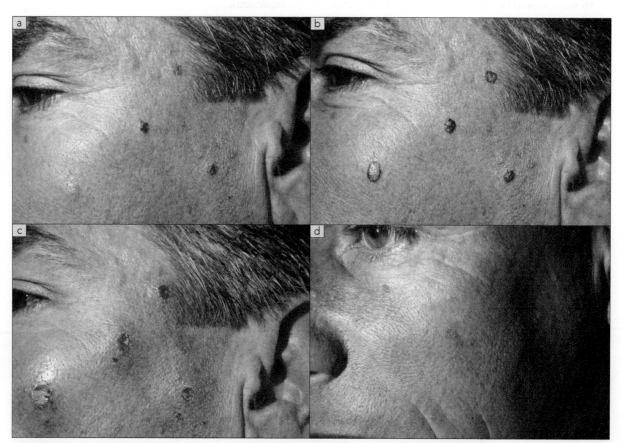

Figure 26.11 (a) Intradermal and compound naevi. The naevi (b) marked and (c) radioshaved. (d) The patient 6 weeks later.

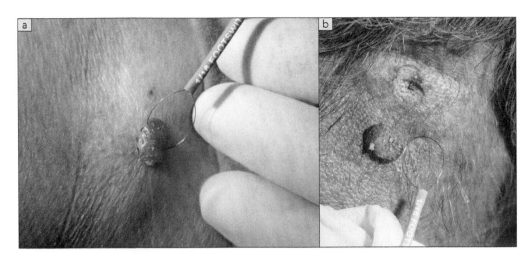

Figure 26.12
The loop (a) passing through a seborrhoeic keratosis and (b) after passing through with the lesion now lying to one side.

10. The remainder of the lesion is trimmed using small, smooth strokes, wiping any charred debris away from the base of the lesion with a moist gauze swab. Finally, the edges are 'feathered' to blend with the adjacent skin.
11. If any bleeding vessels are noticed, they may be sealed with the ball-ended electrode on 'coagulation' (partially rectified).
12. If mild oozing occurs, a cotton bud swab soaked in aluminium chloride (Driclor®) is applied. It can either be pressed onto the bleeding site with gentle pressure, or it may be more effective to roll the bud over the wound.
13. A small 'spot' plaster may be applied or the lesion left exposed to the air.

Telangiectasia and thread veins

Spider naevi and thread veins can be obliterated very successfully using radiosurgery (Figure 26.13). The technique is quick, simple, and easy to learn, and gives excellent results.

⫻ Treatment of telangiectasia

1. The radiosurgical unit is set to partially rectified (coagulation).
2. The power setting is kept low.
3. A fine needle tip is attached to the handpiece and, if necessary, bent to an angle of 45°.
4. With the patient in a comfortable position, the foot switch or finger switch is continuously depressed and each telangiectasis is lightly touched or 'tapped' along its course.
5. Any bleeding points can be treated with a cotton wool bud soaked in aluminium chloride.
6. More than one treatment session may be required.
7. Thread veins are dealt with in the same manner, but in general, facial telangiectasia respond better to radiosurgery than do the thread veins found on the lower limbs.

Radiosurgery (including diathermy)

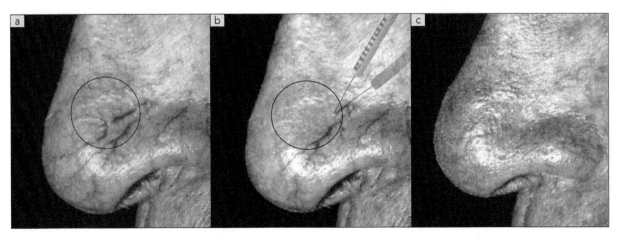

Figure 26.13 (a) Telangiectasia on the nose (circled). (b) Fine wire treating one vessel, and (c) the area after treatment.

// Epilation

Radiosurgery is very effective for epilation (Figure 26.14). Fine, insulated needle electrodes are best.

The needle is inserted to the hair root, parallel to the hair, and the waveform set to the partially rectified (coagulation) lowest setting, 0–1. Gentle traction on the hair will free it.

///// Rhinophyma

This distressing condition (Figure 26.15) can be very effectively treated using radiosurgery and the large wire loop electrode. Local infiltration anaesthesia may be employed and successive layers of excess tissue planed off. Any troublesome bleeding vessels can be coagulated using the ball-ended electrode and partially rectified waveform. Following planing and coagulation, the raw area and adjacent margins may be treated with liquid nitrogen cryospray for 15–20 seconds.

/// Seborrhoeic keratoses

These are generally very superficial and only light 'planing' is needed. The wire loop electrode at a power setting of 2–3 on fully rectified (cut and coagulation) gives very good results (Figure 26.16). It is important to keep the keratosis moistened during treatment. Some dermatologists also give the base a freeze with liquid nitrogen cryospray immediately after radiosurgery.

/// Xanthelasmata

These can be treated either by fulguration using a very fine spark, or by coagulation using the ball-ended electrode. Larger lesions can be planed off using the fully rectified (cut and coagulation) waveform and a wire loop. As these lesions are very superficial, only minimal treatment is needed.

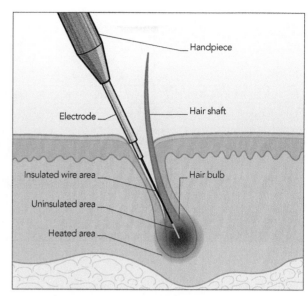

Figure 26.14 Diagrammatic representation of epilation electrode in use.

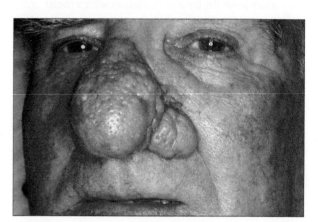

Figure 26.15 Typical appearance of rhinophyma.

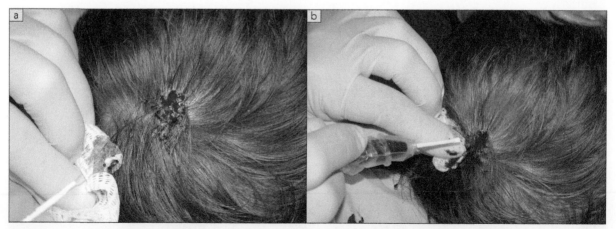

Figure 26.16 Irritated seborrhoeic keratosis on scalp removed by a wire loop, followed by radiocautery of the base.

Cervical dysplasia

For those doctors trained in colposcopy and the treatment of cervical intraepithelial neoplasia, radiosurgery using the specially designed wire-loop electrodes offers a very quick and efficient method of removing suspicious areas of cervix by the 'LLETZ' (large loop excision of the transformation zone) or 'LEEP' (loop electrosurgical excision procedure) technique. A good vacuum extraction system is needed. Any troublesome bleeding can be controlled using the ball-ended electrode and partially rectified (coagulation) waveform. For full details of this technique, the reader should refer to a textbook of gynaecology.

Vasectomy

Radiosurgery can be used for both cutting and coagulation in vasectomy (see Figure 23.8).

Miscellaneous other uses for radiosurgery

Radiosurgery is also widely used in dentistry, plastic and reconstructive surgery, ear, nose and throat surgery, and ophthalmology, but these instances are not covered in this book. The reader who wishes to learn these techniques is advised to refer to the relevant papers or textbooks.

Postoperative care

Various regimes have been advocated for the postoperative management of lesions treated with radiosurgery. The aim is to prevent infection and to keep the area relatively moist to accelerate healing.

Small lesions are probably best left exposed to the air and frequently washed to keep them clean, taking care not to rub the surface too vigorously in case it causes bleeding from capillaries. Larger or deeper wounds are probably best covered with a non-adherent dressing, changed every other day or more frequently if there is much discharge. Any signs of spreading infection should be promptly treated with systemic antibiotics as well as topical antibiotics.

A patient information sheet given at the end of the operation helps to remind the patient how to look after the wound (see Chapter 8 for more details).

REFERENCE

Maness WL, Roeber FW, Clark RE, *et al.* (1978) Histologic evaluation of electrosurgery with varying frequency and waveform. *Journal of Prosthet Dentistry* 40: 304–8.

Index

For Product Safety Concerns and Information please contact our EU
representative GPSR@taylorandfrancis.com Taylor & Francis Verlag GmbH,
Kaufingerstraße 24, 80331 München, Germany

Printed and bound by CPI Group (UK) Ltd, Croydon, CR0 4YY
01/05/2025
01858598-0001